T0206093

Green Coffee Bean Extract in Human Health

Green Coffee Bean Extract in Human Health

Debasis Bagchi
Hiroyoshi Moriyama
Anand Swaroop

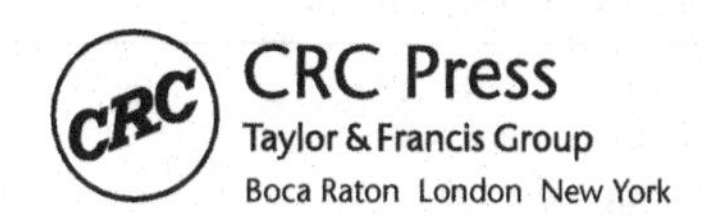

CRC Press is an imprint of the
Taylor & Francis Group, an **informa** business

CRC Press
Taylor & Francis Group
6000 Broken Sound Parkway NW, Suite 300
Boca Raton, FL 33487-2742

First issued in paperback 2021

ISBN 13: 978-1-03-209776-3 (pbk)
ISBN 13: 978-1-4987-1637-6 (hbk)

Publisher's Note
The publisher has gone to great lengths to ensure the quality of this reprint but points out that some imperfections in the original copies may be apparent.

Library of Congress Cataloging-in-Publication Data

Names: Bagchi, Debasis, 1954- , editor. | Moriyama, Hiroyoshi, editor. | Swaroop, Anand, editor.
Title: Green coffee bean extract in human health / editors, Debasis Bagchi, Hiroyoshi Moriyama, and Anand Swaroop.
Description: Boca Raton : Taylor & Francis, 2017. | Includes bibliographical references.
Identifiers: LCCN 2016008201 | ISBN 9781498716376 (hardcover : alk. paper)
Subjects: | MESH: Coffea--chemistry | Seeds | Plant Extracts--pharmacology | Antioxidants--pharmacology | Chlorogenic Acid--pharmacology
Classification: LCC RS160 | NLM QV 766 | DDC 615.3/21--dc23
LC record available at http://lccn.loc.gov/2016008201

Visit the Taylor & Francis Web site at
http://www.taylorandfrancis.com

and the CRC Press Web site at
http://www.crcpress.com

Dedicated to my beloved father,
Mr. Tarak Chandra Bagchi, M.Sc., A.I.C.

Contents

Preface

Green coffee beans are unroasted coffee beans, which are a rich source of novel phenolic antioxidants including chlorogenic acids. It is important to note that *Coffea arabica* contains 3.5%–7.5% (w/w of dry matter) chlorogenic acids, while *Coffea canephora* contains 7.0%–14.0% (w/w of dry matter) chlorogenic acids. Unroasted green coffee beans have a higher level of chlorogenic acids compared to regular, roasted coffee beans. Research demonstrates that chlorogenic acids are novel antioxidants and have potential health benefits in cardiovascular health, hypertension, diabetes, neuroprotection, and metabolic syndrome [1].

The three major classes of chlorogenic acids in green coffee beans are caffeoylquinic acid (CQA), dicaffeoylquinic acid (diCQA), and feruloylquinic acid (FQA), which account for approximately 80% of the total chlorogenic acids in green coffee beans. Moreover, a total of nine chlorogenic acids belong to these three major chlorogenic acids (Table 0.1). These nine chlorogenic acids exhibit varying degrees of efficacy. Furthermore, caffeic acid is another integral constituent of green coffee beans, and exhibits diverse health benefits.

In general, the daily intake of chlorogenic acids in coffee drinkers is 0.5–1.0 g [2]. An epidemiological study conducted by Pellegrini et al. in Italy indicated that coffee has the greatest antioxidant capacity of the commonly consumed beverages [3]. However, a clear distinction in health benefits has been reported between unroasted and roasted green coffee bean extracts, which has been substantiated by structural and compositional analyses.

Scientists have reported significant hypotensive efficacy of chlorogenic acids in hypertensive rats, unique cardioprotective abilities, potent matrix metalloproteinase inhibitory activities, and α-amylase and tyrosinase inhibitory activities. Chlorogenic acids have been demonstrated as potent natural lipase inhibitors [4], which has led researchers to explore the efficacy of green coffee bean extract against diabetes, obesity, and metabolic syndrome.

Green coffee bean extract has brought about a revolution in the nutraceutical marketplace, however, recently there has been some controversies. We have compiled state-of-the-art research studies from eminent scientists around the world in this book, which exhibits the potential and diversified health benefits of green coffee bean extracts. However, it is very important to standardize the appropriate extraction technology, quality control and assurance, broad spectrum safety studies, and human clinical studies to substantiate the claims and position of the product in the marketplace.

Our book focuses on the chemistry, biochemistry, pharmacology, metabolism, safety, and diverse health benefits of green coffee bean extract and its constituents. We extensively discuss chlorogenic acid, caffeoylquinic acid, and caffeic acid in the chapters, which are written by eminent researchers. There are 14 well-defined chapters. The first chapter discusses the chemistry and novel antioxidant benefits of green coffee bean extract and chlorogenic acids. The health and function claims of chlorogenic acids are reviewed in Chapter 2. The standard quality of green coffee bean and extraction methods are reviewed in Chapter 3. The metabolism of chlorogenic acid and

TABLE 0.1
Chlorogenic Acid Classes and Subclasses

Caffeoylquinic Acid (CQA)
3-Caffeoylquinic acid (also known as neochlorogenic acid)
4-Caffeoylquinic acid
5-Caffeoylquinic acid

Dicaffeoylquinic Acid (diCQA)
3,4-Dicaffeoylquinic acid
3,5-Di-O-caffeoylquinic acid (also known as isochlorogenic acid)
4,5-Dicaffeoylquinic acid

Feruloylquinic Acid (FQA)
3-Feruloylquinic acid
4-Feruloylquinc acid
5-Feruloylquinic acid

caffeoylquinic acid is extensively discussed in Chapter 4 by Dr. M. Arnaud, who has been involved in chlorogenic acid research for approximately three decades. Aspects of metabolic syndrome, obesity, and diabetes are elaborated on by three independent research groups in Chapters 5, 6, and 7. Chapter 8 discusses the aspect of hypertension and benefits of green coffee bean extract and chlorogenic acids. Green coffee beans may protect against hepatic fat accumulation and this is demonstrated in Chapter 9. The beneficial efficacy of green coffee bean extract on cognition and brain health are independently discussed in Chapters 10 and 11 by two prestigious research groups in Japan and Australia. Finally, the metabolomics and molecular aspects of green coffee bean extract and chlorogenic acids are discussed in Chapters 12, 13, and 14.

Finally, we sincerely thank all our authors for their valuable contributions to this book and we hope the material will be useful to the readers.

Debasis Bagchi, PhD, MACN, CNS, MAIChE
Hiroyoshi Moriyama, PhD, FACN
Anand Swaroop, PhD, FACN

REFERENCES

1. Kozuma K, Tsuchiya S, Kohori J, Hase T, Tokimitsu I. 2005. Antihypertensive effect of green coffee bean extract on mildly hypertensive subjects. *Hypertens. Res.* 28(9): 711–8.
2. Olthof MR, Hollman PC, Katan MB. 2001. Chlorogenic acid and caffeic acid are absorbed in humans. *J. Nutr.* 131(1): 66–71.
3. Pellegrini N, Serafini M, Colombi B, Del Rio D, Salvatore S, Bianchi M, Brighenti F. 2003. Total antioxidant capacity of plant foods, beverages and oils consumed in Italy assessed by three different *in vitro* assays. *J. Nutr.* 133(9): 2812–9.
4. McCarty MF. 2005. Nutraceutical resources for diabetes prevention—An update. *Med. Hypotheses* 64(1): 151–8.

Editors

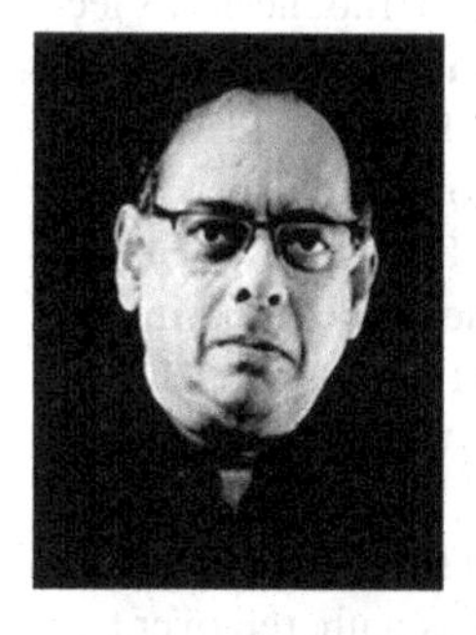

Debasis Bagchi, PhD, MACN, CNS, MAIChE, received his PhD in medicinal chemistry in 1982. He is an adjunct professor in the Department of Pharmacological and Pharmaceutical Sciences at the University of Houston College of Pharmacy, Houston, Texas, and the chief scientific officer of Cepham Research Center, Piscataway, New Jersey. Dr. Bagchi is an adjunct faculty member at Texas Southern University, Houston, Texas. He served as the senior vice president of research and development of InterHealth Nutraceuticals Inc., Benicia, California, from 1998 until February 2011, and then as director of innovation and clinical affairs of Iovate Health Sciences, Oakville, Ontario, until June 2013. Dr. Bagchi received the Master of American College of Nutrition Award in October 2010. He is a past chairman of the International Society of Nutraceuticals and Functional Foods (ISNFF), past president of the American College of Nutrition, Clearwater, Florida, and past chair of the Nutraceuticals and Functional Foods Division of the Institute of Food Technologists (IFT), Chicago, Illinois. He is serving as a distinguished advisor to the Japanese Institute for Health Food Standards (JIHFS), Tokyo, Japan. Dr. Bagchi is a member of the Study Section and Peer Review Committee of the National Institutes of Health (NIH), Bethesda, Maryland. He has 315 papers in peer-reviewed journals, 27 books, and 18 patents. Dr. Bagchi is also a member of the Society of Toxicology, member of the New York Academy of Sciences, fellow of the Nutrition Research Academy, and member of the TCE Stakeholder Committee of the Wright Patterson Air Force Base, Ohio. Dr. Bagchi is an associate editor of the *Journal of Functional Foods*, *Journal of the American College of Nutrition*, and *Archives of Medical and Biomedical Research*, and also serves as an editorial board member of numerous peer-reviewed journals, including *Antioxidants & Redox Signaling*, *Cancer Letters*, *Toxicology Mechanisms and Methods*, *The Original Internist*, and other peer-reviewed journals.

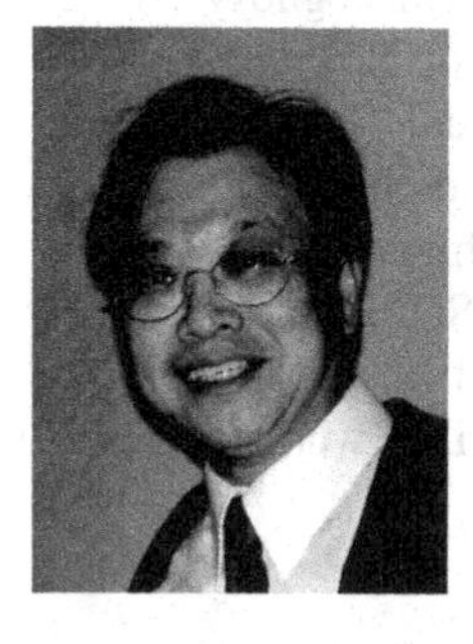

Hiroyoshi Moriyama, PhD, FACN, is a senior technical advisor to Ryusendo Co., Ltd. in Japan. He is also a research fellow at the Laboratory of Drug and Gene Delivery Research, Faculty of Pharmaceutical Sciences, Teikyo University in Tokyo, Japan. He obtained his BS and MS in Chemistry from the University of San Francisco and San Jose State University in 1978 and 1979, respectively. He received his PhD in pharmacognosy from Hoshi University of Pharmaceutical Sciences in Tokyo, Japan. He worked for various multinational companies in the field of pharmaceuticals, cosmetics, and functional foods as product and marketing manager. He has published a number of papers, patents, conference abstracts, and book chapters. He is currently a Board Member of the Japanese Institute for Health Foods Standards (JIHFS). He has been a member of the American Chemical Society (ACS) since 1982. He is also a member of the Japanese Association for Food Immunology (JAFI). He is a fellow of the American College of Nutrition (ACN). He was the special invited speaker of the Ministry of Research and Technology of the Republic of Indonesia to lecture on "Developing Market-Oriented Research Culture on Natural Medicines" at laboratoia pengembangan teknologi industri agro dan biomedika (LAPTIAB) and the Indonesia University in May 2009. He was on the International Advisory Board of the International Society of Nutraceuticals and Functional Foods (ISNFF). His wide array of research interests include Japanese traditional medicine, food immunology, drug delivery systems, and regulatory systems surrounding pharmaceutical, cosmetic, and functional food ingredients in Japan.

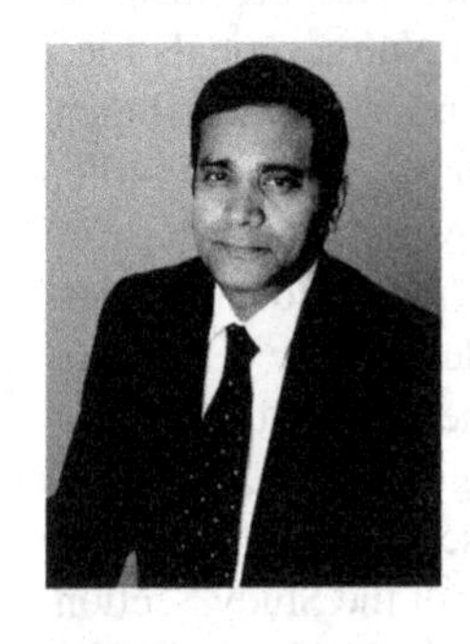

Anand Swaroop, PhD, FACN, obtained his MS in biochemistry and PhD in chemistry in 1997. He has gathered over two decades of diversified global management experience in phytopharmaceuticals, global regulations on nutraceuticals and functional foods, chemicals and pharmaceutical ingredients, outsourcing and supply chain management, business development, market research, and strategic planning. He has worked in various multinational pharmaceutical companies including Alembic Limited (Vadodara, India), Cadila Laboratories Limited (Ahmedabad, India), and Nandesari Rasayanee Limited (Vadodara, India), and in Dai-Ichi Laboratories Limited (Hyderabad, India) and Yag Mag Labs Pvt Limited (Hyderabad, India) in senior management positions. Currently, he is the founder president of a reputable group of companies including Cepham Inc. (Piscataway, NJ), Yag Mag Inc. (Piscataway, NJ), RALLIFE Inc. (Piscataway, NJ), and Cepham Life Sciences Inc. (Piscataway, NJ). Dr. Swaroop has introduced several cutting-edge nutraceutical ingredients for obesity, diabetes, metabolic syndrome, and versatile degenerative conditions in the United States and around the world. He has 12 peer-reviewed publications, 2 books from CRC Press/Taylor & Francis and Wiley-Interscience, and numerous patents. Dr. Swaroop is a Member of the American Chemical Society (ACS), American Association of Pharmaceutical Scientists (AAPS), American Society of Pharmacognosy (ASP), New York Academy of Sciences (NYAS), American College of Nutrition (ACN), Council for Responsible Nutrition (CRN), American Botanical Council (ABC), and Natural Products Association (NPA). He has organized and chaired numerous sessions at the Annual Meetings of the Institutes of Food Technologists (IFT) and International Society of Nutraceuticals and Functional Foods (ISNFF) and other scientific meetings. He has delivered invited lectures and served as session chair at various national and international scientific conferences, organized workshops, and group discussion sessions.

Contributors

Maurice J. Arnaud
Independent Scientific Advisor
Nutrition & Biochemistry
La Tour-de-Peilz, Switzerland

Debasis Bagchi
Department of Pharmacological and Pharmaceutical Sciences
University of Houston College of Pharmacy
Houston, Texas, USA

and

Cepham Inc.
Piscataway, New Jersey, USA

Mirza Sarwar Baig
Department of Biosciences
Jamia Millia Islamia (A Central University)
New Delhi, India

Kuniyo Inouye
Inouye Laboratory of Enzyme Chemistry (i LEC)
Kyoto, Japan

Hiroko Isoda
Faculty of Life and Environmental Sciences and Alliance for Research on North Africa (ARENA)
University of Tsukuba
Tsukuba, Japan

Keiko Iwasa
Suntory Global Innovation Center Ltd.
Osaka, Japan

Raj K. Keservani
School of Pharmaceutical Sciences
Rajiv Gandhi Proudyogiki Vishwavidyalaya
Bhopal, India

Rajesh K. Kesharwani
Faculty of Biotechnology
National Institute of Technology
Telangana, India

Christina Kure
Swinburne Centre for Human Psychopharmacology
Swinburne University
Melbourne, Australia

Takuya Miyakawa
Department of Applied Biological Chemistry
University of Tokyo

Takatoshi Murase
Kao Co., Ltd.
Tokyo, Japan

Hiroyoshi Moriyama
The Japanese Institute for Health Food Standards
Tokyo, Japan

Chifumi Nagai
Hawaii Agriculture Research Center
Honolulu, Hawaii, USA

Rama P. Nair
Nutriwyo LLC
Laramie, Wyoming, USA

Sreejayan Nair
School of Pharmacy and Center for Cardiovascular Research and Alternative Medicine, College of Health Sciences
University of Wyoming
Laramie, Wyoming, USA

Koichi Nakahara
Suntory Global Innovation Center Ltd.
Osaka, Japan

Yusaku Narita
Innovation Center
UCC Ueshima Coffee Co., Ltd.
Osaka, Japan

Karen Nolidin
Swinburne Centre for Human Psychopharmacology
Swinburne University
Melbourne, Australia

Natalia Pandjaitan
Haldin Pacific Semesta PT
Bekasi, Indonesia

Anh Hong Phan
Department of Applied Biological Chemistry
University of Tokyo
Tokyo, Japan

Yuki Sato
Graduate School of Life and Environmental Sciences
University of Tsukuba
Tsukuba, Japan

Andrew Scholey
Swinburne Centre for Human Psychopharmacology
Swinburne University
Melbourne, Australia

Hiroshi Shimoda
R&D
Oryza Oil & Fat Chemical Co., Ltd
Aichi, Japan

Prabhakar Singh
Department of Biochemistry
University of Allahabad
Allahabad, India

Con Stough
Swinburne Centre for Human Psychopharmacology
Swinburne University
Melbourne, Australia

Atsushi Suzuki
Kao Co., Ltd.
Tochigi, Japan

Anand Swaroop
Cepham Inc.
Piscataway, New Jersey

Masaru Tanokura
Department of Applied Biological Chemistry
University of Tokyo
Tokyo, Japan

Ichiro Tokimitsu
Kao Co., Ltd.
Tokyo, Japan

Myra O. Villareal
Faculty of Life and Environmental Sciences
Alliance for Research on North Africa (ARENA)
University of Tsukuba
Tsukuba, Japan

Orie Yoshinari
The Japanese Institute for Health Food Standards
Tokyo, Japan

1 Green Coffee Bean Extract and Chlorogenic Acids

Chemistry and Novel Antioxidant Benefits

Rajesh K. Kesharwani, Prabhakar Singh, and Raj K. Keservani

CONTENTS

ABSTRACT

Coffee is the most widely consumed beverage in the world. Green coffee bean extract (GCBE) is derived from the coffee before it is roasted. It has potential to induce weight loss, stimulate the liver cells to increase fat metabolism, and reduce fat accumulation in the body without causing caloric restriction. The beneficial health effects of green coffee bean extract are attributed to its high antioxidant activity detected in chlorogenic, ferulic, caffeic, and n-coumaric acids. Chlorogenic acid (CGA) ((1*S*,3*R*,4*R*,5*R*)-3-{[(2E)-3-(3,4-dihydroxyphenyl) prop-2-enoyl]oxy}-1,4,5-trihydroxycyclohexanecarboxylic acid), the ester of caffeic acid and (−)-quinic acid, is the most studied bioactive polyphenolic compound of green coffee bean extract. It is derived from cinnamic acid synthesized during lignin biosynthesis, and it has been reported to elicit pleiotropic health-promoting effects due to its antioxidant and anti-inflammatory activities. Antioxidants trap free radicals and protect the body from damage caused by free radical–induced oxidative stress. Epidemiological studies have presented the possibility of chlorogenic acid and green coffee bean extract to be considered as phytomedicine. The objective of this study focused on the chemistry, antioxidant potential status, and various health-promoting effects of chlorogenic acid and green coffee bean extracts.

Keywords: green coffee been extract, chlorogenic acid, antioxidant, obesity, diabetes, bioavailability

List of Abbreviations

CGA chlorogenic acid
GCBE green coffee bean extract
GSH glutathione
SOD superoxide dismutase

1.1 INTRODUCTION

Antioxidants are molecules that inhibit the oxidation of biomolecules. Oxidation is a chemical process that involves the loss of electrons, which leads to an increase of oxidation, resulting in the production of free radicals. The presence of free radicals in the biological system starts a vicious chain reaction of oxidation of biomolecules. Oxidative chain reactions in cells induce the conformation changes in biomolecules, reflecting cellular damage that leads to cell death. Antioxidants mitigate free radical–mediated oxidative damage of biomolecules by directly neutralizing the free radicals or breaking the chain reaction. Antioxidants do this by being oxidized themselves. Antioxidants are often reducing agents such as thiols, ascorbic acid (vitamin C), or polyphenols (Sies 1997).

Plants and their extracts have been used as medicine since ancient times to cure various diseases. Bioactive compounds present in plants and their products have been documented to possess different biological activities that implicate their use as therapeutic agents against several chronic human diseases (Rizvi and Pandey 2009b). Coffee is one of the most popular beverages due to its pleasant flavor and pharmacological properties. Beneficial health effects of GCBE have been attributed to chlorogenic acid (CGA) and other strong antioxidant molecules (Moreira et al. 2005). Green coffee bean extract is derived from the coffee bean before roasting. The two species of coffee plants that have the greatest commercial importance are *Coffea arabica* and *Coffea robusta*. These two species differ in chemical composition and antioxidant potential. *C. robusta* coffee beans exhibited higher antioxidant potential than *C. arabica* coffee. However, after roasting, there was no significant antioxidant potential differences (Ginz et al. 2000). The effects of GCBE and

CGA are multifaceted. An intake of GCBE has been reported to reduce the risk of cardiovascular disease, type 2 diabetes, Alzheimer's disease, and Parkinson's disease (Lindsay et al. 2002, Ascherio et al. 2004, Vinson et al. 2009, Salazar-Martinez et al. 2004), and exhibits antibacterial and anti-inflammatory properties (Almeida et al. 2006; Daglia et al. 2007; Bonita et al. 2007). GCBE extract can reduce blood pressure and prevent the onset of high blood pressure (Watanabe et al. 2006; Kozuma et al. 2005). GCBE is proven to be effective in reducing excess weight and tackling obesity (Vinson et al. 2009). Consuming coffee is reported to reduce fatigue and increase the activity of the nervous system.

The beneficial health effects of GCBE have been attributed to both the antioxidant potential enhanced by various polyphenol constituents as well as a major contribution of CGA. Roasting of coffee has been associated with changes in the antioxidant potential depending on the roasting temperature. Here, we will discuss the antioxidant potential, chemistry and bioavailability, and various health benefits due to the antioxidant potential of GCBE and CGA. Oxidative stress in animal cells is often associated with an overproduction of O_2 or H_2O_2. It causes damage to the biological molecules. The accumulation of this damage is the cause of various diseases. The body has several defenses against oxidative stress, including: enzymes, proteins chelating, and transition metals (Perez-Matute et al. 2012). There are other ways to fight against oxidative stress such as biological antioxidants. These are exogenous biological substances that protect biological systems against the deleterious effects of oxidative stress (Perez-Matute et al. 2012).

Coffee is one of the most widely consumed beverages in the world, and therefore the potential health consequences of coffee consumption are of great public interest. Heavy coffee drinking may result in sleep disorders, hypokalemia, and cardiac arrhythmias (Smith 2002; Appel and Myles 2001; Curatolo and Robertson 1983; Cornelis 2012). At the same time, several epidemiologic studies have reported that the risk of Parkinson's disease, Alzheimer's disease, and certain types of cancer is reduced in regular coffee consumers (Rosso et al. 2008).

1.2 ANTIOXIDANT POTENTIAL OF GREEN COFFEE BEAN EXTRACTS (GCBE)

There have been various studies over the years on the antioxidant potential of coffee beans and its beverages using different detection methods (Figure 1.1). Scientific evidence has proved that green coffee beverages present high antioxidant properties *in vivo* and *in vitro*. Several studies indicate that a high content of polyphenols in coffee leads to higher antioxidant potential, resulting in strong

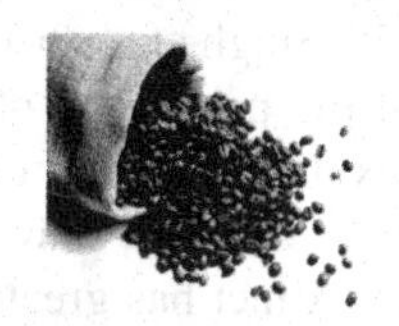

FIGURE 1.1 (See color insert.) Green coffee bean fruit.

antioxidant action. The concentration of active polyphenols in green beans is influenced by the species and its origin; however, in beverages it depends on the process of brewing. During the roasting process, phenolic compounds in green coffee beans are partially degraded and/or bound to polymer structures, depending on roasting conditions.

Antioxidants derived from plants are of interest owing to their observed biological effects such as free radical scavenging ability, inhibition of cellular proliferation, and modulation of various enzymatic activity while also acting as antibiotic, anti-allergic, antidiarrheal, anti-ulcer, and anti-inflammatory agents (Rizvi and Pandey 2009b). The antioxidant effects of GCBE are usually attributed to the presence of chlorogenic, ferulic, caffeic, and n-coumaric acids (Yashin et al. 2013). Green coffee has major antioxidant potential as CGA (5–12 g/100 g), which is an ester formed from cinnamic acid and quinic acid and is also known as 5-ocaffeoylquinnic acid (5-CQA) (Ayelign and Sabally 2013). In GCBE, six antioxidant compounds have been identified as caffeoylquinic acids and dicaffeoylquinic acids with radical scavenging potential; however, depending on the roasting process, roasted coffees could produce up to 16 different antioxidant compounds (Van der Werf et al. 2014). It has been reported repeatedly that light roasted coffee displays higher antioxidant activity and total phenolic content of the coffee beans than dark roasted coffee, but less than unroasted (green) bean (Somporn et al. 2011).

During the roasting process, antioxidant molecules such as citric, malic, and CGA were found to decrease as a result of the reduction in antioxidant potential. CGA is observed to degrade during the roasting process (Nebesny and Budryn 2003). Roasting the green coffee beans at 230°C for 12 min reduced the total CGA content by nearly 50%, while roasting it at 250°C for 21 min reduced the CGA to almost trace levels. According to Hecimovic et al. (2011), CGA content was decreased and affected by the degree of roasting in various coffee samples.

A positive but nonlinear relationship was reported for the amount of CGA after roasting (Keservani et al. 2010). Melanoidins formed via the Maillard reaction during roasting of coffee are also known to be increase the antioxidant potential. Melanoidins exhibit antioxidant potential due to the scavenging ability of hydroxyl radicals and the ability to break radical chain reactions through oxygen radicals scavenging. Melanoidins contribute approximately 25% of the total antioxidant activity of coffee. Up to now, only the influence of the roasting condition on the total antioxidant action of coffee has been investigated. The human body relies on antioxidants, which limit the damaging effects of oxidative stress. Dietary antioxidants include phenolic compounds, whereas alkaloid and steroid activity is generally attributed to the hydrogen donating ability of polyphenols, which intercept the free radical chain of oxidation and form a stable end product that does not initiate or propagate oxidation of biomolecules (Sherwin 1978; Singh et al. 2015).

Recent research has presented the possibility of GCBE or CGA to be considered as phytomedicine. The antioxidant potential of GCBE is believed to be more effective than green tea and grape seed (Wild Flavors n.d.). Research conducted in Italy found that green coffee bean extract has greater antioxidant potential than 34 other beverages (Pellegrini et al. 2003). *In vivo* induction of GCBE against diabetic rats has been reported to increase the antioxidant potential in plasma by increasing the GSH level (Ahmed et al. 2013). The GSH level was found to decrease in the erythrocytes as well as plasma with increasing oxidative stress or decreasing total antioxidant potential in both rats and humans (Rizvi and Pandey 2009a). Regular and decaffeinated coffee intake has been reported to reduce the serum and uric acid concentrations, a product of the catabolism of purines, which increases during oxidative stress, mutagenesis, and probably cancer (Aucamp et al. 1997; Choi and Cyrhan 2007; Kiyohara et al. 1999). Despite inducing the antioxidant molecule level in cell or extracellular fluid, GCBE supplementation also has been reported to modulate the activity of antioxidant enzymes.

The antioxidant potential of caffeine (1,3,7-trimethylxanthine) exhibits levels similar to that of reduced glutathione, which is reported to be significantly higher than ascorbic acid. The antioxidant activity of caffeine was evaluated in a study of oxidative damage in rat liver microsomes. The damage was induced by three reactive oxygen species (ROS) that caused membrane damage *in vivo*, namely: hydroxyl radical (OH), peroxyl radical (ROO), and singlet oxygen ($1O_2$). Caffeine was found to be an effective inhibitor of lipid peroxidation at milimolar concentrations against all three reactive species (Devasagayam et al. 1996).

Raw coffee beans are rich in CGA and caffeine, which significantly decrease during the roasting and decaffeination processes (Moon et al. 2009) (Figure 1.2a). The GCBE used in the present study is prepared from decaffeinated and unroasted coffee beans, making it a novel source of CGA and eliminating the possible side effects of caffeine (Smith 2002; Appel and Myles 2001; Curatolo and Robertson 1983). There have been no reports of toxicological studies on GCBE. In a clinical trial, decaffeinated GCBE induced weight loss in overweight volunteers who were administered 400 mg/day for 60 days (Dellalibera et al. 2006). Concurrent with the rise in obesity is the rise in nutraceuticals that may aid weight loss. GCBE is a nutraceutical that has recently received both media and research attention as a weight loss supplement. GCBE is present in green or raw coffee beans. GCBE contains large amounts of CGA, a polyphenol that has antioxidant properties and influences glucose, fat, and brain energy metabolism (Henry-Vitrac et al. 2010; Ho et al. 2012).

Given the high moisture content and fast decomposition of the coffee pulp, one way to preserve it is by ensiling it with molasses (Ulloa Rojas et al. 2003). On the other hand, coffee based drinks are proven to have a great antioxidant activity (Richelle et al. 2001). This activity is due to the great amount of phenolic compounds present in the coffee grain (Farah et al. 2006), which decreases depending on the type of roasting and also might decrease polyphenol concentrations (Castillo et al.

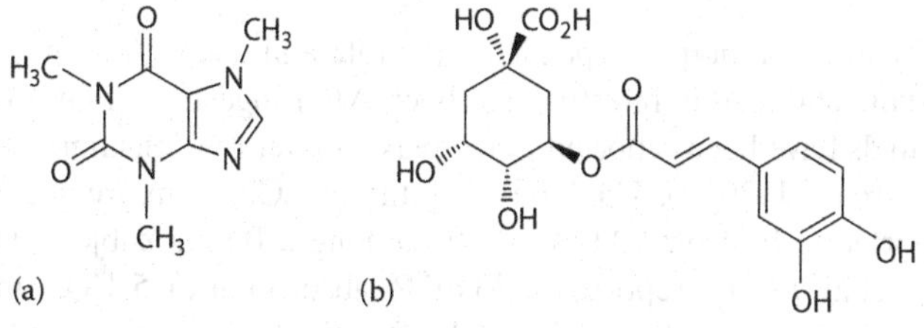

FIGURE 1.2 Structure of (a) caffeine and (b) chlorogenic acids.

2002, Duarte et al. 2005). Like the grain, coffee pulp has been attributed with a few antioxidant properties (Arellano-Gonzalez et al. 2011), and it is possible that some handling practices alter its antioxidant capacity. Recently, the discovery of a new dietary supplement has attracted attention in Western countries, especially the GCBE from *C. arabica*. This was found to contain large amounts of the crucial substance, CGA, which is an antioxidant (Bisht and Sisodia 2010). This can be used as a supplement for weight loss and lead to a reduction of BMI (Onakpoya et al. 2011; Vinson et al. 2012).

1.3 COMPOSITION OF GREEN COFFEE BEAN EXTRACTS (GCBE)

Green coffee is composed primarily of water, carbohydrates, fiber, proteins, free amino acids, lipids, minerals, organic acids, CGA, trigonelline, caffeine, and different volatile compounds. The most important contributors inducing beverage flavor after roasting includeCGA, caffeine, trigonelline, soluble fiber, and diterpenes. Among the various biomolecules and compounds recorded, approximately 100 different volatile compounds have been reported in green coffee including alcohols, esters, hydrocarbons, aldehydes, ketones, pyrazines, furans, and sulfur compounds (Toci and Farah 2008; Flament et al. 1968).

1.4 CHLOROGENIC ACIDS

1.4.1 Chemistry

CGAs are a major class of phenolic compounds, which are derived from esterification of trans-cinnamic acids like caffeic, ferulic, and p-coumaric with (−)-quinic acid. The esters are formed with the hydroxyl of carbon-5, -3, and -4 according to the number of cinnamic substituents and the esterification position in the cyclohexane ring of the quinic acid. The subclasses of CGA are caffeoylquinic acids, dicaffeoylquinic acids, and feruloylquinic acids, which are considered as major compounds; however, the less abundant subclasses include p-coumaroylquinic acids and caffeoyl-feruloylquinic acids. Only caffeoylquinic acids reflect 80% of the total CGA. Among caffeoylquinic acids, 5-caffeoylquinic acid accounts for approximately 60%. The compound 5-caffeoylquinic acid (5-CQA) was identified first and is the most studied isomer. CGA is responsible for the bitterness and acidity in coffee brew (Farah 2012).

1.4.2 Chemistry of Bioavailability

Bioavailability of a compound depends on the rate and concentration at which it is absorbed and metabolized in intestine and liver. After ingestion of GCBE, six major CGA compounds have been reported in the plasma after the consumption of roasted coffee (Monteiro et al. 2007). The bioavailability of CGA from green coffee extract has been reported to be from 7.8% to 72.1% among different subjects (Farah et al. 2008). Olthof et al. (2003) reported a 33.617% absorption of 5-CQA in ileostomy fluids from colostomized subjects for 24 h after the consumption of 2.8 mmol of 5-CQA. Smaller quantities of caffeic, ferulic, isoferulic, and p-coumaric acids were also identified in the plasma after green coffee extract consumption. A higher mean molar ratio of 5-CQA:4-CQA and 3-CQA in the plasma explains the preferential absorption of 5-CQA as well as rapid metabolization and uptake of 3-CQA by organs such as liver (Farah et al. 2005; Olthof et al. 2003) and adipose tissue. Similarly, molar ratio in plasma of 3,4-diCQA:4,5diCQA and 3,5diCQA explain the mechanisms favoring plasma levels.

CGA compounds present in the green coffee matrix are highly bioavailable in humans (Figure 1.2b). CQA and diCQA, the major CGA compounds in coffee, are differentially absorbed and/or metabolized throughout the whole gastrointestinal tract. CGA is absorbed in the small intestine as well as in the colon. CGA is absorbed in the small intestine and appears in the circulatory system as glucuronide, sulfate, and methylated metabolites (Farah et al. 2008). After ingestion of coffee, both free and sulfated conjugates of dihydroferulic acid and dihydrocaffeic acid were detected in highest concentrations in human plasma. Most CGA metabolites are rapidly removed from the circulatory system with a half-life of 0.3–1.9 h. However, dihydroferulic acid-4-O-sulfate, dihydroferulic acid-3-O-sulfate, and ferulic acid-4-O-sulfate are reported to have an extended half-life and to present an unusual biphasic plasma profile with dual Tmax values at 0.6 and 4.3 h.

It was found that the small intestine is the cleavage site of quinic acid, which in turn releases caffeic acid and ferulic acid, metabolizes caffeic acid to its 3- and 4-O-sulfates, and ferulic acid to ferulic acid-4-O-sulfate, and the methylation of caffeic acid to form isoferulic acid and its subsequent 3-O-sulfation and glucuronidation. In addition, the colon is the site for the conversion of ferulic acid to feruloylglycine and dihydroferulic acid, and caffeic acid to dihydrocaffeic acid.

Urine may not be the preferential excretion route for intact CGA and metabolites (Farah 2004; Farah et al. 2006; Choudhury et al. 1999; Gugler et al. 1975). Sinapic, gallic, p-hydroxybenzoic, and dihydrocaffeic acids have been reported as the four major urinary phenolic compounds excreted after green coffee consumption, and are thought to be preferential metabolic products of the cinnamates identified in plasma. Rechner has reported that after ingestion of two cups of coffee at 4 h intervals, free metabolites ferulic acid, isoferulic acid, dihydroferulic acid, 3-methoxy-4-hydroxybenzoic acid, hippuric acid, and 3-hydroxyhippuric acid were found in human urine (Rechner et al. 2001).

1.4.3 Antioxidant Potential and Biological Activities of Chlorogenic Acid

CGA is a highly valuable natural antioxidant used in medicine and industries. Diets rich in CGA content has been reported to prevent various diseases associated with oxidative stress such as cancer, cardiovascular, aging, and neurodegenerative disease (Belay and Gholap 2009). Epidemiologic *in vitro* and animal studies reported the CGA and their metabolites exhibit antimutagenic property, antibacterial and anti-inflammatory activity (Almeida et al. 2006; Daglia et al. 2007; Bonita et al. 2007), antiviral activity mainly against adenovirus and herpes virus (Chiang et al. 2002), hepatoprotective activity in rats (Basnet et al. 1996), and immune-stimulatory activity (Tatefuji et al. 1996).

CGA reduces oxidative stress via neutralizing the free radicals and hydroxyl radicals. Lipid peroxidation is the primary marker of oxidative stress for lipid molecules (Singh and Rizvi 2012). Oxidative stress damages all types of cellular molecules including lipid and proteins, which in turn induces pathological conditions such as cancers, cardiovascular diseases, osteoporosis, and aging (Rizvi and Pandey 2009a). Polyphenols limit the development of cancers, cardiovascular diseases, neurodegenerative diseases, diabetes, and osteoporosis due to their strong antioxidant potential. CGA was also reported to reduce the lipid peroxidation in kidney cells of diabetic rats by modulating the activities of antioxidant enzymes such as superoxide dismutase (SOD) and catalase, indicating its antioxidant potential (Nishi and Kumar 2013). Pharmacologically, CGA has also been reported to inhibit glucose-6-phosphate translocase in the intestine and hence delay glucose absorption. CGA also selectively inhibits glucose-6-phosphatase in the liver, the rate-limiting enzyme involved in gluconeogenesis (Arion et al. 1997). CGAs have health benefits by reducing weight through modulating glucose and fat metabolism while simultaneously contributing to antihyperlipidemic activity (Shimoda et al. 2006).

CGA is an antioxidant, and an ester of caffeic acid and (−)-quinic acid. It is an important biosynthetic intermediate in lignin biosynthesis (Boerjan et al. 2003). CGA has been reported to slow the release rate of glucose into the bloodstream after a meal (Johnston et al. 2003). The term CGA refers to a related family of esters of hydroxycinnamic acids (caffeic acid, ferulic acid, and p-coumaric acid) with quinic acid (Clifford et al. 2003).

Tea (*Camellia sinensis* L., family Theaceae) is a great source of phenolic compounds such as flavonoids (Keservani and Sharma 2014) and phenolic acids, which are responsible for the total antioxidant activity of tea infusion (Kim et al. 2011). *Hibiscus sabdariffa* leaves from different countries have different chemical compositions and different antioxidant potential. The five major antioxidant compounds identified from *H. sabdariffa* leaves are neochlorogenic acid, chlorogenic acid, cryptochlorogenic acid, rutin, and isoquercitrin (Ochani and D'Mello 2009; Essa and Subramanian 2007; Mohd-Esa et al. 2010).

CGA is a well-known antioxidant and has more isomers according to the difference in binding location and number of caffeic or quinic acid. Mullen (2011) studied the antioxidant and CGA profiles of whole coffee fruits that are influenced by extraction procedures and reported that the antioxidant activity in whole coffee fruit extracts was up to 25 times higher than in powders dependent on the radical. Total antioxidant activity of samples displayed a strong correlation to CGA content (Mullen et al. 2011).

Budryn and colleagues studied the correlation between the stability of CGA, antioxidant activity, and acrylamide content in coffee beans roasted in different conditions and demonstrated that the increase of humidity in roasting air reduces acrylamide formation only at the highest used roasting temperature. However, the modification of roasting conditions to achieve a drop in acrylamide concentration resulted in increased degradation of polyphenols and/or deterioration of antioxidant activity. It was found that a temperature of 203°C of dry air, with low velocity of roasting air, reduced the levels of acrylamide and also moderately degraded the polyphenols (Budryn et al. 2015). The optimal roasting parameters were a temperature of 203°C, dry air, and a low velocity of roasting air. Under these conditions, the roasted beans were characterized by a relatively low level of acrylamide and moderate degradation of polyphenols (Budryn et al. 2015). The total antioxidant activity of food snacks has been attributed to the total phenolic content. Ultra performance liquid chromatography (UPLC)-mediated profiling of polyphenols led to the detection of three common biomolecules in all kale foods but with different levels of gallic acid, CGA, and catechin. The amount of CGA in the snacks ranges from 431 μg/g (Yellow Kale) to 1706 μg/g (Happy Kale), whereas gallic acid ranges from 94.7 μg/g (Yellow Kale) to 448 μg/g (Inspiral Kale).

CGAs have been reported to reduce the risk of type 2 diabetes. CGA present in the circulatory system have positive effects on the cardiovascular system (Johnston et al. 2003). *In vivo* studies have proved the antioxidant and the anticarcinogenic properties of CGA. The bioavailability of CGA is lower due to poor absorption in the small intestine, but it is conversely capable of providing higher yields of microbial metabolites and various active compounds responsible for the biological properties attributed to dietary polyphenols (Gonthier et al. 2003).

1.5 HEALTH BENEFIT EFFECTS OF GREEN COFFEE BEAN EXTRACT AND CHLOROGENIC ACID

1.5.1 Obesity

Excess weight and obesity are serious health concerns associated with cardiovascular problems and diabetes. GCBE induces the alteration of plasma adipokine levels and body fat distribution despite downregulating fatty acid and cholesterol biosynthesis. It is also reported to induce the fatty acid oxidation and peroxisome proliferator–activated receptor alpha (PPARα) expression in the liver (Cho et al. 2010). The antiobesity effect of GCBE may be mediated via suppressing the accumulation of hepatic triglycerides (TG) (Shimoda et al. 2006). It was found that supplementation of GCBE for 14 days reduced weight gain and visceral fat accumulation in mice. It was found that intravenous administration of CGA to rats reduced the serum and TG levels; however, the TG levels in the adipose tissue were unaffected (Ayton Global Research 2009). Oral supplementation of CGA was also found to reduce the level of hepatic TG in mice, but the amount of visceral fat was unchanged.

It was found that intake of an adequate amount of coffee polyphenols modulated the fatty acid or glucose metabolism, reduced weight gain, and abdominal and liver fat accumulation, and reduced obesity-associated diseases (Murase et al. 2011). Song et al. (2014) studied the effects of decaffeinated GCBE on diet-induced obesity and insulin resistance in mice, and suggested that 5-CQA, and other polyphenols in GCBE, may bring an additive effect in decreasing body weight gain and increasing insulin sensitivity. These beneficial effects are possibly due to the downregulation of genes associated with adipogenesis and inflammation in the white adipose tissue (WAT) of mice (Song et al. 2014).

1.5.2 Diabetes

Polyphenol-rich plant extracts are reported to control diabetes and its associated complications (Rizvi and Srivastva 2007). The use of natural extracts or plant products are common among diabetic patients due to less, or no, side effects of these medications. There is repeated evidence that coffee components, especially CGA, reduce the risk of type 2 diabetes. A study of Asian men and women in Singapore concluded that regular intake of coffee significantly reduced the risk of type 2 diabetes (Odegaard et al. 2008). CGA value decreased during the roasting process, hence, GCBE consumption might have potential against type 2 diabetes.

Antidiabetic effects of GCBE were found due to the inhibition potential of CGA for glucose-6-phosphatase hydrolysis, and hence led to a downregulation of glucose-producing pathways such as gluconeogenesis and glycogenolysis in the liver (Arion et al. 1997). CGA, caffeoylquinic acids, and dicaffeoylquinic acids competitively inhibited the glucose-6-phosphatase hydrolysis in the microsomes of human liver. Henry-Vitrac (2010) reported these glucose-lowering effects by reducing the hepatic glucose production and making it a potential antidiabetic molecule (Henry-Vitrac et al. 2010).

1.5.3 Cardiovascular Disorders

Polyphenols are reported to contain good antioxidants that help limit cardiovascular diseases (Hertog et al. 1993; Schachinger et al. 2000). Polyphenols in red wine have been attributed to a low mortality rate due to a lack of cardiovascular disorders, even after high consumption of a fat-rich diet. Consumption of tea and red wine are regularly associated to a lower risk of myocardial infarction. Similar effects were observed after the consumption of GCBE. It was found that a daily intake of GCBE reduced blood pressure in hypertensive subjects, and reduced the risk of stroke and coronary heart disease (Kozuma et al. 2005). Ochiai found that GCBE intake improved vasoreactivity through acting on the blood vessels, which in turn reduced hypertension and helped reduce the progression of arteriosclerosis (Ochiai et al. 2004).

1.5.4 Anticancer Effects

It was found that polyphenols are most often protective on human cancer cell lines and reduce the number of tumors or their growth (Yang et al. 2001). Polyphenols acted as halting agents at the initiation stage of cancer development and also inhibited cell proliferation especially against mammary and prostate cancers observed in different animal models (Lamartiniere et al. 2002; Kuntz et al. 1999). The relationship between coffee and cancer is associated with the bioactive molecule in the coffee that could potentially alter the risk of cancer through several biological mechanisms. In recent studies, it was found that coffee consumption significantly reduced the risk of liver, kidney, and to a lesser extent, premenopausal breast and colorectal cancers.

Research studies involving a total of 2,260 cases and 239,146 non-cases indicated that coffee consumption reduced the risk of liver cancer in individuals with and without a history of liver disease (Nkondjock 2009). The antioxidant potential, as a putative mechanism, explained the antiliver cancer effects of coffee. Despite this, antioxidant molecules in coffee maintain a relatively lower iron status and therefore reduce the risk of liver injury (Mascitelli et al. 2008). It also prevents cirrhosis of the liver, which is a major risk factor for the development of hepatocellular carcinoma (La Vecchia et al. 1998). Coffee modulates the transaminases activity which reduces the risk or mortality from liver cirrhosis (Klatsky et al. 2006; Tverdal and Skurtveit 2003). Coffee consumption also reduces the risk of kidney cancer by improving the insulin sensitivity. The prevention of obesity is also associated with a reduction in renal cancer.

Coffee consumption is also associated with a reduction in breast cancer. A Norwegian grouping of 14,593 women who drank >5 cups of coffee per day experienced a statistically significant decrease in breast cancer risk (Vatten et al. 1990). In addition, premenopausal women with the BRCA1 or BRCA2 gene mutation who drank 6 or more cups of coffee per day experienced a significant reduction (70% statistically) in breast cancer risk (Nkondjock et al. 2006).

Consumption of GCBE is associated with a reduction in obesity by increasing the antioxidant potential in the plasma. Mitigating effects of GCBE are still under process, but the preclinical data about the anticancer effects of coffee explain the potential green coffee been extracts has as an anticancer agent. Oxidative stress is reported to contribute to the pathogenesis of Alzheimer's disease, Parkinson's disease, atherosclerosis, amyotrophic lateral sclerosis, ischemia/reperfusion neuronal injuries, cataract formation, degenerative disease of the human temporomandibular-joint, macular degeneration, degenerative retinal damage, rheumatoid arthritis, multiple sclerosis, muscular dystrophy, human cancers, as well as the aging process. A poor diet containing lower amounts of antioxidant may also indirectly result in oxidative stress, which impairs the cellular defense mechanisms. The strong antioxidant potential of GCBE and CGA, the compound found in GCBE, may explain the beneficial health effects based on the scientific evidence. Polysaccharides from coffee decrease the cholesterol levels in blood, control the blood glucose and insulin response, and act as agents against infectious and tumor diseases (Gniechwitz et al. 2007; Simoes et al. 2009).

1.5.5 Multifocal Electroretinography

The antibacterial, anti-inflammatory, antioxidant, and anticarcinogenic activities of CGA have been demonstrated in many studies (DosSantos et al. 2006; Cho et al. 2010; Kim et al. 2010). Shin and Yu (2014) explain that CGA supplementation improved multifocal electroretinography in patients with retinitis pigmentosa and reported that CGA may have a beneficial effect on the peripheral area at the margins of retinal degeneration, and should be considered as an antioxidant for the management of retinitis pigmentosa (Shin et al. 2013; Shin and Yu 2014).

1.5.6 Brain Health

Coffee bean was recently used in a mental health and prevention of mental disorder study (Keservani et al. 2015b). Green tea polyphenols (GTPP) may potentiate nerve growth factor (NGF)-induced neuritogenesis and may serve as an optional therapy for neurodegenerative disease (Gundimeda et al. 2010).

1.6 CONCLUSION

Numerous studies have produced evidence that the polyphenols isolated from natural resources, in particular herbal plants, are key factors for improving health. The health protective role of natural polyphenols as an antioxidant against degenerative diseases is supported by several studies carried out *in vitro* as well as *in vivo*. These studies outline a current understanding of the chemistry, antioxidant, bioavailability, and pleiotropic effects of GCBE and CGA. GCBE and CGA provide significant protection against the development and progression of obesity, diabetes, and associated cardiovascular problems. Epidemiological studies explained the biological effects of GCBE and CGA in relevance to human health, yet some mechanisms of the action are still unknown and not fully understood. The role of GCBE in human health is a fertile area of research and offers great hope for the prevention of various chronic diseases.

REFERENCES

Ahmed, G.M., H.E. El-Ghamery, M.F. Samy. 2013. Effect of green and degree of roasted Arabic coffee on hyperlipidemia and antioxidant status in diabetic rats. *Adv. J. Food Sci. Technol.* 5(5): 619–626.

Almeida, A.A., A. Farah, D.A. Silv, E.A. Nunan, M.B. Gloria. 2006. Anti-bacterial activity of coffee extracts and selected coffee chemical compounds against enterobacteria. *J. Agric. Food Chem.* 54(23): 8738–8743.

Appel, C.C. and T. D. Myles. 2001. Caffeine-induced hypokalemic paralysis in pregnancy. *Obstet Gynecol.* 97(5 Pt 2): 805–807.

Arellano-Gonzalez, M.A., M.A. Ramirez-Coronel, M.T. Torres-Mancera, G.G. Perez-Morales, G. Saucedo-Castaneda. 2011. Antioxidant activity of fermented and nonfermented coffee (*Coffea arabica*) pulp extracts. *Food Technol. Biotech.* 49: 374–378.

Arion, W.J., W.K. Canfield, F.C. Ramos, P.W. Schindler, H.J. Burger, H. Hemmerle, G. Schubert, P. Below, A.W. Herling. 1997. Chlorogenic acid and hydroxynitrobenzaldehyde: New inhibitors of hepatic glucose 6-phosphatase. *Arch. Biochem. Biophys.* 339: 315–322.

Ascherio, A., M.G. Weisskopf, E.J. O'Reilly, M.L. McCullough, E.E. Calle, C. Rodriguez, M.J. Thun. 2004. Coffee consumption, gender, and Parkinson's disease mortality in the cancer prevention study II cohort: The modifying effects of estrogen. *Am. J. Epidemiol.* 160: 977–984.

Aucamp, J., A. Gaspar, Y. Hara, Z. Apostolides. 1997. Inhibition of xanthine oxidase by catechins from tea. *Anticancer Res.* 17: 4381–4385.

Ayelign, A. and K. Sabally. 2013. Determination of chlorogenic acids (CGA) in coffee beans using HPLC. *Am. J. Res. Commun.* 2: 78–91.

Ayton Global Research. 2009. Independent market study on the effect of coffee shape on weight loss: The effect of chlorogenic acid enriched coffee (coffee chape) on weight when used in overweight people. http://pdfsr.com/pdf/the-effect-of-chlorogenic-acid-enriched-coffee-coffee-shape-on-weight-when-used-in-overweight-people.

Basnet, P., K. Matsushige, K. Hase, S. Kadota, T. Namba. 1996. Four di-o-caffeoyl quinic acid derivatives from propolis. Potent hepatoprotective activity in experimental liver injury models. *Biol. Pharm. Bull.* 19: 1479–1484.

Belay, A. and A.V. Gholap. 2009. Characterization and determination of chlorogenic acids (CGA) in coffee beans by UV-Vis spectroscopy. *Afr. J. Pure Appl. Chem.* 3(11): 234–240.

Bisht, S. and S.S. Sisodia. 2010. *Coffee arabica*: A wonder gift to medical science. *J. Nat. Pharm.* 1(1): 1–8.

Boerjan, W., J. Ralph, M. Baucher. 2003. Lignin biosynthesis. *Annu. Rev. Plant Biol.* 54: 519–546.

Bonita, J.S., M. Mandarano, D. Shuta, J. Vinson. 2007. Coffee and cardiovascular disease: *In vitro*, cellular, animal, and human studies. *Pharmacol. Res.* 55(3): 187–198.

Budryn, G., E. Nebesny, J. Oracz. 2015. Correlation between the stability of chlorogenic acids, antioxidant activity and acrylamide content in coffee beans roasted in different conditions. *Int. J. Food Prop.* 18(2): 290–302.

Castillo, M.D., J.M. Ames, M.H. Gordon. 2002. Effect of roasting on the antioxidant activity of coffee brews. *J. Agric. Food Chem.* 50: 3698–3703.

Chiang, L.C., W. Chiang, M.Y. Chang, L.T. Ng, C.C. Lin. 2002. Antiviral activity of *Plantago* major extracts and related compounds *in vitro*. *Antiviral Res.* 55: 53–62.

Cho, A.S., S.M. Jeon, M.J. Kim, J. Yeo, K.I. Seo, M.S. Choi, M.K. Lee. 2010. Chlorogenic acid exhibits anti-obesity property and improves lipid metabolism in high-fat diet-induced-obese mice. *Food Chem. Toxicol.* 48(3): 937–943.

Choi, H.K. and G. Cyrhan. 2007. Coffee, tea and caffeine consumption and serum uric acid level: The third national health and nutrition examination survey. *Arthritis Rheum.* 57: 816–821.

Choudhury, R., S.K. Srai, E. Debnam, C. Rice-Evans. 1999. Urinary excretion of hydroxycinnamates and flavonoids after oral and intravenous administration. *Free Radic. Biol. Med.* 27: 278–286.

Clifford, M. N., K.L. Johnston, S. Knigh, N. Kuhnert. 2003. Hierarchical scheme for LC-MSn identification of chlorogenic acids. *J. Agric. Food Chem.* 51(10): 2900–2911.

Cornelis, M.C. 2012. Coffee intake. *Prog. Mol. Biol. Transl. Sci.* 108: 293–322.

Curatolo, P.W. and D. Robertson. 1983. The health consequences of caffeine. *Ann. Intern. Med.* 98(5 Pt 1): 641–653.

Daglia, M., A. Papetti, P. Grisoli, C. Aceti, V. Spini, C. Dacarro, G. Gazzani. 2007. Isolation, identification, and quantification of roasted coffee anti-bacterial compounds. *J. Agric. Food Chem.* 55(25): 10208–10213.

Dellalibera, O., B. Lemaire, S. Lafay. 2006. Svetol, green coffee extract, induces weight loss and increases the lean to fat mass ratio in volunteers with overweight problem. *Phytotherapie.* 4(4): 194–197.

Devasagayama, T.P.A., J.P. Kamata, H. Mohanb, P.C. Kesavan. 1996. Caffeine as an anti-oxidants: Inhibition of lipid peroxidation induced by reactive O_2 species. *Biochem. Biophys. Acta.* 1282: 63–70.

DosSantos, M.D., M.C. Almeida, N.P. Lopes, G.E. de Souza. 2006. Evaluation of the anti-inflammatory, analgesic and antipyretic activities of the natural polyphenol chlorogenic acid. *Biol. Pharm. Bull.* 29: 2236–2240.

Duarte, S.M.S., C.M.P. Abreu, H.C. Menezes, M.H. Santos, C.M.C.P. Gouvea. 2005. Effect of processing and roasting on the antioxidant activity of coffee brews. *Food Sci. Technol.* 25: 387–393.

Essa, M.M. and P. Subramanian. 2007. Hibiscus sabdariffa affects ammonium chloride-induced hyperammone mic rats. *Evid. Based Complement. Alt. Med.* 4: 321–325.

Farah, A. 2004. Distribuição nos grãos, importância na qualidade da bebida e biodisponibilidade dos ácidos clorogêncios do café. PhD diss., Rio de Janeiro: Universidade Federal do Rio de Janeiro.

Farah, A. 2012. Coffee constituents. In ed. C. Y.-F. Chu, *Coffee: Emerging Health Effects and Disease Prevention*, pp. 21–58. Oxford.

Farah, A., T. de Paulis, L.C. Trugo, P.R. Martin. 2005. Effect of roasting on the formation of chlorogenic acid lactones in coffee. *J. Agric. Food. Chem.* 53(5): 1505–1513.

Farah, A., M. Monteiro, C.M. Donangelo, S. Lafay. 2008. Chlorogenic acids from green coffee extract are highly bioavailable in humans. *J. Nutr.* 138(12): 2309–2315.

Farah, A., M.C. Monteiro, F. Guigon, D.P. Moreira, C.M. Donangelo, L.C. Trugo. 2006. Chlorogenic acids from coffee are absorbed and excreted in human digestive fluids. *Proceedings of the 21st International Conference on Coffee Science*, pp. 58–64.

Flament, I., F. Gautschi, M. Winter, B. Willhalm, M. Stoll. 1968. Les composants furanniques de l'arome cafe: Quelques aspects chimiques et spectroscopiques. *Proceedings of the Third International Conference on Coffee Science*, ASIC, Paris, pp. 197–215.

Ginz, M., H. Balzer, A. Bradbury, H. Maier. 2000. Formation of aliphatic acids by carbohydrate degradation during roasting of coffee. *Eur. Food Res. Technol.* 211: 404–410.

Gniechwitz, D., N. Reichardt, M. Blaut, H. Steinhart, M. Bunzel. 2007. Dietary fiber from coffee beverage: Degradation by human fecal microbiota. *J. Agric. Food Chem.* 55(17): 6989–6996.

Gonthier, M.P., M.A.Verny, C. Besson, C. Remesy, A. Scalbert. 2003. Chlorogenic acid bioavailability largely depends on its metabolism by the gut microflora in rats. *J. Nutr.* 133: 1853–1859.

Gugler, R., M. Leschik, H.J. Dengler. 1975. Disposition of quercetin in man after single oral and intravenous doses. *Eur. J. Clin. Pharmacol.* 9: 229–234.

Gundimeda, U., T.H. McNeill, J.E. Schiffman, D.R. Hinton, R. Gopalakrishna. 2010. Green tea polyphenols potentiate the action of nerve growth factor to induce neuritogenesis: Possible role of reactive oxygen species. *J. Neurosci. Res.* 88: 3644–3655.

Hecimovic, I., A. Belscak-Cvitanovic, D. Horzic, D. Komes. 2011. Comparative study of polyphenols and caffeine in different coffee varieties affected by the degree of roasting. *Food Chem.* 129(3): 991–1000.

Henry-Vitrac, C., A. Ibarra, M. Roller, J.M. Mérillon, X. Vitrac. 2010. Contribution of chlorogenic acids to the inhibition of human hepatic glucose-6-phosphatase activity *in vitro* by Svetol, a standardized decaffeinated green coffee extract. *J. Agric. Food Chem.* 58: 4141–4144.

Hertog, M.G., E.J. Feskens, P.C. Hollman, M.B. Katan, D. Kromhout. 1993. Dietary antioxidant flavonoids and risk of coronary heart disease: The Zutphen Elderly Study. *Lancet.* 342: 1007–1011.

Ho, L., M. Varghese, J. Wang, W. Zhao, W.F. Chen, L.A. Knable, M. Ferruzzi, G.M. Pasinetti. 2012. Dietary supplementation with decaffeinated green coffee improves diet-induced insulin resistance and brain energy metabolism in mice. *Nutr. Neurosci.* 15(1): 37–45.

Johnston, K.L., M.N. Clifford, L.M. Morgan. 2003. Coffee acutely modifies gastrointestinal hormone secretion and glucose tolerance in humans: Glycemic effects of chlorogenic acid and caffeine. *Am. J. Clin. Nutr.* 78: 728–733.

Keservani, R.K., R.K. Kesharwani, A.K. Sharma. 2015a. *Pulmonary and Respiratory Health: Antioxidants and Nutraceuticals.* UK: CRC Press, Taylor and Francis Group.

Keservani, R.K., R.K. Kesharwani, N. Vyas, S. Jain, R. Raghuvanshi, A.K. Sharma. 2010. Nutraceutical and functional food as future food: A review. *Der Pharmacia. Lett.* 2: 106–116.

Keservani, R.K. and A.K. Sharma. 2014. Flavonoids: Emerging trends and potential health benefits. *J. Chin. Pharm. Sci.* 23(12): 815–822.

Keservani, R.K., S. Singh, V. Singh, R.K. Kesharwani, A.K. Sharma. 2015b. *Nutraceuticals and Functional Foods in the Prevention of Mental Disorder.* UK: CRC Press, Taylor & Francis.

Kim, C., H.G. Yu, J. Sohn. 2010. The anti-angiogenic effect of chlorogenic acid on choroidal neovascularization. *Korean J. Ophthalmol.* 24: 163–168.

Kim, Y., K.L. Goodne, J.D. Park, J. Choi, S.T. Talcott. 2011. Changes in antioxidant phytochemicals and volatile composition of Camellia sinensis by oxidation during tea fermentation. *Food Chem.* 129: 1331–1342.

Kiyohara, C., S. Kono, S. Honjo, I. Todoroki, Y. Sakurai, M. Nishiwaki, H. Hamada, et al. 1999. Inverse association between coffee drinking and serum uric acid concentrations in middle-aged Japanese males. *Br. J. Nutr.* 82: 125–130.

Klatsky, A.L., C. Morton, G.D. Udaltsova, G.D. Friedman. 2006. Coffee, cirrhosis, and transaminase enzymes. *Arch. Intern. Med.* 166: 1190–1195.

Kozuma, K., S. Tsuchiya, J. Kohori, T. Hase, I. Tokimitsu. 2005. Antihypertensive effect of green coffee bean extract on mildly hypertensive subjects. *Hypertens. Res.* 28(9): 711–718.

Kuntz, S., U. Wenzel, H. Daniel. 1999. Comparative analysis of the effects of flavonoids on proliferation, cytotoxicity, and apoptosis in human colon cancer cell lines. *Eur. J. Nutr.* 38: 133–342.

La Vecchia, C., E. Negri, L. Cavalieri d'Oro, S. Franceschi. 1998. Liver cirrhosis and the risk of primary liver cancer. *Eur. J. Cancer Prev.* 7: 315–320.

Lamartiniere, C.A., M.S. Cotroneo, W.A. Fritz, J. Wang, R. Mentor-Marcel, A. Elgavish. 2002. Genistein chemoprevention: Timing and mechanisms of action in murine mammary and prostate. *J. Nutr.* 132(3): 552S–558S.

Lindsay, J., D. Laurin, R. Verreault, R. Hebert, B. Helliwell, G.B. Hill, I. McDowell. 2002. Risk factors for Alzheimer's disease: A prospective analysis from the Canadian study of health and aging. *Am. J. Epidemiol.* 156: 445–453.

Mascitelli, L., F. Pezzetta, J.L. Sullivan. 2008. Putative hepatoprotective effects of coffee. *Aliment. Pharmacol. Ther.* 27: 90–91.

Mohd-Esa, N., F.S. Hern, A. Ismail, C.L. Yee. 2010. Antioxidant activity in different parts of roselle (Hibiscus sabdariffa L.) extracts and potential exploitation of the seeds. *Food Chem.* 122: 1055–1060.

Monteiro, M., A. Farah, D. Perrone, L.C. Trugo, C. Donangelo. 2007. Chlorogenic acid compounds from coffee are differentially absorbed and metabolized in humans. *J. Nutr.* 137(10): 2196–2201.

Moon, J.K., H.S. Yoo, T. Shibamoto. 2009. Role of roasting conditions in the level of chlorogenic acid content in coffee beans: Correlation with coffee acidity. *J. Agric. Food Chem.* 57(12): 5365–5369.

Moreira, D.P., M.C. Monteiro, M. Ribeiro-Alves, C.M. Donangelo, L.C. Trugo. 2005. Contribution of chlorogenic acids to the iron reducing activity of coffee beverages. *J. Agric. Food Chem.* 53: 1399–1402.

Mullen, W., B. Nemzer, B. Ou, A. Stalmach, J. Hunter, M. N. Clifford, and E. Combet. 2011. The antioxidant and chlorogenic acid profiles of whole coffee fruits are influenced by the extraction procedures. *J. Agric. Food Chem.* 59(8): 3754–3762.

Murase, T., K. Misawa, Y. Minegishi, M. Aoki, H. Ominami, Y. Suzuki, Y.Shibuya, T. Hase. 2011. Coffee polyphenols suppress diet-induced body fat accumulation by down regulating SREBP-1c and related molecules in C57BL/6 J mice. *Am. J. Physiol. Endocrinol. Metab.* 300(1): E122–E133.

Nebesny, E. and G. Budryn. 2003. Antioxidative activity of green and roasted coffee beans as influenced by convection and microwave roasting methods and content of certain compounds. *Eur. Food Res. Technol.* 217: 157–163.

Nishi, A. A., P. Kumar. 2013. Protective effect of chlorogenic acid against diabetic nephropathy in high fat diet/streptozotocin induced type-2 diabetic rats. *Int. J. Pharm. Pharm. Sci.* 5(2): 489–495.

Nkondjock, A. 2009. Coffee consumption and the risk of cancer: An overview. *Cancer Lett.* 277: 121–125.

Nkondjock, A., P. Ghadirian, J. Kotsopoulos, J. Lubinski, H. Lynch, C. Kim-Sing, D. Horsman, et al. 2006. Coffee consumption and breast cancer risk among BRCA1 and BRCA2 mutation carriers. *Int. J. Cancer* 118: 103–107.

Ochani, P.C. and P. D'Mello. 2009. Antioxidant and antihyperlipidemic activity of Hibiscus sabdariffa Linn. leaves and calyces extracts in rats. *Indian J. Exp. Biol.* 47: 276–282.

Ochiai, R., H. Jokura, A. Suzuki, I. Tokimitsu, M. Ohishi, N.Komai, H. Rakugi, T. Ogihara. 2004. Green coffee bean extract improves human vasoreactivity. *Hypertens. Res.* 27: 731–737.

Odegaard, A.O., M.A. Pereira, W.P. Koh, K. Arakawa, H.P. Lee, M.C. Yu. 2008. Coffee, tea, and incident type 2 diabetes: The Singapore Chinese Health Study. *Am. J. Clin. Nutr.* 88(4): 979–985.

Olthof, M.R., P.C. Hollman, M.N. Buijsman, J.M. van Amelsvoort, M.B. Katan. 2003. Chlorogenic acid, quercetin-3-rutinoside and black tea phenols are extensively metabolized in humans. *J. Nutr.* 133(6): 1806–1814.

Onakpoya, I., R. Terry, E. Ernst. 2011. The use of green coffee extract as a weight loss supplement: A systematic review and meta-analysis of randomised clinical trials. *Gastroenterol. Res. Pract.*. 382852: 1–6.

Pellegrini, N., M. Serafini, B. Colombi, D. Del Rio, S. Salvatore, M. Bianchi, F. Brighenti. 2003. Total antioxidant capacity of plant foods, beverages and oils consumed in Italy assessed by three different *in vitro* assays. *J. Nutr.* 133: 2812–2819.

Perez-Matute, P., A.B. Crujeiras, M. Fernandez-Galilea, P. Prieto-Hontoria. 2012. Compounds with antioxidant capacity as potential tools against several oxidative stress related disorders: Fact or artifact? In *Oxidative Stress and Diseases*, V.I. Lushchak and D.V. Gospodaryov (eds), pp. 545–584.

Rechner, A.R., J.P.E. Spencer, G. Kuhnle, U. Harn, C.A. Rice-Evans. 2001. Novel biomarkers of the metabolism of caffeic acid derivatives *in vivo. Free Radic. Biol. Med.* 30: 1213–1222.

Richelle, M., I. Tavazzi, E. Offord. 2001. Comparison of the antioxidant activity of commonly consumed polyphenolic beverages (coffee, cocoa, and tea) prepared per cup serving. *J. Agric. Food Chem.* 49: 3438–3442.

Rizvi, S.I. and K.B. Pandey. 2009a. Current understanding of dietary polyphenols and their role in health and disease. *Curr. Nutr. Food Sci.* 5: 249–263.

Rizvi, S.I. and K.B. Pandey. 2009b. Plant polyphenols as dietary antioxidants in human health and disease. *Oxid. Med. Cell. Longev.* 2(5): 270–278.

Rizvi, S.I. and N. Srivastva. 2007. Diabetes mellitus: Etiology, complications and treatment. *Herbal Med. Hum. Dis.* 3: 178–215.

Rosso, A., J. Mossey, C.F. Lippa. 2008. Caffeine: Neuroprotective functions in cognition and Alzheimer's disease. *Am. J. Alzheimer's Dis. Other Demen.* 23(5): 417–422.

Salazar-Martinez, E., W.C. Willett, A. Ascherio, J.E. Manson, M.F. Leitzmann, M.J. Stampfer, F.B. Hu. 2004. Coffee consumption and risk for type 2 diabetes mellitus. *Ann. Intern. Med.* 140: 1–8.

Schachinger, V., M.B. Britten, A.M. Zeiher. 2000. Prognostic impact of coronary vasodilator dysfunction on adverse long-term outcome of coronary heart disease. *Circulation.* 101: 1899–1906.

Sherwin, E.R. 1978. Oxidation and antioxidants in fat and oil processing. *J. Am. Oil Chem. Soc.* 55: 809–814.

Shimoda, H., E. Seki, M. Aitani. 2006. Inhibitory effect of green coffee bean extract on fat accumulation and body weight gain in mice. *BMC Complement. Altern. Med.* 6: 1–9.

Shin, J.Y. and H.G. Yu. 2014. Chlorogenic acid supplementation improves multifocal electroretinography in patients with retinitis pigmentosa. *J. Korean Med. Sci.* 29: 117–121.

Shin, J.Y., J. Sohn, K.H. Park. 2013. Chlorogenic acid decreases retinal vascular hyper permeability in diabetic rat model. *J. Korean Med. Sci.* 28: 608–613.

Sies, H. 1997. Oxidative stress: Oxidants and antioxidants. *Exp. Physiol.* 82(2): 291–295.

Simoes, J., P. Madureira, F.M. Nunes, M. Rosário Domingues, M. Vilanova, M.A. Coimbra. 2009. Immunostimulatory properties of coffee mannans. *Mol. Nutr. Food Res.* 53(8): 1036–1043.

Singh, P. and S.I. Rizvi. 2012. Anti-oxidative effect of curcumin against tert- butyl hydroperoxide induced oxidative stress in the human erythrocytes. *Nat. Prod. J.* 2: 69–73.

Singh, P. and S.I. Rizvi. 2015. Role of curcumin in modulating plasma PON1 arylesterase activity and susceptibility to LDL oxidation in oxidatively challenged wistar rats. *Lett. Drug Des. Discov.* 12(4): 319–323.

Smith, A. 2002. Effects of caffeine on human behavior. *Food Chem. Toxicol.* 40(9): 1243–1255.

Somporn, C., A. Kamtuo, P. Theerakulpisut, S. Siriamornpun. 2011. Effects of roasting degree on radical scavenging activity, phenolics and volatile compounds of Arabica coffee beans (*Coffea arabica* L. cv.Catimor). *Int. J. Food Sci. Tech.* 46: 2287–2296.

Song, S.J., S. Choi, T. Park. 2014. Decaffeinated green coffee bean extract attenuates diet-induced obesity and insulin resistance in mice. *Evid. Based Complement. Alternat. Med.* 718379: 1–14.

Tatefuji, T., N. Izumi, T. Ohta, S. Arai, M. Ikeda, M. Kurimoto. 1996. Isolation and identification of compounds from Brazilian propolis which enhance macrophage spreading and mobility. *Biol. Pharm. Bull.* 19: 966–970.

Toci, A.T. and A. Farah. 2008. Volatile compounds as potential defective coffee seeds' markers. *Food Chem.* 108: 1133–1141.

Tverdal, A. and S. Skurtveit. 2003. Coffee intake and mortality from liver cirrhosis. *Ann. Epidemiol.* 13: 419–423.

Ulloa Rojas, J.B., J.A.J. Verreth, S. Amato, E.A. Huisman. 2003. Biological treatments affect the chemical composition of coffee pulp. *Bioresour. Technol.* 89: 267–274.

Van der Werf, R., C. Marcic, A. Khalil, S. Sigrist, E. Marchioni. 2014. ABTS radical scavenging capacity in green and roasted coffee extracts. *LWT: Food Sci. Technol.* 58: 77–85.

Vatten, L.J., K. Solvoll, E.B. Loken. 1990. Coffee consumption and the risk of breast cancer: A prospective study of 14,593 Norwegian women. *Br. J. Cancer* 62: 267–270.

Vinson, J.A., B.R. Burnham, V.M. Nagendran. 2012. Randomized, double-blind, placebo-controlled, linear dose, crossover study to evaluate the efficacy and safety of a green coffee bean extract in overweight subjects. *Diabetes Metab Syndr Obes.* 5: 21–27.

Vinson, J.A., H. Al Kharrat, D. Shuta. 2009. Investigation of an amylase inhibitor on human glucose absorption after starch consumption. *Open Nutraceuticals J.* 2: 88–91.

Watanabe, T., Y. Arai, Y. Mitsui, T. Kusaura, W. Okawa, Y. Kajihara, I. Saito. 2006. The blood pressure-lowering effect and safety of chlorogenic acid from green coffee bean extract in essential hypertension. *Clin. Exp. Hypertens.* 28(5): 439–449.

Yang, C.S., J.M. Landau, M.T. Huang, H.L. Newmark. 2001. Inhibition of carcinogenesis by dietary polyphenolic compounds. *Annu. Rev. Nutr.* 21: 381–406.

Yashin, A., Y. Yashin, J.Y. Wang, B. Nemzer. 2013. Antioxidant and antiradical activity of coffee. *Antioxidants.* 2: 230–245.

Wild Flavors. n.d. The health benefits of green coffee extract. Wild Flavors, Erlanger, KY. http://www.foodprocessing.com/assets/knowledge_centers/WILD_Flavors/assets/Green_Coffee_Extract_White_Paper_Mktg.pdf.

2 Chlorogenic Acids in Green Coffee Bean Extract Are the Key Ingredients in Food with Health and Function Claims

Hiroyoshi Moriyama, Orie Yoshinari, and Debasis Bagchi

CONTENTS

2.1 INTRODUCTION

After World War II, many Japanese people, particularly children, suffered from malnutrition due to food shortages and restrictions. To alleviate the food crisis, Japan imported food from other countries. Through the government policy, consuming Western-style diets was encouraged to help regulate the health of the Japanese people [1]. Malnutrition rates decreased when Japan experienced rapid economic growth in the postwar 1960s. The westernization of diets led to high-calorie eating habits, including the consumption of high-fat-content meals, and resulted in an imbalance of the daily recommended nutritional intake, as shown in Figure 2.1. It is apparent that the daily diets played a role in the imbalance of nutrient consumption

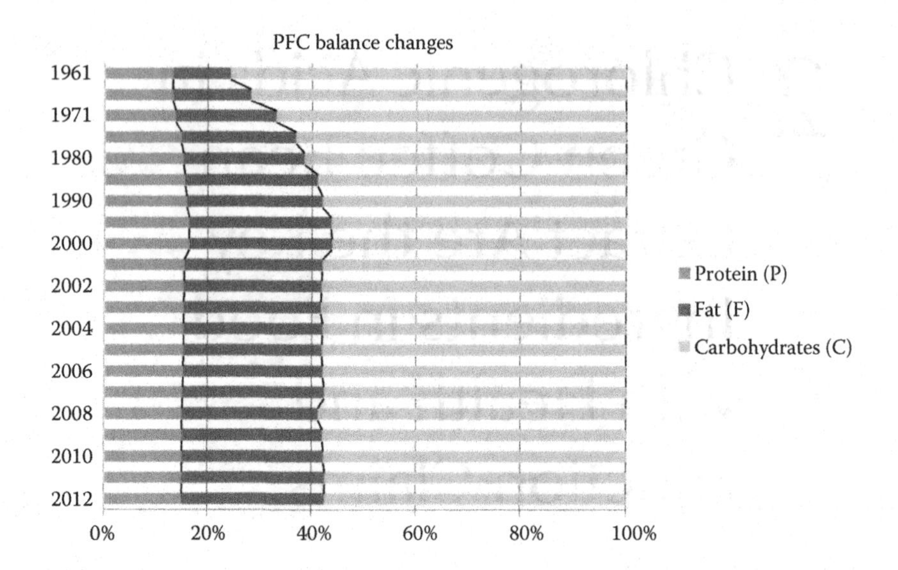

FIGURE 2.1 (See color insert.) The changing dietary structure of the Japanese. (From MHLW (Ministry of Health, Labor, and Welfare), National health and nutrition survey, MHLW, Tokyo, 2012 [2].)

of the Japanese, and elevated the levels of fat intake (Figure 2.1). Other daily lifestyle factors and behaviors such as smoking, lack of physical exercise, sedentary work, and excessive alcohol consumption possibly contribute to the development of lifestyle-related diseases (LSRD) including cancer, cardiovascular and cerebrovascular diseases, and diabetes. According to statistical data on the mortality rates associated with these diseases published by the Ministry of Health, Labor, and Welfare (MHLW), cancer is the leading death-related disease, followed by cardiovascular and cerebrovascular diseases (Figure 2.2), and the mortality rates of all three diseases are steadily increasing.

In 1996, the term *LSRD* was proposed by the Ministry of Health and Welfare's Council on Public Health. The government first attempted to prevent and combat the occurrence of LSRD by encouraging improvements in daily lifestyle. Although this seems to be a relatively simple solution to the problem, the causes of LSRD consist of many complex factors that have not yet been fully investigated; it is obvious that genetic factors play a pivotal role. More recently, the term *metabolic syndrome* (MS), which has become recognized and complementarily used as a specific target of LSRD by the food sellers, health-care providers, and consumers in Japan [3], is described as visceral or abdominal obesity or excessive fat tissue in and around the abdomen with signs or associations of hyperglycemia, hyperlipidemia, and hypertension [4].

Dietary habits likely contribute to the risk of developing LSRD. In recent years, many studies have shown that properly modified dietary habits might be beneficial in preventing LSRD as part of the measures established in the area of preventive medicine aiming to reduce health-care expenditure [5]. Furthermore, the measures not

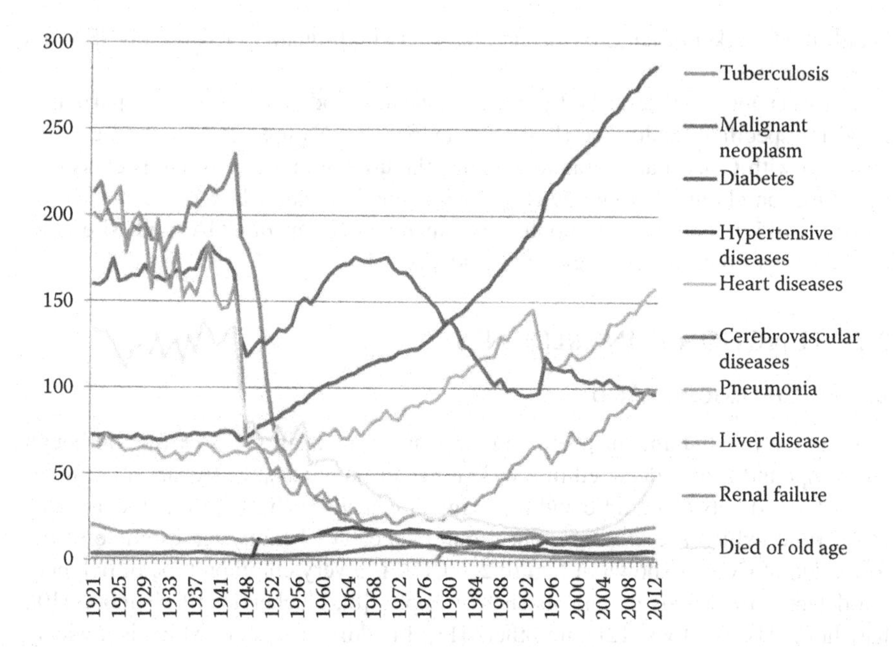

FIGURE 2.2 Changes in mortality rates from principal causes of death per 100,000 population. The principal causes of death among the Japanese have changed from infections to lifestyle-related diseases such as cancer, heart diseases, and cardiovascular diseases. (From MHLW (Ministry of Health, Labor, and Welfare), Vital statistics, MHLW, Tokyo, 2012 [6].)

only promote well-balanced nutritional diets, but also encourage the research and ingestion of food ingredients with physiological effects on human health and function. The new concept is to promote the health benefits and well-being by consuming functional dietary ingredients. The traditional Japanese diet is commonly low in animal fat, and contains plenty of fish, fruits, and vegetables including soybeans that are rich in polyphenols. In the last decade, research has shown that polyphenols, ubiquitous in plants, possess antioxidant properties, which have been extensively studied in the prevention of degenerative diseases such as cancers and cardiovascular diseases [4].

Many plants and botanicals that are traditionally part of our diet, such as turmeric, green tea, and coffee, are all highly beneficial to human health if the recommended daily amount is consumed. Coffee is derived from green coffee beans (GCB), which are commonly referred to as the seeds in the fruits of the coffee tree. Two of the most commercially important species are *Coffea arabica* and *Coffea canephora*, which are first roasted and then prepared as coffee beverages. The GCB is a good source of polyphenols, especially chlorogenic acid (CGA), which is the most abundant compound. Historically, the intake of these traditional food materials as part of the daily diet is considered to be safe.

As a consequence, supplements of GCB extract with a high content of CGA in various forms such as capsules, tablets, and beverages have become popular in the health-food market because of the easy access to high-quality GCB in the USA and other countries.

In this chapter, we describe the Japanese health-food claim system, in particular Food for specified health use (FOSHU), as per the example of a coffee beverage enriched with CGA that claims to enhance the utilization of body fat as energy. A new function claim labeling law (Food with function claim: FFC) was enacted on April 1, 2015, which will potentiate new functional claims of CGA in GCB extract on the basis of their nonbias scientific evidence [7].

2.2 FUNCTIONAL INGREDIENTS

2.2.1 Chlorogenic Acid

CGA is the most abundant phenolic compound present in GCB extract, although the compound is also detected in a wide range of botanicals. CGAs are a family of esters formed between quinic and transcinnamic acids such as caffeic, *p*-coumaric, and ferulic, which are an important group of dietary phenols. An example of the formation of CGA is shown in Figure 2.3. CGA is a very common type of polyphenol detected in various botanicals such as apples [8], blueberries [9], bamboo [10], hawthorn [11], potatoes [12], and others [13]. In addition, coffee, which is a widely consumed drink around the world and is popular for both its aroma and flavor, is derived from GCB and is one of the best botanical sources of CGA. Furthermore, the most dominant CGA identified in GCB extract are 5-O-caffeoquinic acid (5-CQA), 4-O-caffeoquinic acid (4-CQA), and 3-O-caffeoquinic acid (3-CQA), along with the presence of different isomers [14]. The content of CGA in a Colombian GCB extract shows significant differences between the 3-CQA, 4-CQA, and 5-CQA isomers of CGA (mg/g) when compared with roasted coffee bean (RCB); the respective GCB shows 2.45 ± 0.18, 3.73 ± 0.24, and 29.64 ± 2.08, while RCB exhibits 0.78 ± 0.03, 0.86 ± 0.04 and 1.42 ± 0.01 [15]. This study shows that 5-CQA is the predominant CGA in both samples and that the levels of all CQAs decrease remarkably during the roasting process [15].

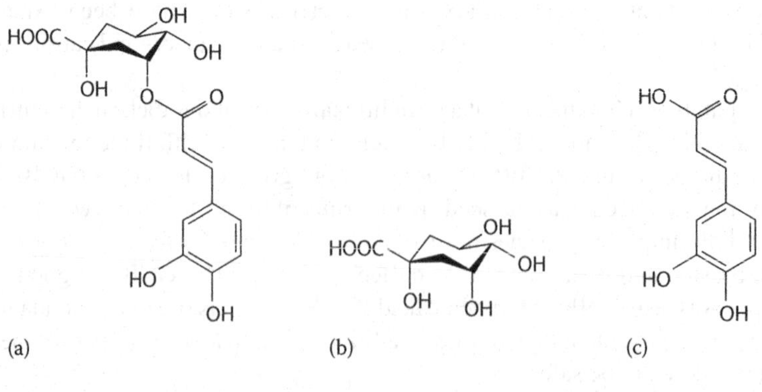

HOOC OH OH OH O O HO OH
(a)

HOOC OH OH OH OH
(b)

HO O HO OH
(c)

FIGURE 2.3 Structural example of (a) 5-O-caffeoquimic (5-CQA) as the major CGA formed from (b) quinic acid and (c) caffeic acid.

2.2.2 Biological Properties

Although the biological properties of CGA are highly dependent on absorption and metabolism, detailed discussion—which is still disputable—on the fate of CGA has been reported using animal models and humans in various studies [16–20]. However, when CGA is ingested orally, a wide spectrum of potential biological activities relating to LSRD-associated MS has been demonstrated, thereby suggesting potential human health benefits. The biological properties include antioxidant [21], anti-inflammatory [22], analgesic [22], antipyretic [22], antihepatitis B virus [23], hypoglycemic [24], hypotensive [25–28], vasorelaxant [29], neuroprotection [30] antiobesity [31,32], and anticancer activities [33].

Consequently, the biological effects of CGA are expected to decrease the incidence of, for example, hyperlipidemia, hypertension, hyperglycemia, and obesity as well-recognized risk factors for the occurrence of cardiovascular diseases. For example, the effect of CGA on obesity, which will be examined in detail, is of significant importance as we have seen a global rise in the rates of obesity in recent years, leading to a socioeconomic health issue in aged-population groups regardless of gender. It is also a determining risk factor for coronary heart disease, type 2 diabetes, and stroke.

For those subjects who are at the very early stages of LSRD, for example, dietary intervention is highly recommended compared with drug intervention due to the serious side effects of various drugs used for the therapy of these subjects. Dietary intervention advocates eating fruits and vegetables rich in polyphenols, and increasing fiber intake, which controls the metabolism of ingested high-calorie food materials, and assists weight management. Polyphenols derived from GCB extract, or CGA, help reduce oxidative stress, which is a possible cause of the aforementioned diseases, and can be easily taken as a daily supplement in tablet or hard capsule form.

Furthermore, the antiobesity effect of GCB has been examined in both preclinical and human clinical studies [31,32]. Based on a systematic review (SR) and a meta-analysis of randomized clinical trials (RCTs), the efficacy of GCB was evaluated on weight loss [34]. The study examined the findings of several reports and data from human clinical trials on the efficacy of GCB extract to aid weight loss and also a literature review was conducted using databases such as MEDLINE, EMBASE, CINAHL, AMED, and the Cochrane Library [35]. In the study [34], even though the results of the evaluated studies may demonstrate efficacy, the quality of the methodology according to the SR is poor, and a study needs to be carried out over a longer time frame in order to examine the full effects of GCB extract on body weight. The importance of SR is emphasized when FFC is discussed since it forms part of the data requirements.

2.3 FOOD WITH HEALTH CLAIM

The term *functional food* (FF) was first used in a project led by the Ministry of Education (now the Ministry of Education, Culture, Sports, Science, and Technology or MECSI). Recently, terms such as *nutraceuticals* have been used to describe FF or ingredients that have a high nutritional value and can provide enhanced health benefits to humans [4]. Specifically, they can target the symptoms of higher blood pressure, higher blood glucose, and higher blood lipid levels diagnosed in healthy or borderline people. In the last decade, there has been a dramatic increase in the rates of LSRD related to MS, which is further complicated by the increase in the aged population. The rate at which the aged groups are increasing is higher than that forecasted by academia and government, and consequently, the aforementioned project had a significant influence on the development of FF. Interestingly, the term *function* has never been used or approved as an official term due to its implication of drug-like effects; therefore, a different term was assigned, which is now commonly known as FOSHU.

2.4 FOOD FOR SPECIFIED HEALTH USE

The implementation of the FOSHU system started in 1991, emerging from health foods such as those shown in Figure 2.4. In the last 20 years, over 400 FOSHU products have been introduced into the Japanese marketplace, and these can be accessed at any retail store including supermarkets, convenience stores, and drug stores, and even from vending machines. As of 2015, nine categories of health claims and benefits associated with FOSHU products have been established. Fulfilling the safety and efficacy requirements to move from SCHF as "Food" to FOSHU has been previously reported in detail [4], while it should be noted that all subjects taking the final formulated product must be in a nondiseased state or borderline for the required RCT. Safety is a major challenge to the approval system since FOSHU is easily procured by consumers for their health benefits. Under such circumstances, the panel of the Food Safety Commission plays a pivotal role in determining the safety of relative (active) ingredients, to protect the health of consumers in light of the potential hazard of such ingredients. Details of the mandated safety requirements have been previously described [7].

One such safety requirement is a clinical overdose trial using healthy Japanese subjects of both genders, which analyzes the data of blood samples. The subjects take a fivefold dosage of the recommended daily dose for 28 days (4 weeks). The trial is only required when the dosage is in tablet or capsule form. Similarly, a second control is performed to test a threefold dosage of the recommended daily intake amount where the relative or active ingredient is added to conventional food and beverages. The results of the data from the blood chemistry clinical trial based on the 4-week ingestion period prove that CGA is a safe, functional ingredient for human use [4].

The health claims of FOSHU target the risk factors associated with cardiovascular diseases. The government, the medical industry, as well as consumer groups have paid a lot of attention to these FOSHU with the aim of reducing the risk factors including high blood pressure and high blood cholesterol, and abdominal fat. FOSHU products can support Japanese people with borderline levels of such risk factors, helping them regulate the symptoms. Obviously, lack of physical exercise and poor lifestyle choices such as smoking and excessive consumption of alcohol will have negative health effects, and it should be controlled by adjusting to a healthy diet that includes FOSHU and FFC products.

Only one CGA FOSHU product, a beverage, is available in the Japanese marketplace, but other CGA SCHF products are available in tablet and capsule form

(a)

	Food with health claim (FHC)						
		Food for specified health use (FOSHU)					
"Drug"	Food for nutrient function claim (FNFC)	Ordinary	Standardized	Disease risk reduction claim	Qualified	"So-called health food" (SCHF)	"Food"

(b)

	Food with health claim (FHC)						
		Food for specific health use (FOSHU)				Food with function claim (FFC)	
"Drug"	Food for nutrient function claim (FNFC)	Ordinary	Standardized	Disease risk reduction claim	Qualified	Evidence-based function claims	"Food" + SCHF

FIGURE 2.4 The FFC emerging from the SCHF. (a) Before March 30, 2015 and (b) after April 1, 2015. FHC belongs to the Food category. Note (b) shows that "Food" = SCHF + FFC + FOSHU + FNFC.

and are sold without any health claims. According to the "Drug and Food" classification, GCB extract is classed as a "Food." A major Japanese health and beauty care company launched the first FOSHU product in the form of a coffee beverage in a steel 185 g can enriched with 270 mg CGA, mainly 5-CQA. The product was launched on April 4, 2013, and is now available at multiple retail outlets such as convenience stores, drug stores, supermarkets, and other consumer accessible retail outlets. Its health benefit is attributed to its effect on utilizing body fat as energy. The final formula contains 90 mg of caffeine. Although caffeine has various physiological effects, caffeine is not the active agent in FOSHU. A basic study in developing a CGA beverage is described by Watanabe et al. [36]. The study assessed the feasibility of drinking a CGA-rich beverage or ready-to-drink coffee in daily life to aid abdominal fat reduction with body weight loss in humans.

The results of the study supported the claim that consuming the CGA-rich coffee generates health benefits, and as a result the first CGA-enriched coffee came onto the Japanese marketplace. Thus far, no adverse reaction has been found; however, the concentration of caffeine in GCB extract should be kept lower for consumers who are sensitive to caffeine.

2.5 NEW REGULATORY FRAMEWORK

As of April 1, 2015, a new food function labeling law aimed at the health-conscious consumer was enacted, outlining on the packaging the specific health benefits of FFC products. The new framework of the "Drug and Food" scheme is shown in Figure 2.4b. FFC has partially replaced SCHF or foods in various forms without any scientific evidence, which has not been fully subjected to safety and efficacy studies.

As described in Figure 2.4, "Drug" and "Food" are available for those ingested by humans. "Food" is further classified into Food with nutrient function claim (FNFC), FOSHU (disease risk reduction claim), and SCHF. With the emergence of FFC, three basic categories are now authorized to make claims. Because FOSHU is the only category that requires the approval of the CAA relating to its health claims, thus the labels differ significantly. An obvious difference on the labels are the disclaimers; FOSHU's statement indicates that the health claims have received government approval, while the FFC guideline states that the health claims are not approved like FOSHU but are primarily based on safety and efficacy data provided by sellers.

2.6 FOOD WITH FUNCTION CLAIM

At a regulatory meeting in February 2013, the cabinet came to a decision to promote food, including SCHF, and vegetables that exhibit a wide range of beneficial health claims in order to stimulate the Japanese food industry. The CAA established an investigative committee to frame the new labeling regulation associated with SCHF. Its basic concept is rooted in the Dietary Supplement Health and Education Act (DSHEA) in the USA. The latest requirements in the guideline are outlined on the updated website of the CAA [7], but part of the requirements of FFC are quite similar to FOSHU, in particular the safety requirements. To sell FFC products in the marketplace requires no approval from the CAA, but sellers as well as manufacturers must pay close attention to any negative side effects experienced by consumers in order to protect themselves from developing a poor reputation. Because of the nonapproval system, a notification with the required documentation is mandated to be filed 60 days prior to the launch of FFC products in the marketplace. Currently, there are significant delays in issuing the registration numbers, implying some changes in the review system will be required.

To better understand these systems, a comparison between FOSHU and FFC if CGA is present in the formulation is shown in Table 2.1. The main difference is that FOSHU is regulated under the CAA approval system. The basic safety requirement of FFC is almost the same as FOSHU, but to prove any function claims there are two existing ways to generate supporting evidence. One is to conduct an RCT on a finished product, and the other is to conduct an SR on the relative or active ingredients using appropriate keywords to exclude and include all literature for final evaluation on how claims can be labeled based on the results of the outcome.

Since FFC is not an approval system but a notification system, sellers or distributors named on the product label are responsible for filing the correct information on all documents.

TABLE 2.1
Comparison of Major Different Aspects between FOSHU and FFC Systems

Difference in Regulatory	Health Claims (FOSHU)	Functional Food Claims (FFC)
Safety assessment	History of food use (preclinical and human overdose studies) [4]	History of food use (if quantifiable) (preclinical and human overdose studies) [7]
Efficacy assessment	RCT	RCT or SR
Application	Addition to food/drink and dietary supplement	Addition to food/drink and dietary supplement
Type of claim	See [4]	Structure/function [7]
Level of evidence supporting efficacy	Finished products (RCT)	RCT or SR
Deciding body	Approval by the CAA (government)	Notification to the CAA by sellers
Public closure	Closed	Via website [7]

Note: RCT: randomized controlled trial; SR: systematic review.

2.7 DISCUSSION

FOSHU has been enacted and implemented for over 20 years, creating about 10 health claims that include risk reduction claims. During the past two decades, a wide variety of relative (active or key) ingredients have been tested and added to FOSHU products. The most popular ingredient used in FOSHU products is ingestible dextrin due to the data supporting its safety and efficacy. However, some claims that support knee joint health, the immune system, skin care, and eye care are yet to be tested for their consumer health benefits. Although the turnover of FOSHU has significantly contributed to the health-food market, an in-depth study has not yet been conducted. For example, in-depth study is designed to assess the statistical data whether affecting the reduction of LSRD. Moreover, FOSHU has not aggressively explored any new health claims that can be identified with the new regulatory system, such as immune and joint health-care claims.

Furthermore, CGA has a wide variety of biological properties, some of which have been extensively studied for their health claims, for example, body fat loss as a result of consuming a CGA-enriched coffee beverage. The supplementation of CGA with the aforementioned health benefit may support the established FFC, based on an RCT or an SR in accordance with the FFC labeling guideline, as agents for reducing many of the risk factors associated with LSRD. Unlike FOSHU, it is less costly to register FFC if evidence supporting these claims can be prepared using an SR. CGA has great potential to provide a range of FFC products that target issues such as hypertension, hyperlipidemia, weight loss, and many others.

Using the example of the effect that CGA has on hypertension, an SR can claim "the active agent of the product contains CGA which has been reported to lower blood pressure, or control or manage blood pressure." Similarly, CGA has the physiological effects of controlling the high blood lipid level or on body weight. The other potential claims relate to the control of the proper glucose level in the blood. The vasorelaxant effect of CGA [29] may contribute a unique function claim such as regulating or managing the blood flow. All of these claims contribute to reducing the risk of LSRD. Apparently, if new physiological effects are identified to have potential human health benefits, then it is possible to generate new functions, which can be registered as FFC.

However, reported biological properties such as antidiabetes and anticancer effects should not be connected to the antioxidant and to FFC as they belong to the category of diseases. Although antioxidant properties are intrinsic to polyphenols or CGA, the underlying mechanism of their effect is difficult to confirm in humans. In consideration of all these, polyphenols or a group of constituents such as CGA in nonroasted coffee or GCB extract are safe to consume as they are found in diets in most advanced countries.

On the other hand, small- and medium-sized companies encounter a challenge to register FFC products since they may not be able to ensure functional ingredients with scientific evidence based on an RCT, that is costly to conduct, or has an SR evaluation of RCTs that mostly involves nonhealthy subjects. As stated previously, the RCT requirements for FOSHU and FFC must be conducted on healthy or borderline subjects. Another SR-related issue that is disputed is how to prove whether the subjects in the RCT are healthy or borderline cases. Obviously, BMI may be utilized as a standard to determine the borderline subjects. Areas such as knee joint health care is another good example. What if subjects visited physicians for mild knee joint discomfort, are they nonhealthy?

2.8 CONCLUSION

The LSRD population has continued to increase along with changes in lifestyle and the increase in the number of aged people. It has been suggested that the poor nutritional intake in recent years can be improved with the aid of supplements. Polyphenols, such as CGA derived from GCB extract, have been proved to be effective in reducing some of the risk factors related to MS such as hyperlipidemia, hypertension, hyperglycemia, and obesity with a daily supplement of CGA. Coffee is one of the most consumed beverages globally and GCB is accessible in supplement form to health-oriented consumers in the USA, Japan, and other countries around the world. In Japan, a widely consumed FOSHU food with beneficial health claims is a beverage containing 270 mg of total CGA. With the introduction of FFC, it is anticipated that more supplements, or other dose forms, with new function claims attributed to CGA will be introduced in the coming years if FFC indeed helps reduce the population of LSRD-related MS.

REFERENCES

1. Nakamura T. The integration of school nutrition program into health promotion and prevention of lifestyle-related diseases in Japan. *Asia Pac J Clin Nutr* 2008;17(S1):349–351.
2. MHLW (Ministry of Health, Labor, and Welfare). National health and nutrition survey. Raw data. http://www.mhlw.go.jp/seisakunitsuite/bunya/kenkou_iryou/kenkou/kenkounippon21/en/eiyouchousa/.

3. Matsuzawa Y. Metabolic syndrome: Definition and diagnostic criteria in Japan. *J Jpn Soc Int Med* 2005;94:188–203.
4. Debasis B. (Ed.). *Nutraceutical and Functional Food Regulations in the United States and Around the World* (2nd Ed.), Academic Press, London, UK, 2014.
5. Yazaki Y. Preventive medicine efforts in Japan focusing on metabolic syndrome. *J Jpn Med Assoc* 2008;51:317–321.
6. MHLW (Ministry of Health, Labor, and Welfare), Summary of vital statistics, http://www.mhlw.go.jp/english/database/db-hw/populate/dl/03.pdf (accessed on 10 April 2016).
7. Consumer Affairs Agency. Government of Japan. FFC Registration Guideline http://www.caa.go.jp/foods/pdf/food_with_function_clains_guideline_shinkyu.pdf _ (accessed on 10 April 2016).
8. Aminor MJ, Tacchini M, Aubert S, et al. Phenolic composition and browning susceptibility of various apple cultivars at maturity. *J Food Sci* 1992;57:958–962.
9. Gao L, Mazza G. Quantification and distribution of simple and acylated anthocyanins and others phenolics in blueberries. *J Food Sci* 1994;59:1057–1059.
10. Kwaeon M-H, Hwang H-J, Sung H-C. Identification of antioxidant activity of novel chlorogenic acid derivatives from bamboo (*Phyllostachys edulis*). *J Agric Food Chem* 2001;49:4646–4655.
11. Ozturk N, Tuncel M. Assessment of phenolic acid content and in vitro antiradical characteristics of hawthorn. *J Med Food* 2011;14:665–669.
12. Dao L, Friedman M. Chlorogenic acid content of fresh and processed potatoes determined by ultraviolet spectrophotometry. *J Agric Food Chem* 1992;40:2152–2156.
13. Clifford MN. Chlorogenic acids and other cinnamates: Nature, occurrence and dietary burden. *J Sci Food Agric* 1999;79:362–372.
14. Jaiswal RM, Patras MA, Eravuchira PJ. Profile and characterization of the chlorogenic acids in green robusta coffee beans by LC-MS^n: Identification of seven new classes of compounds. *J Agric Food Chem* 2010;87:22–37.
15. Moon JK, Yoo HS, Ahibamoto T. Role of roasting conditions in the level of chlorogenic acid content in coffee beans: Correlation with coffee activity. *J Agric Food Chem* 2009;54:374–381.
16. Olthof MR, Hollman PCH, Katan MB. Chlorogenic acid and caffeic acid are absorbed in humans. *J Nutr* 2001;131:66–71.
17. Gonhier M-P, Verny M-A, Besson C, et al. Chlorogenic acid bioavailability largely depends on its metabolism by the gut microflora in rats. *J Nutr* 2003;133:1853–1859.
18. Azuma K, Ippoushi K, Nakayama M, et al. Absorption of chlorogenic acid and caffeic acid in rats after oral administration. *J Agric Food Chem* 2000;48(11):5496–5500.
19. Lafay S, Gil-Izquierdo A, Manach C, et al. Absorption and metabolism of caffeic acid and chlorogenic acid in the small intestine of rats. *J Nutr* 2006;136:1192–1197.
20. Farah D, Monteiro M, Donagelo CM, Lafay S. Chlorogenic acids from green coffee extract and highly bioavailable in humans. *J Nutr* 2008;138:2309–2315.
21. Saito Y, Itagaki S, Kurosawa T, et al. *In vitro* and *in vivo* antioxidant properties of chlorogenic acid and caffeic acid. *In J Pharm* 2011;403:136–138.
22. dos Santos MD, Aleida MC, Lopes NP. Evaluation of the anti-inflammatory, analgesic and antipyretic activities of the natural polyphenol chlorogenic acid. *Biol Pharm Bull* 2006;29:2236–2240.
23. Wang GF, Shi LP, Ren YD, et al. Anti-hepatitis B virus activity of chlorogenic acid, quinic acid and caffeic acid *in vivo* and *in vitro*. *Antiviral Res* 2009;83:186–190.
24. Bassoli BK, Cassola P, Boarba-Murad GR, et al. Chlorogenic acid reduces the plasma glucose peak in the oral glucose tolerance test: Effects on hepatic glucose release and glycaemia. *Cell Biochem Funct* 2008;3:320–328.

25. Suzuki A, Kagawa D, Ochiai R, Tokumitsu I, Saito I. Green coffee bean extract and its metabolites have a hypotensive effect in spontaneously hypertensive rats. *Hypertens Res* 2002;25:99–107.
26. Saito I, Tsuchida T, Watanabe T, et al. Effect of coffee bean extract in essential hypertension. *Jpn J Med Pharm Sci* 2002;47:67–74 (in Japanese).
27. Kozuma K, Tsuchiya S, Kohori J, Hase T, Tokimitsu I. Antihypertensive effect of green coffees bean extract on mildly hypertensive subjects. *Hypertens Res* 2005;28:711–718.
28. Watanabe T, Arai Y, Mitsui Y, et al. The blood pressure-lowering effect and safety of chlorogenic acid from green coffee bean extract in essential hypotension. *Clin Exp Hypertens* 2006;28:439–449.
29. Ochiai R, Jokura H, Suzuki A, et al. Green coffee bean extract improves human vasoreactivity. *Hypertens Res* 2004;27:731–737.
30. Shen W, Qi R, Wang Z, et al. Chlorogenic acid inhibits LPS-induced microgial activation and improves survival of dopaminergic neurons. *Brain Res Bull* 2012;88:487–494.
31. Shimoda H, Seki E, Aitani M. Inhibitory effect of green coffee bean extract on fat accumulation and body weight gain in mice. *BMC Complement Altern Med* 2006;6:19.
32. Cho AS, Jeon SM, Kim MJ, et al. Chlorogenic acid exhibits anti-obesity property and improves lipid metabolism in high-fat diet-induced obese mice. *Food Chem Toxicol* 2010;48:937–943.
33. Kang TY, Yang HR, Zhang J, et al. The studies of chlorogenic acid antitumor mechanism by gene chip detection: The immune pathway gene expression. *J Anal Methods Chem* 2013;Article ID617243.
34. Onakpoya I, Terry R, Ernst E. The use of green coffee extract as a weight loss supplement: A systematic review and meta-analysis of randomised clinical trials. *Gastroenterol Res Pract.* 2011, 10.1155/2011/382852, (August 31, 2010).
35. Higgins JPT, Green S. *Cochrane Handbook for Systematic Reviews of Interventions.* The Cochrane Collaboration and Wiley, London, UK, 2008.
36. Watanabe K, Yamaguchi TF, Kusaura T, et al. Consumer health benefits of habitual consumption of chlorogenic-enriched coffee: A large single-arm study. *Nutrafoods* 2014;13:103–111.

3 Chlorogenic Acids from Green Coffee Beans

Standard Quality and Extraction Methods

Natalia Pandjaitan

CONTENTS

ABSTRACT

The health effects of green coffee bean extract has stimulated the production of this valuable product. A minimum content of chlorogenic acids, measured by high-performance liquid chromatography (HPLC) analysis, is needed for the standardization of a green coffee bean extract. The raw quality of green coffee as the starting material, as well as different processing methods, affect the concentration of the active ingredients—chlorogenic acids— in the extract.

Today, coffee is considered a functional food, primarily due to its high content of compounds that exert antioxidant and other beneficial biological properties. Coffee is known as one of the most important daily sources of antioxidants. The most prevalent antioxidants are phenolic acids of which the chlorogenic acids accumulate to high levels in crop plants. The antioxidants in coffee include chlorogenic acids, caffeic acid, tannic acid, eugenol, scopoletin, quinines, and so on, which are purported to have health benefits against heart disease, diabetes, weight loss, and others.

Coffee contains a number of compounds that contribute to its bioactivity. To obtain a functional coffee extract with optimum health benefits, it is important to consider every aspect of coffee production, starting with high-quality seeds, preferably processed at low to medium temperatures. The green coffee bean is rich in chlorogenic acid and its related compounds (Clifford, 1999). Chlorogenic acid compounds, which constitute 5%–8% of green coffee, are one of the water-soluble constituents of the bean (Moores et al., 1948). Green *Coffea robusta* beans contain a significantly higher amount of total chlorogenic acids when compared with *Coffea arabica* (Daglia et al., 2000). The 5-caffeoylquinic acid compound is the most abundant of the chlorogenic acids and is present in half of the total chlorogenic acids found in green coffee beans (Koshiro et al., 2007).

The nonvolatile fraction of green coffee is composed primarily of water, carbohydrates, fiber, proteins and free amino acids, lipids, minerals, organic acids, chlorogenic acids, trigonelline, and caffeine. Chlorogenic acids comprise a major class of phenolic compounds, which are primarily derived from esterification of transcinnamic acids. The main subclasses of chlorogenic acid in green coffee are caffeoylquinic acids, dicaffeoylquinic acids, feruloylquinic acids, and less abundantly are *p*-coumaroylquinic acids and caffeoyl-feruloylquinic acids. The 5-caffeoylquinic acid is the most abundant compound in green coffee, and constitutes about 56%–62% of total chlorogenic acids (Farah and Donangelo, 2006), followed by 4-caffeoylquinic acid and 3-caffeoylquinic acid. Perrone et al. (2008) analyzed Brazilian coffee cultivars and concluded that the second most abundant chlorogenic acid was the dichloroquinic acids (11%–15%), followed by feruloylquinic acids (FQA) (4%–7%), while the remaining minor chlorogenic acids were the *p*-coumaroylquinic acids and caffeoylferuloylquinic acids.

C. arabica and *C. robusta* beans differ in many ways, including their ideal growing climates, physical properties, and chemical composition. After harvesting, coffee fruits undergo primary processing to separate the seeds. Secondary processing such as decaffeination and steam treatment are performed before roasting. Conditions including the degree of coffee maturation and avoiding mold contamination during the harvesting, drying, and storage of the seeds are especially critical to producing good quality coffee.

3.1 COFFEE PLANT CULTIVATION PRACTICES

Growing conditions such as light have a significant effect on the biochemical contents of green coffee beans. Sun-grown beans have higher trigonelline and chlorogenic acids. Vaast et al. (2006) found that not only did shade reduce coffee productivity and increase bean size, but coffee grown in 45% shade had significantly lower chlorogenic acids than coffee grown in full sun.

Coffee fruits are typically harvested in one of three ways: picking, stripping, or mechanical harvesting. In the first method, the ripe fruits known as cherries are picked one at a time. As coffee fruits usually do not ripen simultaneously, this method is time-consuming and is expensive as a large workforce is required to carry out the picking. Nevertheless, picking tends to produce better-quality coffee seeds, in term of both taste and health, than other methods. Manual stripping of the twigs collects immature, ripe, and overripe seeds, along with leaves. Mechanical harvesting is performed by shaking the trees or by stripping the branches with an apparatus similar to a flexible comb. Stripping and mechanical harvesting yield defective fruits with different degrees of maturation and fermentation. Defective seeds such as immature, black, sour, black-immature, insect-damaged, and bored seeds are relevant to cup quality and health. Ramalakshmi et al. (2007) found that chlorogenic acids in defective coffee beans were undamaged.

Harvested green coffee beans are normally sorted by eliminating beans with defects in color, odor, form, and maturity. Low-quality green coffee beans that contain a high fraction of immature beans have lower chlorogenic acids when compared with commercial green coffee beans (Iwai et al., 2004). Immature beans have a higher content of 5-caffeoylquinic acid and soluble phenols when compared with immature black beans and nondefective beans (Mazzafera, 1999). De Menezes (1994) found differences in the monocaffeoylquinic acid to dicaffeoylquinic acid ratio in green coffee at different maturity stages. Koshiro et al. (2007) also evaluated the content of chlorogenic acids in green *C. canephora* seeds at different maturity stages, and found that the seed contained more chlorogenic acids at the fully ripened (red) stage than at the ripening (pink) stage. Ohiokpehai (1982) also found that the chlorogenic acids content increased in both *C. canephora* and *C. arabica* beans during development to full maturity.

Robusta coffee trees are more robust, which means that they are stronger, more resistant to pests and disease, and less demanding than *C. arabica* trees with regard to climate. *Robusta* coffee also contains higher amounts of antioxidant compounds and caffeine (Budryn and Nebesny, 2008). For decades, hybridization efforts have attempted to combine the resistance of *robusta* trees with the organoleptic quality found in *C. arabica* trees, but it is likely that the traits responsible for pest resistance in *robusta* plants are partially responsible for its lower organoleptic taste.

The higher chlorogenic acid content in *Robusta* coffee protects the plant more against microorganisms, insects, and UV radiation as compared with *C. arabica* coffee. *C. canephora* also contains a few secondary metabolites (e.g., minor chlorogenic acids, isomers, and diterpenes) that are not present in *C. arabica* (Ky et al., 2001). Other theories pointed out the possibility of a synthesis of chlorogenic acid compounds specifically to control seed germination and cell growth through unknown mechanisms.

3.2 POSTHARVEST PRACTICES

Harvested coffee fruits undergo pulp extraction to produce green coffee seeds. The most common methods of pulp extraction are the dry and wet methods. Alternatively, they may be decaffeinated or steam treated before the roasting process.

3.2.1 Decaffeination

Coffee decaffeination usually reduces caffeine content from 1–2 to 0.02–0.30 g/100 g (Balyaya and Clifford, 1995). The loss of other coffee components depends on the decaffeination method. Water tends to remove many soluble components, but the use of various organic solvents tends to produce more specific results. Two different water decaffeination processes in *Arabica* green coffee reported 1.5% gain and 20% loss in chlorogenic acids (Farah et al., 2006a).

Loss of chlorogenic acids during decaffeination with dichloromethane has been reported as 16% for *arabica* and 11% for *robusta* coffees (Toci et al., 2006). Simultaneous loss of caffeine and chlorogenic acids during the decaffeination process is to be expected since the two compounds normally form a complex in coffee beans (Hamidi and Wanner, 1964).

Supercritical carbon dioxide decaffeination appears to be more selective in removing caffeine, sparing the compounds that are responsible for aroma and bioactivity such as chlorogenic acids (Machmudah et al., 2008). The application of the supercritical method reported a 1.2% loss of chlorogenic acids in green *arabica* coffee beans. Although the relative increase of chlorogenic acids in water-decaffeinated coffees may be due to lixiviation of highly soluble compounds, the supercritical carbon dioxide method appears to reduce chlorogenic acid losses while maintaining the integrity of the seeds.

3.2.2 Dry Processing

The dry processing technique is generally used in areas with little or no access to water. The whole cherry (bean, mucilage, pulp) is exposed to the sun or air dryers immediately after harvest. A final moisture content of 10%–12% is crucial to obtain good quality green coffee beans. The separation of ripe fruits from unripe, overripe, and damaged fruits is done manually with the help of a sieve. If air dryers are not available, low rainfall during harvesting is needed to ensure good quality coffee. In Brazil and Africa, where sun and space are abundant and fruits are harvested by stripping, the seeds are mechanically and electronically sorted to separate defected seeds from the high-quality seeds. Strip-picking of coffee beans from branches means that there is little attention given to the fruit ripeness, and hence many imperfect beans slip through the process and need to be sorted out manually (Selmar, 2006). The greater possibility of a mixture of fruit from any stage of development in the dry process means that immature fruits with low chlorogenic acids content are included.

After drying, fruits are cleaned and dehulled, and the dried skin and pulp are removed leaving a mucilaginous material (silver skin) adhering to the seed surface. The dry process produces a lower ratio of monocaffeoylquinic acid to dicaffeoylquinic acid compared with the wet process of *C. arabica* (De Menezes, 1994). The degradation of the chlorogenic acids could be caused by sun heat exposure.

A variation of the wet method commonly done in Brazil and Indonesia is the semidry method, also called the wet-hulled or semi-washed or pulped natural process. Coffee processed by the semidry method showed a lower content of chlorogenic acids and trigonelline compared with the wet method (Duarte et al., 2010). In this semidry process, a small amount of water is used to separate ripe and unripe cherries. The coffee fruits are depulped but the fermentation process occurs directly on the platform. The distribution of individual chlorogenic acid compounds is similar between the semidry and the wet method. Although both the wet and semidry methods involve a depulping step, the semidry process is more similar to the dry method due to mucilage removal by drying and hulling. Mucilage equates to approximately 17% by mass of a coffee berry, and is rich in pectin and sugars. Murthy and Naidu (2011) investigated the composition of *C. robusta* coffee pulp and mucilage and found that the pulp contained most of the chlorogenic acids while the mucilage contained none. This could be the reason why the dry process produced far less chlorogenic acids when compared with the semidry and wet methods. Coffee seeds that undergo the natural process are often used in espresso coffee blends, as they tend to add more body to the beverage than the wet-processed seeds because the polysaccharides in the silver skin are not fermented, but remain on the seeds.

3.2.3 Wet Processing

The wet processing method is more sophisticated and generally produces a higher-quality brew with a more consistent flavor compared with other methods. Before dehulling and separating the seeds, cherry selection takes place in flotation tanks, followed by soaking and fermentation. Ripe red fruits that sink in water immersion are selected, whereas the unripe cherries that float on water are not included in the process. During fermentation, enzymes may be added, the silver skin is removed and as the acidity level increases, the pH balance may be reduced to 4.5. The seeds (parchment coffee) are then extensively washed, polished, sun dried and/or air dried. Wet processing is frequently used in countries where coffee is harvested by picking, such as Columbia, Asia, and Central America.

The fermentation step in the wet process may affect the chlorogenic acids in coffee due to the loss of other water-soluble components. Uniformity in berry size is important as removal of the pulp around the coffee bean is carried out by a machine calibrated to size and any smaller beans would escape having their pulp removed. If the mucilage is not removed, it can cause the beans to ferment, and a slight fermentation causes the mucilage to dissolve. Water-soluble phenolic acids, including chlorogenic acids, can easily be lost during underwater fermentation.

The wet method produced significantly higher total chlorogenic acids than the semidry method with the exception of dicaffeoylquinic acids (Duarte et al., 2010). The primary difference between the processing methods is that wet-processed seeds are separated from the pulp and skin before drying. The wet processing method generates a better consistency of ripe fruits by floating sorting; this may influence the total chlorogenic acids content.

3.2.4 Steaming

Commercial processing of *robusta* coffee beans may involve a steaming step to obtain milder flavor profiles and to improve digestibility. With steam-treated coffees, differences in their volatile compositions are mainly due to the partial hydrolysis of chlorogenic acids, and either a loss or change of low-molecular-weight compounds caused by humidity. The steaming of coffee beans before roasting eliminates stomach-upsetting substances, including the chlorogenic acids (Schrader et al., 1996). Increasing the water uptake, and the high temperatures during steaming, could be responsible for the loss of the water-soluble chlorogenic acids.

3.2.5 Roasting

After the seeds are dried, they are sized and graded, and mechanically, manually, and/or electronically sorted to eliminate defective seeds. This process may be followed by ultraviolet excitation, which separates defective seeds produced during processing that are difficult to detect except by fluorescence. The green coffee seeds are then ready for the roasting process, in which the coffee will develop its organoleptic character by the formation of aromatic compounds. Many studies have confirmed that roasting significantly reduced the total chlorogenic acids content of coffee beans (Trugo and Macrae, 1984; Moon et al., 2009). Nebesny and Budryn (2003) reported that more than 60% of total chlorogenic acids is lost during roasting. Green coffee beans contain higher amount of the compounds of chlorogenic acids in comparison with regular roasted coffee beans.

Roasting produces chlorogenic acid lactones with the 3-caffeoylquinic-1,5-lactone as the most abundant compound in both *C. arabica* and *C. robusta* (Farah et al., 2005). Approximately 30% of the original chlorogenic acids were converted to their lactone counterparts. Schrader et al. (1996) found that keeping the coffee brewing at 80°C caused a decrease in most of the 5-caffeoylquinic acid, but not in the 3-caffeoylquinic acid and 4-caffeoylquinic acid.

3.3 ANALYSIS METHOD OF CHLOROGENIC ACIDS

Quantification of chlorogenic acids as a group is well established. Phenolic acids such as chlorogenic acids showed characteristic absorbances in the ultraviolet-visible section at 324 nm (Moores et al., 1948). HPLC with a photodiode array detector is normally used for measuring chlorogenic acids at their maximum absorption of 325 nm. Isomers of chloroquinic acids, feruloylquinicacids, coumaroylquinicacids, and dichloroquinicacids are normally identified in coffee samples (Farah et al., 2008).

The separation of chlorogenic acid isomers can be accomplished with gradient elution during chromatographic analysis using acidified water containing methanol, and acidified methanol. In order to get a fine chromatographic separation, Ky et al. (1997) used a gradient condition of 5% methanol in a phosphoric acid solution, and 5% phosphoric acid solution in methanol. Figure 3.1 shows eight chlorogenic acid peaks from green coffee bean extract without separation between the 4- and 5-chloroquinic acids peaks. Relative precision measured by the coefficient of variation was low (1%–7%), while the highest value for standard deviation was 0.286 for total chlorogenic acids using this method.

Quantification is normally achieved by peak area measurement and by comparison with either the 5-chloroquinic acid or the 3-chloroquinic acid standard, the total

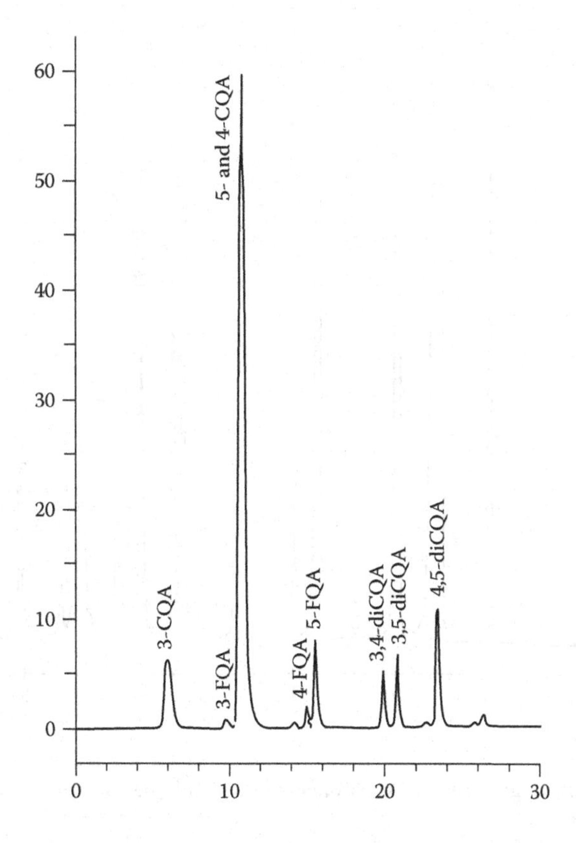

FIGURE 3.1 Binary gradient HPLC chromatogram of chlorogenic acids of a green *robusta* coffee.

chloroquinic acids, total feruloylquinicacids, total dicaffeoylquinic acids, and total chlorogenic acids. Bicchi et al. (1995) found 22 chlorogenic acids from green coffee using a 15%–45% methanol solution in a citrate–hydrochloric acid buffer in a linear gradient. Figure 3.2 shows the separation of 22 isomers of chlorogenic acid along with 11 unidentified chlorogenic acid compounds using this analysis method. Peak areas of the target compounds were within the linear range of the curve.

3.4 STANDARDIZED GREEN COFFEE EXTRACTS

In 2002, Berkem published a patent for a green coffee extract with the precise composition of its chlorogenic acids. The patent included the effect of the green coffee extract on body weight management and control. A minimum of 45% of total chlorogenic acids content and 400 mg of daily dosage were also recorded in the document. Studies have proven that chlorogenic compounds from green coffee are easily absorbed and metabolized in humans (Farah et al., 2008). After the acquisition of Berkem by Naturex in 2008, a specific composition of decaffeinated green coffee extract, named Svetol, quickly became the number one slimming ingredient in the USA. Svetol, which is standardized in chlorogenic acids, is shown to inhibit

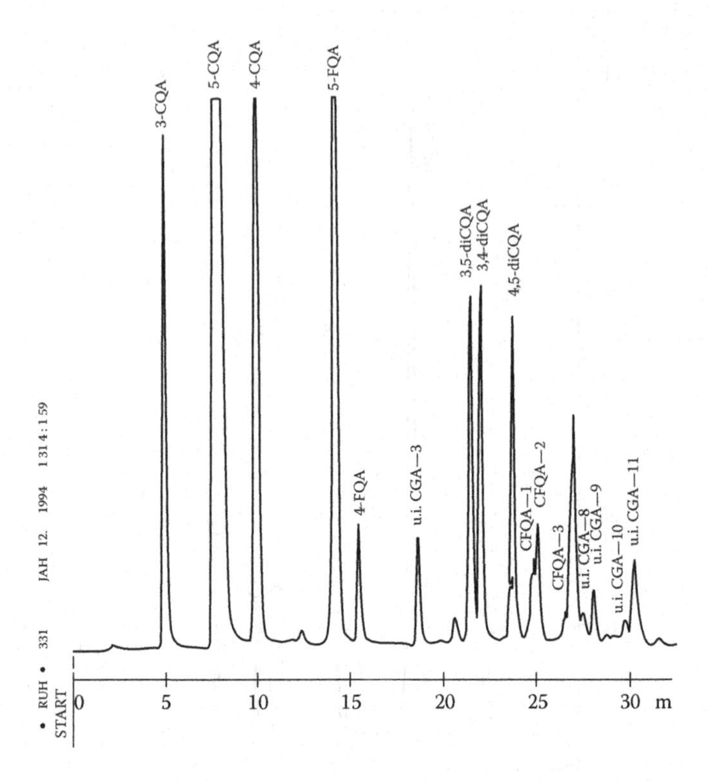

FIGURE 3.2 Linear gradient HPLC chromatogram of chlorogenic acids of a green *robusta* coffee.

gluconeogenesis and glycogenolysis reactions (Henry-Vitrac et al., 2010), and has a significant effect in reducing body mass and body fat (Thom, 2007).

Another well-known standardized green coffee extract is produced by Applied Food Sciences Inc., which gives the option of 40%–50% chlorogenic acids content. Their green coffee extract, commercially named Green Coffee Antioxidant (GCA), contains 4%–40% of caffeine in contrast to a maximum of 2% of caffeine in the Svetol product. The standardized Svetol extract also contains more than 10% of 5-caffeoylquinic acid, whereas GCA extract does not mention the proportion of this specific compound.

Other green coffee extract manufacturers usually adhere to the 45%–50% total chlorogenic acids content as a standard. Since the Svetol patent (Lemaire et al., 2008) also mentioned that the green coffee extract in particular contains a ratio of 5-caffeoylquinic acid to total chlorogenic acids (5-CQA/tCGA) in the range of 0.2–0.3, other green coffee extract manufacturers normally avoid stating the proportion of 5-CQA in their extract to the total chlorogenic acids amount. Since the typical amount of 5-caffeoylquinic acid in *C. canephora* is 50% of the total chlorogenic acids, it is easy to get green coffee extracts with a higher proportion of 5-caffeoylquinic acid. Svetol also laid claim to a well-balanced composition of 3-, 4-, and 5-caffeoylquinic acids as opposed to a much higher 5-caffeoylquinic acid level compared with other caffeoylquinic acids in alternative green coffee extracts.

Svetol is included in the product Coffee Slender, a popular weight loss product sold in many countries but first sold in Norway. Several other supplement products such as Europharma followed. It is sold as an ingredient with more than one benefit including to help manage weight, to reduce blood pressure, and to decrease blood sugar levels. While Svetol has a dose recommendation for both high blood pressure and weight loss, GCA only has a dose recommendation for weight loss. In comparison, the suggested daily dose for weight loss for GCA is 700–1050 mg daily whereas the dose for Svetol is only 80–200 mg daily.

While the minimum concentration of chlorogenic acids needed in green coffee extract for weight loss has been established, the concentration of chlorogenic acids for other positive benefits was shown to be lower. Watanabe et al. (2006) used 140 mg/day of chlorogenic acids supplementation to investigate the effects on blood pressure and found that there was a significant hypertension lowering effect. The daily dose recommendation for high blood pressure treatment is 93–185 mg of the standardized Svetol. Blum et al. (2007) used a daily dose of 3×200 mg of Svetol for glucose metabolism regulation.

3.5 CHLOROGENIC ACIDS EXTRACTION METHODS

The basic chemical composition depends primarily on genetic aspects, especially species, and on physiological aspects such as the degree of maturation. External factors such as soil composition, climate, agricultural practices, and storage conditions also affect seed physiology and chemical composition, but to a lesser extent. Therefore, these aspects should be considered when comparing the chemical compositions of coffees.

Each of the subclasses of chlorogenic acids consists of at least three major positional isomers in addition to minor compounds, except for the latter class, which contains six major isomers. Caffeoylquinic acids, which are esters of caffeic acid with quinic acid, account for approximately 80% of the total chlorogenic acid content (Clifford and Kazi, 1987). In particular, 5-caffeoylquinic acid is the first of these compounds identified (Moores et al., 1948). Other minor compounds identified include dicaffeoylquinic acids, acyl dicaffeoylquinic acids, dimethoxycinnamoylquinic acids, sinapoylquinic acids, and sinapoyl-caffeoylquinic acids. The most studied isomer is 5-caffeoylquinic acid and it is commonly called *chlorogenic acid.*

Chlorogenic acids content in *C. canephora* is generally 1–2.5 times higher than in *C. arabica*, but this concentration varies considerably between species. In the last few years, a series of epidemiologic and clinical studies have reported that coffee consumption, independent of caffeine intake, is associated with health benefits such as lower risk of type 2 diabetes, Parkinson's disease, Alzheimer's disease, and liver cancer.

The compound chlorogenic acid (5-caffeoylquinic acid) is not soluble in nonpolar solvents, but is partially soluble in ethanol and methanol (Lu et al., 2004). Chlorogenic acid alone is easily and freely soluble in water. In addition to the 45%–50% of total chlorogenic acids found in Svetol, the specific composition also mentioned 10%–15% of 5-caffeoylquinic acid in the product. Belay and Gholap (2009) dissolved chlorogenic acids in ethanol, methanol, water, and acetonitrile, and found that chlorogenic acids can be dissolved in all four solvents.

3.5.1 Traditional Organic Solvent Extraction of Chlorogenic Acids

Phenolic compounds exhibit a wide range of solubilities in polar solvents and are often more soluble in solvents less polar than water (Zuorro and Lavecchia, 2013). Phenolics are commonly extracted in an aqueous solution mixed with alcohol or acetone. The solution containing phenolic acids and soluble esters is then fractionated using ethyl acetate or diethyl ether. The total free phenolic acids are then quantified after the phenolic acid esters in the aqueous phase are hydrolyzed with acid or alkali (Krygier et al., 1982). Water extraction of phenolic compounds from spent coffee showed that alkaline water (pH 9.5) extracted the most antioxidants (Bravo et al., 2013). The addition of carbonate compounds to coffee brewing water has been found to increase antioxidant compounds including chlorogenic acids in mocha and espresso coffee (Perez-Martinez et al., 2010). Acidified solvents can also be used to extract phenolic acids (Robbins, 2003).

Naidu et al. (2008) extracted antioxidant components of green coffee with aqueous isopropanol. They obtained the best yield (27%–29%) using a 60:40 ratio of isopropanol to water with both *C. arabica* and *C. robusta*. Both varieties showed increasing total chlorogenic acids concentration with increasing water ratio, and increasing the water content from 20% to 40% resulted in a 29.7% increase of total chlorogenic acids concentration in a *C. robusta* extract. The concentration of chlorogenic acids in extracts from both varieties obtained with a 60:40 ratio of isopropanol to water solvent was 30%.

Dibert et al. (1989) investigated the effects of temperature, particle diameter, and solvent to mass ratio, in green coffee extraction. Concentrations of chlorogenic acids obtained with this extraction were in the range of 3.7%–18.1%. They examined 70% methanol–water as the solvent for extracting chlorogenic acids from oil-free green coffee beans. Using this solvent, 20%–40% of chlorogenic acids were extracted in the first 10 min. Raising the extraction temperatures from 30°C to 50°C increased the extraction yield. The effect of the temperature was diminished with the increasing mass ratio of ground coffee to the solvent. The variation in the mass ratio of ground coffee to the solvent showed that equilibrium was reached faster with a higher mass ratio.

Suarez-Quiroz et al. (2014) found no significant differences in the chlorogenic acids content of extracts using hot water, aqueous methanol, and aqueous isopropanol. Green coffee extract from *C. arabica* obtained by water extraction at 80°C was ultimately purified further using activated carbon as an alternative to organic solvents for isolation of chlorogenic acids. A minimum of 97% purity was verified with each of the final chlorogenic acids isolated in this study.

An evaluation of purification methods of chlorogenic acids was carried out by Ky et al. (1997) to determine the most accurate procedure for the quantification of the compounds by HPLC. They compared the five different procedures after first extracting chlorogenic acids from green coffee beans with 70% methanol in water. The isolation method treated with Carrez reagents gave the highest content and approximately twice the value of total chlorogenic acids compared with the isolation method using organic solvents. Since the inclusion of chemical reagents such as the ingredients of the Carrez reagents is not suitable for the production of green coffee extract with a high concentration of chlorogenic acids, the use of organic solvents is still the main method used to obtain a standardized extract with 50% chlorogenic acids.

3.5.2 Alternative Extraction of Chlorogenic Acids

Mullen et al. (2011) compared the chlorogenic acids contents in a multistep extract, a single-step extract, a freeze-dried extract, and an air-dried extract of whole green coffee fruits. The levels of total chlorogenic acids measured in an extract from freeze-dried whole coffee fruits powder extracted with a 50% ethanol:water solvent was 4.5%, whereas the application of the same extraction procedure on freeze-dried fruits powder gave 8.8% total chlorogenic acids. Two different whole coffee fruits extracted with ethanol, followed by purification, had 42% and 88% total chlorogenic acids contents, respectively.

Upadhyay et al. (Food chem., 2012) obtained 32.7%–61.9% of total chlorogenic acids using a microwave-assisted extraction. They evaluated water, ethanol, and methanol to extract chlorogenic acids. Each solvent used the same 800 W on the microwave at 50°C for 5 min. Variation in temperatures (30°C–90°C) showed that 50°C was the ideal temperature for extracting chlorogenic acids. Time variation (2, 5, and 10 min) showed the highest yield of chlorogenic acids at 5 min. The wattage used on the microwave was also investigated, and the 800 W gave the highest result of extracted chlorogenic acids. The microwave-assisted extraction was also compared with the conventional extraction method, using a hot water bath at 50°C for 5 min, and the yield for chlorogenic acids from microwave extraction showed more than twice the value from conventional extraction. Water extraction had the highest yield in both chlorogenic acids and caffeine; however, the extract showed lower concentration levels of total chlorogenic acids (46.4%) as compared with the methanol extract (61.9%).

Supercritical carbon dioxide extraction has gained popularity as a safer alternative to flammable and toxic organic solvent extraction for the decaffeination of green coffee. The application of supercritical carbon dioxide to extract chlorogenic acids was achieved only when isopropyl alcohol was used as the cosolvent (De Avezedo et al., 2008). With the addition of isopropyl alcohol, the highest concentration observed was below 0.01% in dried green coffee beans. Carbon dioxide extraction can be done with ethanol as a cosolvent, but isopropyl alcohol has lower polarity when compared with ethanol. Machmudah et al. (2008) also extracted chlorogenic acids and caffeine with supercritical carbon dioxide and found that increasing the pressure from 15 to 25 MPa increased the chlorogenic acids concentration, whereas increasing the temperature from 40°C to 60°C had no major effect on the extracted chlorogenic acids. The application of elevated pressure at 10 MPa resulted in four times the amount of chlorogenic acid extracted from mate leaves when compared with pressure at 5 MPa (Grujic et al., 2012) using 40% ethanol as cosolvent.

Budryn et al. (2009) reviewed water and ethanolic extraction solvents in green and roasted *C. arabica* and *C. robusta* beans for chlorogenic acids, and found that the ethanolic extracts contained lower chlorogenic acids compared with water extracts. Water extracts of *C. robusta* beans gave a higher antioxidant content than *C. arabica* beans, and the dry extracts contained up to 36% of chlorogenic acids. Three water extract preparations were conducted: brewing with boiling water, boiling in water, and boiling in water using a pressure cooker. Water extracts using boiling water under elevated pressure gave the highest concentration of chlorogenic acids. Ethanol extracts gave lower chlorogenic acids and pigment concentration when compared with the water extracts.

Nebesny and Budryn (2003) studied the antioxidant activity of green coffee extracted with convection and microwave roasting techniques. The roasted coffee extract prepared with microwave rather than the usual convection heating resulted in higher antioxidant property. A decreasing concentration of the main phenolics in coffee (chlorogenic acids) is most likely the reason for the lower antioxidative effects of coffee beans that have undergone microwave roasting.

3.6 CONCLUSION

The quality of green coffee beans is influenced by the chemical properties and composition of the crop. Factors such as maturity, defects, and processing have significant effects on chlorogenic acids—the functional chemical compound most abundant in coffee. The *C. robusta* variety is a better material for chlorogenic acids extraction when compared with the *C. arabica* variety. Primary processing of green coffee beans through wet processing is the best method to obtain mature seeds with the highest content of chlorogenic acids. Secondary processing aspects have an effect on the health benefits of green coffee products. The decaffeination process with supercritical CO_2 gave the least loss of chlorogenic acids. The roasting process degrades almost all chlorogenic acids in the coffee beans.

The identification and quantification of chlorogenic acid and its derivatives are attainable with HPLC at 325 nm for greatest sensitivity analysis. A binary HPLC solvent system based on methanol/water can give adequate separation of chlorogenic acid and its derivatives. More than 20 chlorogenic acids have already been identified and 9 of their isomers are normally measured in coffee samples using HPLC.

Green coffee beans that have not gone through secondary processing are the best starting material for extraction or purification of chlorogenic acids. For food-grade solvent extraction of chlorogenic acids, water is a comparable solvent when compared with alcohol. A standard minimum of 45% chlorogenic acids concentration in green coffee extract can only be achieved using either mechanical-assisted extraction such as a microwave with elevated pressure to enhance molecular interaction, or by purification using organic solvents.

REFERENCES

Balyaya, K. J., Clifford, M. N. 1995. Individual chlorogenic acids and caffeine contents in commercial grades of wet and dry processed Indian green *robusta* coffee. *Journal of Food Science and Technology* 32: 104–108.

Belay, A., Gholap, A. V. 2009. Characterization and determination of chlorogenic acids (CGA) in coffee beans by UV-Vis spectroscopy. *African Journal of Pure and Applied Chemistry* 3: 234–240.

Bicchi, C. P., Binollo, A. E., Pellegrino, G. M., Vanni, A. C. 1995. Characterization of green and roasted coffees through the chlorogenic acid fraction by HPLC-UV and principal component analysis. *Journal of the Agricultural and Food Chemistry* 43: 1549–1555.

Blum, J., Lemaire, B., Lafay, S. 2007. Effect of a green decaffeinated coffee extract on glycaemia. *Nutrafoods* 6: 13–17.

Bravo, J., Monente, C., Juaniz, I., de Pena, M. P., Cid, C. 2013. Influence of extraction process on antioxidant capacity of spent coffee. *Food Research International* 50: 610–616.

Budryn, G., Nebesny, E. 2008. Antioxidant properties of *Arabica* and *Robusta* coffee extracts prepared under different conditions. *Deutsche Lebbensmittel Rundschau* 104: 69–78.

Budryn, G., Nebesny, E., Podsedek, A., Zyzelewicz, D., Materska, M., Jankowski, S., Janda. B. 2009. Effect of different extraction methods on the recovery of chlorogenic acids, caffeine and Maillard reaction product in coffee beans. *European Food Research and Technology* 228: 913–922.

Clifford, M. N. 1999. Chlorogenic acids and other cinnamates-nature, occurrence and dietary burden. *Journal of the Science of Food and Agriculture* 79: 362–372.

Clifford, M. N., Kazi, T. 1987. The influence of coffee bean maturity on the content of chlorogenic acids, caffeine, and trigonelline. *Food Chemistry* 26: 56–59.

Daglia, M., Papetti, A., Gregotti, C., Berte, F., Gazzani, G. 2000. *In vitro* antioxidant and *ex vivo* protective activities of green and roasted coffee. *Journal of Agricultural and Food Chemistry* 48: 1449–1454.

De Avezedo, A. B. A., Mazzafera, P., Mohamed, R. S., Vieira de Melo, S. A. B., Kieckbush, T. G., 2008. Extraction of caffeine, chlorogenic acids and lipids from green coffee beans using supercritical carbon dioxide and co-solvents. *Brazilian Journal of Chemical Engineering* 25: 543–552.

De Menezes, H. C. 1994. The relationship between the state of maturity of raw coffee beans and the isomers of caffeoylquinic acid. *Food Chemistry*. 293–296.

Dibert, K., Cros, E., Andrieu, J. 1989. Solvent extraction of oil and chlorogenic acid from green coffee. Part II: Kinetic data. *Journal of Food Engineering* 10: 199–214.

Duarte, G. S., Pereira, A. A., Farah, A. 2010. Chlorogenic acids and other relevant compounds in Brazilian coffees processed by semi-dry and wet post-harvesting methods. *Analytical Methods* 118: 851–855.

Farah, A., de Paulis, T., Moreira, D. P., Trugo, L.C., Martin, P. R. 2006a. Chlorogenic acids and lactones in regular and water-decaffeinated *Arabica* coffees. *Journal of Agricultural and Food Chemistry* 54: 374–381.

Farah, A., de Paulis, T., Trugo, L. C., Martin, P. R. 2005. Effect of roasting on the formation of chlorogenic acid lactones. *Journal of Agricultural and Food Chemistry* 53: 1505–1513.

Farah, A., Donangelo, C. M. 2006b. Phenolic compounds in coffee. *Brazilian Journal of Plant Physiology* 18: 23–36.

Farah, A., Monteiro, M., Donangelo, C. M., Lafay, S. 2008. Chlorogenic acids from green coffee extract are highly bioavailable in humans. *Journal of Nutrition* 138: 2309–2315.

Grujic, N., Lepojevic, Z., Srdjenovic, B., Vladic, J., Sudji, J. 2012. Effects of different extraction methods and conditions on the phenolic composition of mate tea extracts. *Molecules* 17: 2518–2528.

Hamidi, A., Wanner, H. 1964. The distribution pattern of chlorogenic acid and caffeine in *Coffea Arabica*. *Planta* 61: 90–96.

Henry-Vitrac, C., Ibarra, A., Roller, M., Merillon, J.-M., Vitrac, X. 2010. Contribution of chlorogenic acids to the inhibition of human hepatic glucose-6-phosphatase activity *in vitro* by svetol, a standardized decaffeinated green coffee extract. *Journal of Agricultural and Food Chemistry* 58: 4141–4144.

Iwai, K., Kishimoto, N., Kakino, Y., Mochida, K., Fujita, T. 2004. *In vitro* antioxidative effects and tyronase inhibitory activities of seven hydroxycinnamoyl derivatives in green coffee beans. *Journal of Agricultural and Food Chemistry* 52: 4893–4898.

Koshiro, Y., Jackson, M.C., Katahira, R., Wang, M., Nagai, C., Ashihara, H. 2007. Biosynthesis of chlorogenic acids in growing and ripening fruits of *Coffea Arabica* and *Coffea Canephora* plants. *Zeitschrift für Naturforschung C* 62: 731–742.

Krygier, K., Sosulsky, F., Hogge, L. 1982. Free, esterified, and insoluble-bound phenolic acids. 1. Extraction and purification procedure. *Journal of Agricultural and Food Chemistry* 30: 330–334.

Ky, C., Louarn, J., Dussert, S., Guyot, B., Hamon, S., Noirot, M. 2001. Caffeine, trigonelline, chlorogenic acids, and sucrose diversity in wild *Coffea arabica* L. and *C. canephora* P. accessions. *Food Chemistry* 75: 223–230.

Ky, C., Noirot, M., Hamon, S. 1997. Comparison of five purification methods for chlorogenic acids in green coffee beans (*Coffea* sp.). *Journal of Agricultural and Food Chemistry* 45: 786–790.

Lemaire, B., Lafay, S., Nardon, K., Ibarra, A., Roller, M., Dikansky, J. 2008. Effects of a decaffeinated green coffee extract on body weight control by regulation of glucose metabolism. U.S. Patent Application 12/263,292, filed October 31, 2008.

Lu, H. T., Jiang, Y., Chen, F. 2004. Application of preparative high-speed counter-current chromatography for separation of chlorogenic acid from Flos Lonicerae. *Journal of Chromatography* 1026: 185–190.

Machmudah, S., Kitada, K., Goto, M., Sasaki, M. 2008. Caffeine and chlorogenic acid separation from raw coffee beans using supercritical CO_2 in water. *Industrial & Engineering Chemistry Research* 50: 2227–2235.

Mazzafera, P. 1999. Chemical composition of defective coffee beans. *Food Chemistry* 64: 547–554.

Moon, J.-K., Yoo, H. S., Shibamoto, T. 2009. Role of roasting conditions in the level of chlorogenic acids content in coffee beans: Correlation with coffee acidity. *Journal of Agricultural and Food Chemistry* 57: 5365–5369.

Moores, R. G., McDermott, D. L., Wood. T. R. 1948. Determination of chlorogenic acid in coffee. *Analytical Chemistry* 20, 620–624.

Mullen, W., Nemzer, B., Ou, B., Stalmach, A., Hunter, J., Clifford, M. N., Combet, E. 2011. The antioxidant and chlorogenic acid profiles of whole coffee fruits are influenced by the extraction procedures. *Journal of Agricultural and Food Chemistry* 59: 3754–3762.

Murthy, P. S., Naidu, M. M. 2011. Improvement of *robusta* coffee fermentation with microbial enzymes. *European Journal of Applied Sciences* 3: 130–139.

Naidu, M. M., Sulochanamma, G., Sampathu, S. R., Srinivas, P. 2008. Studies on extraction antioxidant potential of green coffee. *Food Chemistry* 107: 377–384.

Nebesny, E. Budryn, G. 2003. Antioxidative activity of green and roasted coffee beans as influenced by convection and microwave roasting methods and content of certain compounds. *European Food Research and Technology* 217: 157–163.

Ohiokpehai, O. 1982. Chlorogenic Acid Content of Green Coffee Beans. Diss. Faculty of Biological and Chemical Sciences, University of Surrey, Guilford.

Perez-Martinez, M., Caemmerer, B, Paz de Pena, M., Cid, C., Kroh, L. W. 2010. Influence of the brewing method and acidity regulators on the antioxidant capacity of coffee brews. *Journal of Agricultural and Food Chemistry* 58: 2958–2965.

Perrone, D., Farah, A., Donangelo, C. M., de Paulis, T., Martin, P. R. 2008. Comprehensive analysis of major and minor chlorogenic acids and lactones in economically relevant Brazilian coffee cultivars. *Food Chemistry* 106: 859–867.

Ramalakshmi, K., Kubra, I. R., Rao, L. J. M. 2007. Physicochemical characteristics of green coffee: Comparison of graded and defective beans. *Journal of Food Science* 72: S333–S337.

Robbins, R. J. 2003. Phenolic acids in foods: An overview of analytical methodology. *Journal of Agricultural and Food Chemistry* 51: 2866–2887.

Schrader, K., Kiehne, A., Engelhardt, U. H., Maier, H. G. 1996. Determination of chlorogenic acids with lactones in roasted coffee. *Journal of the Science of Food and Agriculture* 71: 392–398.

Selmar, D., Bytof, F., Knopp, S. E., Breitenstein, B. 2006. Germination of coffee seeds and its significance for coffee quality. *Plant Biology* 8: 260–264.

Suarez-Quiroz, M. L., Campos, A. A., Alfaro, G. V., Gonzalez-Rios, O., Villeneuve, P., Figueroa-Espinoza, M. L. 2014. Isolation of green coffee chlorogenic acids using activated carbon. *Journal of Food Composition and Analysis* 33: 55–58.

Thom, E. 2007. The effect of chlorogenic acid enriched coffee on glucose absorption in healthy volunteers and its effect on body mass when used long-term in overweight and obese people. *Journal of International Medical Research* 35: 900–908.

Toci, A., Farah, A., Trugo, L. C. 2006. Effect of decaffeination using dichloromethane on the chemical composition of *arabica* and *robusta* raw and roasted coffees. *Quimica Nova* 29: 965–971.

Trugo, L. C., Macrae, R. 1984. A study of the effect of roasting on chlorogenic acid composition of coffee using HPLC. *Food Chemistry* 15: 219–227.

Upadhyay R., Ramalakshmi, K., Rao, L. J. M. 2012. Microwave-assisted extraction of chlorogenic acids from green coffee beans. *Food Chemistry* 130: 184–188.

Vaast, P., Bertrand, B., Perriot, J., Guyot, B., Genard, M. 2006. Fruit thinning and shade improve bean characteristics and beverage quality of coffee (*Coffea arabica* L.) under optimal conditions. *Journal of the Science of Food and Agriculture* 86: 197–204.

Watanabe, T., Arai, Y., Mitsui, Y., Kusaura, T., Okawa, W., Kajihara, Y., Saito, I. 2006. The blood pressure-lowering effect and safety of chlorogenic acid from green coffee bean extract in essential hypertension. *Clinical and Experimental Hypertension* 28: 439–449.

Zuorro, A., Lavecchia, R. 2013. Influence of extraction conditions on the recovery of phenolic antioxidants from spent coffee grounds. *American Journal of Applied Sciences* 10: 478–486.

4 Occurrence in Plants and *In Vitro*, Animal and Human Metabolism of Chlorogenic Acids

Maurice J. Arnaud

CONTENTS

ABSTRACT

Chlorogenic acid, a depside of caffeic with quinic acid, exhibits large variations in plant contents according to cultivars and varieties, part of the plant, maturation and ripening, and processing such as roasting. A dietary survey showed that coffee is often the best source of chlorogenic acid followed by bread, cereals, tea, fruits, and vegetables, reaching 1 g of daily intake.

During the last two decades, major progress has been made in the identification of new compounds in plants and the investigation of the bioavailability of chlorogenic acid. From 1950 to 1990, only 13 metabolites of chlorogenic acid were reported, while today 35 metabolites have been identified. Our understanding of the metabolic cycle of chlorogenic acid has improved with the major impact of colonic flora, the formation of bacterial metabolites, their absorption into the bloodstream, their hepatic metabolism, and urinary elimination. The contribution of bacterial and cellular metabolism may explain individual variations reported in metabolic balance and the difficulty in measuring pharmacokinetic parameters.

More research is needed to identify intestinal absorption transporters, the relative contribution of bacterial metabolism from Phase I and II tissue metabolism. Studies on the physiological and health effects of these metabolites are needed for scientific substantiation of health claims.

Keywords: coffee, phenolic acids, chlorogenic acids, caffeic acid, ferulic acid, metabolism

4.1 CHEMICAL STRUCTURE AND OCCURRENCE OF CHLOROGENIC ACIDS IN PLANTS

Among the important classes of phenolic compounds, which constitute a large and widely distributed group of secondary metabolites ubiquitous to all plants, are the depsides of transcinnamic acids (Figure 4.1) such as caffeic, ferulic, and *p*-coumaric acid with quinic acid. Chlorogenic acids are depsides of caffeic with quinic acid (Figure 4.2). Chlorogenic acid is the 5-caffeoylquinic acid according to the IUPAC-IUB (IUPAC, 1976) nomenclature, while chlorogenic acids often refer to 5-caffeoylquinic acid and its isomers, 3-caffeoylquinic acid (neochlorogenic acid) and 4-caffeoylquinic acid (cryptochlorogenic acid). In some studies, the di-esters, 3,4-, 3,5-, and 4,5-dicaffeoylquinic acid, are also included. These hydroxycinnamic acids esters are found in all parts of fruits and vegetables with higher concentrations in the outer part of mature fruits. Decreased concentrations during ripening and extensive hydrolysis of hydroxycinnamic derivatives to free acids during long storage period were reported (Manach et al., 2004; Rapisarda et al., 2001). Instead of using IUPAC numbering, it has been reported that the pre-IUPAC nomenclature is still used by research groups as well as chemical commercial suppliers, causing confusion (Ludwig et al., 2014).

4.1.1 Chlorogenic Acids in Vegetables, Fruits, Cereals, and Beverages

The concentration of chlorogenic acids in some fruits, vegetables, and beverages are shown in Table 4.1. Many other plants and beverages contain chlorogenic acids such as black chokecherry, thyme, sage, spearmint, spices, basil, aniseed, caraway, rosemary, tarragon, marjoram, savory, sage, dill, absinthe, sunflower seeds, tobacco, spinach, red peppers, plums, ligonberry, coconut, barley, and rye grain as well as

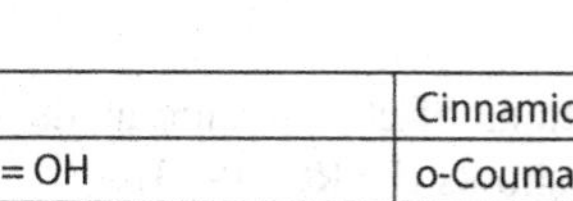

$R_1, R_2, R_3, R_4 = H$	Cinnamic acid
$R_2, R_3, R_4 = H; R_1 = OH$	o-Coumaric acid
$R_1, R_3, R_4 = H; R_2 = OH$	m-Coumaric acid
$R_1, R_2, R_4 = H; R_3 = OH$	p-Coumaric acid
$R_1, R_4 = H; R_2, R_3 = OH$	Caffeic acid
$R_1, R_4 = H; R_2 = OCH_3; R_3 = OH$	Ferulic acid
$R_1, R_4 = H; R_3 = OCH_3; R_2 = OH$	Isoferulic acid
$R_1 = H; R_2, R_4 = OCH_3; R_3 = OH$	Sinapic acid

FIGURE 4.1 Chemical structures of the main hydroxycinnamic acids.

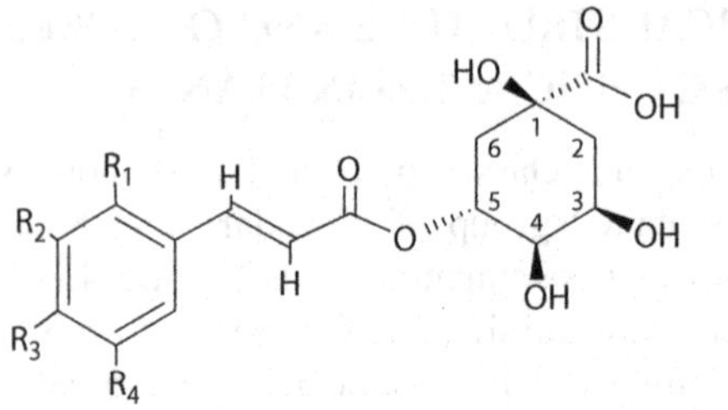

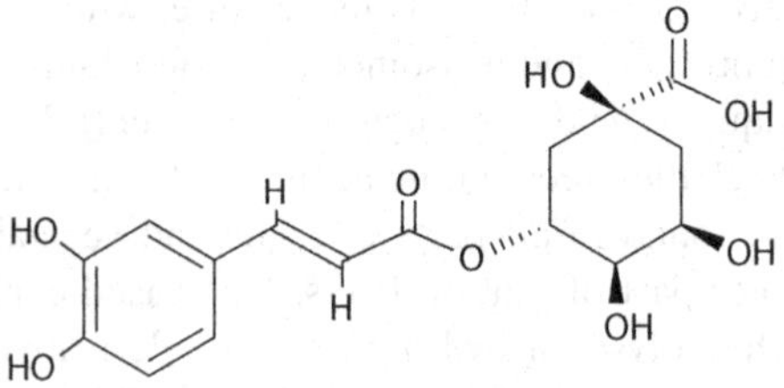

5-Caffeoylquinic acid

5-Caffeoylquinic acid (chlorogenic acid) R_2, R_3 = OH; R_1, R_4 = H
3-Caffeoylquinic acid
4-Caffeoylquinic acid
1,5-Dicaffeoylquinic acid
1,3-Dicaffeoylquinic acid
3,4-Dicaffeoylquinic acid
3,5-Dicaffeoylquinic acid
4,5-Dicaffeoylquinic acid

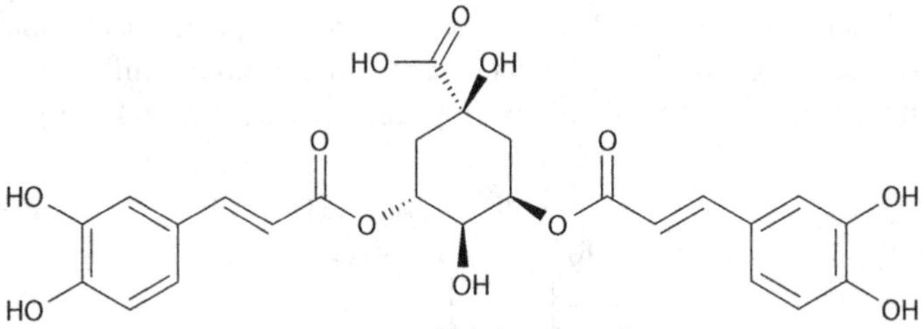

3,5-Dicaffeoylquinic acid

FIGURE 4.2 Chemical structures of esters of hydroxycinnamic acids and quinic acid (chlorogenic acids).

wine. In tea, high concentrations of chlorogenic acids were reported, in the range 5590–6740 mg/kg of dry tea shoots (IARC, 1993).

Chlorogenic acid is present at concentrations ranging from approximately 50–500 mg/kg in apples, pears, peaches, apricots, plums, cherries, Brussels sprouts, kale, cabbage, and broccoli (Ames et al., 1991). The average concentration of caffeic acid–derived products was 2.5 mg/L in 50 samples of commercial white wines. German Riesling wines contained the highest concentration at 4.1 mg/L, Chardonnay wine contains 1.7 mg/L, and Sémilon wine the lowest at 0.9 mg/L. Most hydroxycinnamic acids were found to be in combined form with tartaric acid in wine (Okamura and Watanabe, 1981).

TABLE 4.1
Content of Hydroxycinnamic Acids and Chlorogenic Acid in Plant Food and Beverages

Hydroxycinnamic Acids	Content (mg/100 g Fresh Weight)				
Foods	Chlorogenic Acids	p-Coumaric Acid	Caffeic Acid	Ferulic Acid	Sinapic Acid
Green coffee beans	1158–2741/2300–11000[b]	—	141–33[b]	6–35[b]	—
Roasted coffee beans	1500–3800[b]	—	—	—	—
Coffee drink	96/7–160[a]/8.6–11.0[b]	—	—	9	—
Tea shoots	559–674	—	—	—	—
Tea beverage	0.2	—	—	—	—
Mate	2.8–9.7[b]/5.9–13.9	—	—	—	—
Sweet cherries	3.2–12.0/7.7–48.6	1.0–6.8/1.0–26.6	—	—	—
Sour cherries	0.6–5.8	0.9–4.1	—	—	—
Apricot	3.0–16.5	—	—	—	—
Nectarines	2.3–27.7	—	—	—	—
Orange juice	—	7.9–4.46	—	3.07–6.37[a]	0.78–3.59[a]
Citrus[c]	—	1.8–19.3[b]	—	3.6–158[b]	3.0–95.4[b]
Peaches	2.4–24.2	—	—	—	—
Prunes	41.1–43.6	—	—	—	—
Apples	1.93–119.5	—	—	—	—
Pear	6–59	—	—	—	—
Quince pulp	0.56–18.71	—	—	—	—
Blackberries	—	—	1.38–3.64	2.99–3.51	—
Blueberries	—	2.4–15.8	0–6.32	3.02–16.97	—
Cranberries	—	2.2–25.4	0.38–15.6	0.8–8.8	0–21.18
Tomato	8.5	—	—	—	—
Potato	0.35–18.71	—	3.6	—	—
Sweet potato	4.6–13.6	—	0.3–2.2	—	—
Broccoli	—	130.6 ± 42	—	105.9	—
Eggplant	—	173.3 ± 40	—	93.6	—
Asparagus	—	18.3 ± 16	—	46.1	—
Artichoke heads	389[b] (cynarin)	—	—	—	—
Carrot	—	—	14	1.57	—
Lettuce	—	—	4–55	—	—
Black carrot root	65.7[b]	—	—	—	—
Chicory root	10[b]	—	—	—	—
Beet root	—	—	—	1.3–14.3	—

Source: Adapted from Andrés-Lacueva et al., 2009, Phenolic compounds: Chemistry and occurrence in fruits and vegetables, in *Fruit and Vegetable Phytochemicals: Chemistry, Nutritional Value, and Stability* eds L. A. de la Rosa, E. Alvarez-Parrilla and G. A. González-Aguilar, Wiley-Blackwell, Oxford, 53–88; Willeman et al., 2014, *Scientific World J.*, 2014, 11; Kammerer et al., 2004, *Rapid Commun Mass Spectrom.*, 18(12), 1331–40; Schütz et al., 2004, *J Agric Food Chem.*, 52(13), 4090–6; Ballistreri et al., 2013, *Food Chem.*, 140(4), 630–8; IARC, 1993, *Some Naturally Occurring Substances: Food Items and Constituents, Heterocyclic Aromatic Amines and Mycotoxines*, Geneva: World Health Organization, Vol. 56: Caffeic acid 115–34; Clifford et al., 1990, *Food Chem.*, 35, 13–21; Alonso-Salces et al., 2009, *J Agric Food Chem.*, 57(10), 4224–35; Mills et al., 2013, *Food Chem.*, 141(4), 3335–40; Farah, 2012, Coffee constituents, in *Coffee: Emerging Health Effects and Disease Prevention*, ed., Y.-F. Chu, Wiley, and the Institute of Food Technologists, Wiley-Blackwell, Oxford, 21–58.

[a] Per100 mL.
[b] Per100 g dry weight.
[c] Peel and seeds.

In many studies, the plant content of chlorogenic acid is presented as its aglycones obtained after hydrolysis so that the chlorogenic acid cannot be quantified (Mattila et al., 2006; Wang and Zuo, 2011). In addition, some studies reported concentrations of phenolic acids expressed in milligram per wet or fresh weight (FW) and others in milligram per dry weight (DW), with water losses not evaluated, making a comparison between studies difficult.

4.1.2 Chlorogenic Acids Distribution in Plant, Effects of Cultivars, Maturation, and Fermentation

4.1.2.1 Cultivars and Varieties

The determination of hydroxycinnamic acids performed in 82 orange juices derived from the more popular blood and blond varieties grown in Italy showed that ferulic acid was the major component in all cases, but the distribution of the four acids (ferulic, caffeic, *p*-coumaric, and sinapic) was typical in each variety (Rapisarda et al., 1998).

In several varieties of potato, the chlorogenic acid content ranged from 34 to 140 mg/kg FW (IARC, 1993).

There are large differences in the concentrations of chlorogenic acids among various cultivars. When 17 cultivars of Oriental pear were compared with 5 cultivars of Occidental pear, the mean concentration of chlorogenic acid in the Oriental pear was lower at 0.163 mg/g FW than that found in the Occidental pear at 0.309 mg/g FW (Cui et al., 2005).

In 33 different sour cherry cultivars, the same hydroxycinnamic acid compounds were present in each cultivar, but there were differences in their relative levels. In almost all cultivars, 3-caffeoylquinic acid (47%) was the major hydroxycinnamic acid, followed by 5-caffeoylquinic acid (30%) and *p*-coumaroylquinic acid (19%), with smaller amounts of 3,5-dicaffeoylquinic acid (4%) present (Wojdyło et al., 2014).

4.1.2.2 Plant Parts

There are large differences in the concentrations of chlorogenic acids between the peel, leaves, and the fruit pulp or tuber. In sweet potatoes, chlorogenic acid has its highest concentrations in the leaves (126–143 mg/100 g FW), then the peel (27–42 mg/100 g FW), and the lowest concentrations in the root tissues (5–9 mg/100 g FW), while 3,5-, 4,5-, and 3,4-dicaffeoylquinic acids were predominant in the leaves (305 mg/100 g FW) when compared with the root (40 mg/100 g FW) and peel (60 mg/100 g FW) (Truong et al., 2007).

Because of the industrial interest in these phenolic compounds, it has been suggested to valorize citrus peels and seeds, which are a by-product of the juice extraction industry, by the extraction of these natural antioxidants (Bocco et al., 1998).

In potato plants, chlorogenic acid and its isomers contribute more than 95% to the total phenolic acid content. Concentrations expressed in g/100 g FW in the peels of five potato varieties grown in Korea ranged from 6.5 to 42.1 compared with that of the flesh (pulp) from 0.5 to 16.5, with peel/pulp ratios ranging from 2.6 to 21.1 (Im et al., 2008).

4.1.2.3 Maturation/Ripening

The concentration of chlorogenic acid in Yali pears was highest in young fruit at 3.72 mg/g FW, and then swiftly declined with fruit growth to less than 0.226 mg/g FW in mature fruit (Cui et al., 2005).

It has been demonstrated that enzymatic browning of peach and nectarine skin tissue depends on the presence of polyphenol oxidase activity and chlorogenic acids, which are major contributors to enzymatic browning. In these fruits, only chlorogenic acids had a significant positive correlation with browning potential (Cheng and Crisosto, 1995).

In 15 Mate teas, sun-exposed (plantation grown) Mate teas exhibited higher levels of all polyphenols as compared with shaded (forest grown) Mate teas (Heck et al., 2008).

4.1.2.4 Process

Chlorogenic acid concentrations were 890 mg/kg FW in mature apples, and the juice produced concentrations of 120–310 mg/L (IARC, 1993). Apple juice contains 0–10 mg/L caffeic acid (Kusnawidjaja et al., 1969) and 20–60 mg/L chlorogenic acid, but higher levels of up to 200 mg/L were found, especially in fermented juice (Kusnawidjaja et al., 1969; Brause and Raterman, 1982; Ciliers et al., 1990).

Chlorogenic acid, which constitutes up to 90% of the total phenolic content in potato tubers, was studied during processing: storage, dry lyophilization into powder, steam cooking, frying, boiling, and microwaving, showing that up to 50% and even 75% of the initial concentration can be lost (Tudela et al., 2002; Truong et al., 2007).

4.1.3 Caffeic Acid

Caffeic acid, both free and esterified, is generally the most abundant phenolic acid and represents between 75% and 100% of the total hydroxycinnamic acid content in fruit (Manach et al., 2004).

Caffeic acid is the most abundant hydroxycinnamic acid occurring in berries, fruits, and coffee. This globally consumed beverage provides a significantly high daily phenolic intake, thus making it a primary dietary polyphenol, the daily intake of which may reach 1 g in coffee drinkers (El-Seedi et al., 2012).

4.1.4 Ferulic Acid

Cereal grains provide the main dietary intake of ferulic acid. The ferulic acid content of wheat grain is 0.8–2 g/kg DW, corresponding to up to 90% of total polyphenols (Sosulski et al., 1982; Lempereur, 1997). Ferulic acid is found in the outer parts of the grain, the aleurone layer, and the pericarp of wheat grain contains 98% of the total ferulic acid, suggesting that ferulic acid content is directly related to levels of sieving, with bran being the main source of polyphenols (Hatcher and Kruger, 1997). Similar amounts of phenolic acids are found in rice, oat, and wheat flours (63 mg/kg) but a threefold higher level was reported in maize flour. Several dimers of ferulic acid are also found in cereals and form bridge structures between chains of hemicellulose (Manach et al., 2004). Recent studies have shown the suppression of hydroxycinnamate network formation in the cell walls of rice shoots grown under microgravity conditions in space (Wakabayashi et al., 2015). Postharvest toughening of asparagus spears is associated with the formation of pectic–xylan–phenolic complexes as shown by a large increase in monomeric and diferulic acids attached to the xylan component in the cell walls of stem tissues (Rodríguez-Arcos et al., 2004).

4.1.5 Caffeic Acid Derivatives

In addition to chlorogenic acid and 3,5-di-*O*-caffeoylquinic acid, tests conducted on vegetables including five varieties of lettuce and one variety of escarole identified other caffeic acid derivatives including *O*-caffeoylmalic acid, di-*O*-caffeoyltartaric acid, *O*-caffeoyltartaric acid, and *meso*-di-*O*-caffeoyltartaric acid (Llorach, 2008). In glycosylated kaempferol derivatives from cabbage leaves, caffeic and ferulic acids derivatives were identified including: the diacyl derivatives kaempferol 3-*O*-(methoxycaffeoyl/caffeoyl)sophoroside-7-*O*-glucoside, kaempferol 3-*O*-(sinapoyl/caffeoyl)sophoroside-7-*O*-glucoside, and kaempferol 3-*O*-(feruloyl/caffeoyl)sophoroside-7-*O*-glucoside, and the monoacylated derivatives kaempferol 3-*O*-(sinapoyl)-sophoroside, kaempferol 3-*O*-(feruloyl)sophorotrioside, and kaempferol 3-*O*-(feruloyl)sophoroside (Ferreres et al., 2005).

4.1.6 Dietary Intake of Phenolic Acids

The absolute intake of the polyphenols and the corresponding food sources were calculated on the basis of 48 h dietary recalls of 2007 Finnish adults: 1095 women and 912 men. The mean total intake of polyphenols was 863 mg/day with the phenolic acids corresponding to 75% of this intake or 647 mg/day. Coffee was the best source of phenolic acids and represented 67.9% of total phenolic acids intake from the diet of Finnish adults, followed by bread and cereals (12.3%), tea (9.7%), fruits (2.2%), and vegetables (2.1%). Caffeic acid intake in women and men was 359 ± 271 and 487 ± 368 mg/day, respectively ferulic acid was 103 ± 47 and 139 ± 67 mg/day, *p*-coumaric acid was 15 ± 6.5 and 17 ± 8.5 mg/day, and sinapic acid was 10 ± 5.3 and 12 ± 7.6 mg/day. Significantly higher dietary intakes of phenolic acids were observed in men (Ovaskainen et al., 2008).

In FINDIET 2002, from the Finnish food composition database, 86% of women and 91% of men consumed coffee with a mean intake of 450 and 600 mL/day, respectively (Fineli, 2007).

Previously, a survey performed in Germany estimated the daily intake of phenolic acids at 222 mg, which was lower than the Finnish intake (Radtke et al., 1998). Another study included participants in the Polish arm of the HAPIEE (Health, Alcohol and Psychosocial factors In Eastern Europe) cohort with a total of 10,477 participants (45–69 years) of an urban population of Krakow, Poland, who were available for the final analyses. The mean intake of phenolic acids was 800 mg/day, and the individual compounds with the highest intake were isomers of chlorogenic acid (5- and 4-caffeoylquinic acid) among hydroxycinnamic acids with an average intake of 150 mg/day, which largely originated from coffee (Grosso et al., 2014).

4.2 CHLOROGENIC ACIDS IN COFFEE BEANS AND COFFEE BEVERAGE

The chemical composition of the two main commercial species of coffee, *Coffea arabica* L., 1753 and *Coffea canephora* Pierre ex Froehner, 1897 show both quantitative and qualitative differences. The two main varieties of *Coffea canephora* are *Coffea robusta* and *Coffea nganda.*

4.2.1 Green Coffee Beans

5-Caffeoylquinic acid (chlorogenic acid) content, which amounts to 2% DM and 3-caffeoylquinic acid at 1% DM, are quantitatively the most important in green coffee beans. Other phenolic acids such as 4-caffeoylquinic correspond to 0.2% DM, and the three isomers 3,4-, 3,5-, and 4,5-dicaffeoyl to 0.11% DM, while feruloylquinic acids as well as free acids moieties, caffeic, ferulic, and quinic acids are also present (Clifford, 1985; Arnaud, 1992).

4.2.1.1 Robusta and Arabica

Green beans of *C. robusta* contain more chlorogenic acid at 10% DM than *C. arabica* L. at 6.5% DM. Quinic acid content is similar between *C. robusta* and *C. arabica* at 0.4% DM (Clark, 1987; IARC, 1991).

More than 45 chlorogenic acids have been reported in *Arabica* and 85 in *Robusta* green coffee beans, and this number increases with roasting (Table 4.2). In green *Robusta* coffee beans, the acids are characterized as 3,4-di-*p*-coumaroylquinic acid, 3,5-di-*p*-coumaroylquinic acid, and 4,5-di-*p*-coumaroylquinic acid; 3-*p*-coumaroyl-4-caffeoylquinic acid, 3-*p*-coumaroyl-5-caffeoylquinic acid, 4-*p*-coumaroyl-5-caffeoylquinic acid, 3-caffeoyl-4-*p*-coumaroyl-quinic acid, 3-caffeoyl-5-*p*-coumaroyl-quinic acid, and 4-caffeoyl-5-*p*-coumaroyl-quinic acid; 3-p-coumaroyl-4-feruloylquinic acid, 3-*p*-coumaroyl-5-feruloylquinic acid, and 4-*p*-coumaroyl-5-feruloylquinic acid; 4-dimethoxycinnamoyl-5-*p*-coumaroylquinic acid; three isomeric dimethoxycinnamoylquinic acids, three caffeoyl-dimethoxycinnamoylquinic acids, three diferuloylquinic acids, and three feruloyl-dimethoxycinnamoylquinic acids (Clifford et al., 2006a,b).

Genotype is shown to be a determinant characteristic in the bioactive compound content of total chlorogenic acid: 22.9–37.9 g/100 g of green coffee extract, with *C. canephora* (34.5 g/100 g) and *C. kapakata* (33.4 g/100 g) having 30% higher chlorogenic acid contents when compared with *C. arabica* (24 g/100 g) and *C. racemosa* (24.7 g/100 g). There were also significant differences in the distribution of various chlorogenic acid isomers: total caffeoylquinic acid (3-, 4-, and 5-caffeoylquinic acid), total feruoylquinic acid (3-, 4-, and 5-feruoylquinic acid), total *p*-coumaroylquinic acid (3-, 4-, and 5-*p*-coumaroylquinic acid), total dicaffeoylquinic acid (3,4-, 3,5-, and 4,5-caffeoylquinic acid), and

TABLE 4.2
Chlorogenic Acids and Phenolic Compounds Identified in Green and Roasted Coffee Beans

Phenolic acids	
Caffeic acid	3-*O*-Feruloyl-4-*O*-caffeoylquinic acid
Caffeoylhexose	3-*O*-Caffeoyl-4-*O*-feruloylquinic acid
Caffeoyl-*N*-phenylalanine	3-*O*-Feruloyl-5-*O*-caffeoylquinic acid
Caffeoyl-*N*-tryptophan	3-*O*-Caffeoyl-5-*O*-feruloylquinic acid
Caffeoyl-*N*-tyrosine	4-*O*-Feruloyl-5-*O*-caffeoylquinic acid
p-Coumaroyl-*N*-tyrosine	4-*O*-Caffeoyl-5-*O*-feruloylquinic acid
p-Coumaroyl-*N*-tryptophan	3-*O*-Dimethoxycinnamoyl-4-*O*-caffeoylquinic acid
Feruloyl-*N*-tryptophan	3-*O*-Dimethoxycinnamoyl-5-*O*-caffeoylquinic acid
Feruloyl-*N*-tyrosine	4-*O*-Dimethoxycinnamoyl-5-*O*-caffeoylquinic acid
Dicaffeoylhexose	3-*O*-Caffeoyl-4-*O*-dimethoxycinnamoylquinic acid
Ferulic acid	3-*O*-Caffeoyl-5-*O*-dimethoxycinnamoylquinic acid
Feruloyl-*N*-tryptophan	4-*O*-Caffeoyl-5-*O*-dimethoxycinnamoylquinic acid
1-*O*-Caffeoylquinic acid	3-*O*-Dimethoxycinnamoyl-4-*O*-feruloylquinic acid
1-*O*-Feruloylquinic acid	3-*O*-Dimethoxycinnamoyl-5-*O*-feruloylquinic acid
1-*O*-p-Coumaroylquinic acid	4-*O*-Dimethoxycinnamoyl-5-*O*-feruloylquinic acid
1-*O*-Dimethoxycinnamoylquinic acid	3-*O*-*p*-Coumaroyl-4-*O*-caffeoylquinic acid
1,3-di-*O*-Caffeoylquinic acid	3-*O*-Caffeoyl-4-*O*-*p*-coumaroylquinic acid
1,4-di-*O*-Caffeoylquinic acid	3-*O*-*p*-Coumaroyl-5-*O*-caffeoylquinic acid
1,5-di-*O*-Caffeoylquinic acid	3-*O*-Caffeoyl-5-*O*-*p*-coumaroylquinic acid
1-*O*-Caffeoyl-3-O-feruloylquinic acid	4-*O*-Caffeoyl-5-*O*-*p*-coumaroylquinic acid
1-*O*-Caffeoyl-4-O-feruloylquinic acid	4-*O*-*p*-Coumaroyl-5-*O*-caffeoylquinic acid
3-*O*-Caffeoylquinic acid	3-*O*-*p*-Coumaroyl-4-*O*-feruloylquinic acid
4-*O*-Caffeoylquinic acid	3-*O*-*p*-Coumaroyl-5-*O*-feruloylquinic acid
5-*O*-Caffeoylquinic acid	4-*O*-*p*-Coumaroyl-5-*O*-feruloylquinic acid
3-*O*-Feruloylquinic acid	4-*O*-Dimethoxycinnamoyl-5-*O*-*p*-coumarolyquinic acid
4-*O*-Feruloylquinic acid	3-*O*-*p*-Coumaroyl-4-*O*-dimethoxycinnamoylquinic acid
5-*O*-Feruloylquinic acid	3-*O*-*p*-Coumaroyl-5-*O*-dimethoxycinnamoylquinic acid
3-*O*-*p*-Coumaroylquinic acid	3-*O*-Caffeoyl-4-O-sinapoylquinic acid
4-*O*-*p*-Coumaroylquinic acid	4-*O*-Feruloyl-5-O-dimethoxycinnamolyquinic acid
5-*O*-*p*-Coumaroylquinic acid	1-*O*-Caffeoyl-4-O-dimethoxycinnamolyquinic acid
p-Coumaroyl-N-tryptophan	1-*O*-Caffeoyl-3-O-sinapoylquinic acid
3-*O*-Dimethoxycinnamoylquinic acid	1-*O*-Caffeoyl-4-O-sinapoylquinic acid
4-*O*-Dimethoxycinnamoylquinic acid	1-*O*-Feruloyl-3-O-sinapoylquinic acid
5-*O*-Dimethoxycinnamoylquinic acid	1-*O*-Caffeoyl-3-O-trimethoxycinnamolyquinic acid
5-*O*-Dimethoxycinnamoylhexose	3-*O*-Sinapoyl-5-*O*-caffeoylquinic acid
3,4-Di-*O*-caffeoylquinic acid	3-*O*-Sinapoyl-4-*O*-caffeoylquinic acid
3,5-Di-*O*-caffeoylquinic acid	4-*O*-Sinapoyl-3-*O*-caffeoylquinic acid
4,5-Di-*O*-caffeoylquinic acid	3-*O*-(3,5-dihydroxy-4-methoxy)cinnamoyl-4-*O*-feruloylquinic acid
3,4-Di-*O*-feruloylquinic acid	3-*O*-Sinapoyl-5-*O*-feruloylquinic acid
3,5-Di-*O*-feruloylquinic acid	3-*O*-Feruloyl-4-*O*-sinapoylquinic acid
4,5-Di-*O*-feruloylquinic acid	4-*O*-Sinapoyl-5-*O*-feruloylquinic acid

TABLE 4.2 (CONTINUED)
Chlorogenic Acids and Phenolic Compounds Identified in Green and Roasted Coffee Beans

Phenolic acids	
3-*O*-Sinapoylquinic acid	4-*O*-Trimethoxycinnamoyl-5-*O*-caffeoylquinic acid
4-*O*-Sinapoylquinic acid	3-*O*-Trimethoxycinnamoyl-5-*O*-caffeoylquinic acid
5-*O*-Sinapoylquinic acid	5-*O*-Feruloyl-3-*O*-trimethoxycinnamoylquinic acid
3,4-Di-*O*-*p*-Coumaroylquinic acid	3-*O*-Trimethoxycinnamoyl-4-*O*-feruloylquinic acid
3,5-Di-*O*-*p*-Coumaroylquinic acid	4-*O*-Trimethoxycinnamoyl-5-*O*-feruloylquinic acid
4,5-Di-O-*p*-Coumaroylquinic acid	3-*O*-Trimethoxycinnamoyl-5-*O*-feruloylquinic acid

Source: Adapted from Clifford et al., 2004, *Food Chem.*, 87, 457–463; Farah et al., 2005, *J Agric Food Chem.*, 53(5), 1505–13; Clifford et al., 2006a, *J Agric Food Chem.*, 54(6), 1957–69; Clifford et al., 2006b, *J Agric Food Chem.*, 54(12), 4095–101; Stalmach et al., 2009, *Drug Metab Dispos.*, 37(8), 1749–58; Alonso-Salces et al., 2009, *J Agric Food Chem.*, 57(10), 4224–35; Jaiswal et al., 2010, *J Agric Food Chem.*, 58(15), 8722–37; Del Rio et al., 2010, *Nutrients.*, 2(8), 820–33; Kuhnert et al., 2011, *Anal. Methods* 3, 144–55; Jaiswal 2011, Synthesis and analysis of the dietary relevant isomers of chlorogenic acids, their derivatives and hydroxycinnamates, PhD Thesis, Jacobs University, School of Engineering and Science, Germany; Rodrigues et al., 2015, *J Agric Food Chem.*, 63(19), 4815–26.

total caffeoylferuloylquinic acid (3-caffeoyl,4-feruoylquinic acid, 3-caffeoyl,5-feruoylquinic acid, 4-feruoylquinic acid,5-caffeoyl quinic acid, and 4-caffeoyl,5-feruoylquinic acid) represented, on average, 79%, 6.7%, 1.3%, 12%, and 0.4% of the total chlorogenic acid contents of the *C. arabica* extracts, whereas they represented, on average, 64%, 17%, 0.4%, 14%, and 3.6% of the *C. canephora* extracts (Rodrigues et al., 2015).

4.2.1.2 Botanical and Geographical Characterization

Several attempts have been made to develop analytical procedures for the botanical characterization of green coffee beans. The analysis of caffeic acid, 3-feruloylquinic acid, 5-feruloylquinic acid, 4-feruloylquinic acid, 3,4-dicaffeoylquinic acid, 3-caffeoyl-5-feruloylquinic acid, 3-caffeoyl-4-feruloylquinic acid, 3-*p*-coumaroyl-4-caffeoylquinic acid, 3-caffeoyl-4-dimethoxycinnamoylquinic acid, 3-caffeoyl-5-dimethoxycinnamoylquinic acid, *p*-coumaroyl-*N*-tryptophan, feruloyl-*N*-tryptophan, caffeoyl-*N*-tryptophan, and caffeine enabled the unequivocal botanical characterization of green coffee beans. Some free phenolic acids and cinnamate conjugates of green coffee beans showed great potential as a means for the geographical characterization of coffee, such as *C. robusta* green coffee beans from Uganda, Cameroon, Vietnam, and Indonesia (Alonso-Salces et al., 2009). However, chlorogenic acid content including caffeoylquinic acid, feruloylquinic acid, and dicaffeoylquinic acid, in economically important Brazilian cultivars of *C. arabica*, did not vary significantly across four or five crops, but varied in different years (Monteiro and Farah, 2012).

4.2.1.3 Maturation/Ripening

As shown previously for fruits, changes occur in coffee beans during maturation. It is reported that the chlorogenic acid content in unprocessed coffee beans decreases with the maturation of the coffee fruit, and that there is a difference between the ripe and fully ripe fruit. In the identification of chemical markers differentiating between degrees of ripeness, the different degrees of ripeness can be attributed to an increase in 3-caffeoylquinic acid and a decrease in 5-caffeoylquinic acid and dicaffeoylquinic acids (Smrke et al., 2015).

4.2.2 Decaffeination Process

Caffeine extraction may result in losses of other compounds such as chlorogenic acids and consequently their 1,5-γ-quinolactones in roasted coffee. Decaffeination produced a 16% average increase in the levels of total chlorogenic acids in green coffee (DM), along with a 237% increase in 1,5-γ-quinolactones. Chlorogenic acids levels in roasted coffee were 3%–9% lower in decaffeinated coffee compared with regular coffee. The study concluded that these differences in chlorogenic acids and 1,5-γ-quinolactones contents of regular and decaffeinated roasted coffees appear to be relatively small (Farah et al., 2006).

4.2.3 Roasted Coffee Beans

As a result of the high temperature of roasting, the hydrolysis of chlorogenic acids releases quinic acid that is transformed into quinic acid lactone. Other transformations during the roasting process are dehydration, lactonization, acyl migration, trans-cis-isomerization, and epimerization.

4.2.3.1 Effects of Temperature and Time

Chlorogenic acids content is altered by roasting as moisture is reduced by heating and chemical transformations occur with the formation of volatile substances and polymeric pigments corresponding to weight losses ranging from 13% to 20%. Expressed as percentage DM, chlorogenic acid content in roasted coffee beans was 3.1% for *C. robusta* and 2.7% for *C. arabica.* The feruloylquinic and dicaffeoylquinic acids content in roasted beans are also higher in *robusta* than in *arabica* coffee beans (Spiller, 1984).

Due to light, medium, and dark roasting, chlorogenic acids content decreases by 2.5-, 3.5-, and 40-fold, respectively, and in some conditions as much as 90% of chlorogenic acid is destroyed. The percentage of chlorogenic acid content of roasted coffee ranges from 0.2% to 3.8% with lower values found in dark roasted samples (Viani, 1988).

New studies confirm these observations with a direct comparison of green and roasted beans. The total chlorogenic acids of nine isomers from seven commercial green and roasted coffee beans ranged from 34.43 ± 1.50 to 41.64 ± 3.28 mg/g and from 2.05 ± 0.07 to 7.07 ± 0.16 mg/g, respectively. The total chlorogenic acids present was reduced in accordance with the intensity of the roasting conditions. When green beans were roasted at 230°C for 12 min and at 250°C for 21 min, total chlorogenic acid content was reduced to nearly 50% and to almost trace levels, respectively (Moon et al., 2009).

Robusta coffee beans roasted for various lengths of time and at various temperatures were analyzed for total phenolic acid and chlorogenic acid content. The amount of total phenolics decreased linearly over the roasting temperature from 63.51 ± 0.77 mg chlorogenic acid equivalent/gram of coffee beans (roasted at 200°C) to 42.56 ± 0.33 mg/g coffee beans (roasted at 240°C). The total chlorogenic acid content decreased when the roasting time was increased from 78.33 ± 1.41 to 4.31 ± 0.23 mg/g (roasted for 16 min at 250°C) (Sulaiman et al., 2011).

4.2.3.2 Chemical Changes

With the reduction in moisture during roasting, quinic acid content increases from 1.3% in green beans to a maximum of 3.5% on roasting (Spiller, 1984). In commercial coffee extracts, concentrations of 20–50 g/kg quinic acid were determined. The losses of chlorogenic acids during roasting were confirmed by the release of both quinic and caffeic acid (Arnaud, 1988, 1993; IARC, 1991).

Quantitative analysis of caffeoylquinic acids in a large set of 113 roasted *arabica* and 38 *robusta* coffees revealed that the concentrations of caffeoylquinic acids significantly correlated with the roasting color. Light roasted coffees were rich in caffeoylquinic acids, and during coffee brewing caffeoylquinic acids was nearly quantitatively extracted in the brew (Lang et al., 2013a).

Caffeoylquinic acid lactones and feruloylquinic acid lactones, produced during roasting, can also occur in coffee in significant amounts. Seven chlorogenic acid lactones were identified: 3-caffeoylquinic-1,5-lactone, 4-caffeoylquinic-1,5-lactone, 3-coumaroylquinic-1,5-lactone, 4-coumaroylquinic-1,5-lactone, 3-feruloylquinic-1,5-lactone, 4-feruloylquinic-1,5-lactone, and 3,4-dicaffeoylquinic-1,5-lactone. 3-Caffeoylquinic-1,5-lactone was the most abundant lactone in *C. arabica* and *C. canephora*, reaching peak values of 230 ± 9 and 254 ± 4 mg/100 g DW, respectively (Farah et al., 2005).

It was shown for the first time, by comparison with authentic reference standards obtained by chemical synthesis, that chlorogenic acids follow four distinct reaction pathways, during roasting, including epimerization, acyl migration, lactonization, and dehydration. In addition, two new classes of compounds are formed from chlorogenic acids during roasting. Chlorogenic acid acetates, O-phenolic quinoyl, and shikimoyl esters of chlorogenic acids were identified. Following roasting, around 50% of the original chlorogenic acid content of the green coffee bean is lost (Jaiswal et al., 2012).

Acyl migration was shown to be an important reaction pathway in both coffee roasting and brewing, altering the structure of chlorogenic acid initially present in the green coffee bean. This evidence for transesterification phenomena was demonstrated indirectly by the presence of a series of 1-substituted CGA derivatives in roasted coffee, which are absent in the green bean. In dry roasting conditions, acyl migration competes with dehydration to form 3-caffeoylquinic acid lactone (Deshpande et al., 2014).

The chemical characterization of purified melanoidin populations has provided increasing evidence that polysaccharides, proteins, and chlorogenic acids are involved in the formation of coffee melanoidins. When a mixture of chlorogenic acid from green coffee beans and (α1 → 5)-L-arabinotriose was submitted to dry thermal processing, this treatment promoted the formation of several hybrid compounds composed of one or two chlorogenic acids covalently linked with a variable number of pentose residues as well as other compounds bearing a sugar moiety but composed exclusively of the quinic or caffeic acid moiety of chlorogenic acids. These results highlight the structural complexity of compounds that can be formed between chlorogenic acids and carbohydrates during coffee roasting (Moreira et al., 2015).

4.2.4 Coffee Beverages

While the total content of chlorogenic acid isomers expressed as the percentage of dry matter in roasted coffee samples ranges from 0.2% to 4%, in dry instant coffee this content increases up to 4%–10% (Trugo and Macrae, 1984).

Coffee drinking was shown to be a significant dietary source of phenolic acids in human intake. It was estimated that a cup of brewed coffee prepared with 10 g of roasted and ground coffee at 85% recovery provides between 15 and 325 mg chlorogenic acids (Maier and Grimsehl, 1982; Clifford, 1999). Actual data from the USA give an average of 190 mg total chlorogenic acids per cup of brewed coffee (Clinton, 1985). Coffee drinkers consume particularly high amounts of chlorogenic acids, up to 1 g or more per day (Clifford, 1999).

5-Caffeoylquinic acid was present at the highest levels, between 25% and 30% of total chlorogenic acids in ground and instant coffees. The intake of the other isomers in increasing quantities was: 4-caffeoylquinic acid > 3-caffeoylquinic acid > 5-feruoylquinic acid > 4-feruoylquinic acid > dicaffeoylquinic acid (sum of 3,4-, 3,5-, and 4,5-dicaffeoylquinic acid) (Mills et al., 2013).

Unextracted phenolic acids are detected in spent coffee grounds after brewing. Spent coffee extract showed a lower content of free chlorogenic acids than the coffee brew, whereas the concentration of free dicaffeoylquinic acids was 1.8-fold higher in the spent coffee. Spent coffee had a twofold higher content of total phenolics in comparison with free compounds. Approximately 54% of the phenolic acids detected with one or more caffeic acid is linked to macromolecules such as melanoidins, mainly by noncovalent interactions. The rest of the quantitated phenolic acids were mainly attached to other structures by covalent bonds (Monente et al., 2015a).

4.3 METABOLISM OF CHLOROGENIC ACIDS IN ANIMAL AND HUMANS

4.3.1 *In Vitro* Studies

4.3.1.1 Absorption

Mucosal uptake of radioactively labeled cinnamic acid as a model substance in the rat jejunum using an *in vitro* mucosal uptake technique, indicates the existence of a Na(+)-dependent saturable transport mechanism for the uptake of cinnamic acid across the jejunal brush border membrane. Na+ appears to directly stimulate mucosal cinnamate uptake, most likely by Na+ cinnamate cotransport. Absorption is increased by the lower pH of the incubation medium and is influenced by intracellular HCO_3- and/or pH (Wolffram et al., 1995). In another study, the transport kinetics of the mucosal uptake of labeled cinnamic acid was determined under various conditions using a short-term mucosal uptake technique. In addition, the transfer of cinnamic acid across the jejunal wall was investigated using everted intestinal sacs. It was shown that the kinetics of cinnamic acid uptake by the mid-jejunal mucosa had two transport components, a diffusive Na(+)-independent mechanism and a saturable Na(+)-dependent mechanism. With everted sacs, further evidence of the existence of an active Na+ gradient–driven transport of cinnamic acid across the intestinal epithelium was demonstrated. A significant accumulation of cinnamate inside the serosal compartment in the presence of Na+ was observed, which was strongly inhibited by serosal ouabain. A decrease in extracellular pH stimulated mucosal cinnamate uptake by increasing the apparent affinity. The kinetics of cinnamate transport in the absence or presence of a surplus of either unlabeled cinnamate or unlabeled butyrate indicate a reduction in the apparent affinity of the Na(+)-dependent mechanism involved in cinnamate uptake. These results may be explained not only by a modification of the mechanism by the intracellular pH but also by a competitive inhibition of cinnamate uptake by substances structurally related to cinnamic acid (Ader et al., 1996).

A study investigated the absorption and metabolism of hydroxycinnamates in the gastrointestinal tract by using an isolated preparation of jejunum and ileum from the small intestine and monitoring unchanged compound, conjugates, and metabolites. The absorption of the hydroxycinnamates through the ileum was much lower than that observed through the jejunum. Over the 90 min perfusion, the absorption of ferulic acid through the ileum was 10-fold lower than through the jejunum. After perfusion with caffeic acid, two glucuronides were detected in the serosal fluid. The levels of glucuronide detected were approximately twofold higher than caffeic acid. Significant amounts of ferulic acid glucuronide were observed; however, these were low compared with the amount of the ferulic acid itself. In contrast to the other hydroxycinnamates, no glucuronide of chlorogenic acid was observed at any time point (Spencer et al., 1999).

Esterase activity toward diferulate esters was observed in cell-free extracts from human and rat small intestine mucosa. In conclusion, esterified diferulates can be released from cereal brans by intestinal enzymes, and free diferulic acids can be absorbed and enter the circulatory system (Andreasen et al., 2001a). Wheat and rye brans are rich sources of the hydroxycinnamates ferulic acid, sinapic acid, and p-coumaric acid, which are esters linked to the main polymers in the plant cell wall and cannot be absorbed in this complex form. However, esterases with activity toward these esters are distributed throughout the intestinal tract of mammals. In rats, the cinnamoyl esterase activity in the small intestine is derived mainly from the mucosa, whereas in the large intestine the esterase activity was found predominantly in the luminal microflora. In human, mucosa cell-free extracts obtained from the duodenum, jejunum, and ileum efficiently hydrolyzed various hydroxycinnamoyl esters, providing evidence of human cinnamoyl esterase(s). Hydrolysis by intestinal esterases may be the major route for release of hydroxycinnamic acids *in vivo* (Andreasen et al., 2001b).

Using an *in vitro* guinea pig stomach cell model, with an acidic apical pH, the relative permeability coefficients and metabolic fate of a series of chlorogenic acids were investigated. The results showed intact absorption by passive diffusion of feruloylquinic acids and caffeoylquinic acid lactones across the gastric epithelium. It was suggested that a potential carrier-mediated component may be involved in the uptake of certain 4-acyl of chlorogenic acid isomers. For another compound, di-*O*-caffeoylquinic acids, the absorption was rapid but nonlinear. Methylation occurs in gastric mucosa, and isoferulic acid, dimethoxycinnamic acid, and ferulic acid were identified as novel gastric metabolites of chlorogenic acid biotransformation (Farrell et al., 2011).

In a recent publication, the authors point out that in 2014 no data on structure–absorption relationships for chlorogenic acids have been published, despite this being the most consumed group of polyphenols in the Western diet. Using *ex vivo* absorption experiments with pig jejunal mucosa and the Ussing chamber model, caffeoylquinic acid, feruloylquinic acid, caffeic acid, dicaffeoylquinic acid, and D-(–)-quinic acid, were incubated in individual experiments to study the relationship between the structure/dose of chlorogenic acids and their absorption from the mucosal to the serosal side of pig mucosa. Some interesterification reactions were observed in the mucosal compartment and a metabolite, 5-caffeoylquinic acid glucuronide, was identified in the serosal compartment. Secretion occurred at a significantly higher rate than absorption and the percentages of chlorogenic acids that were absorbed were, in increasing order: trace of dicaffeoylquinic acid, ~1% caffeoylquinic acid, ~1.5% caffeic acid, ~2% feruloylquinic acid, and ~4% quinic acid. Although these absorption values are very low, they suggest a passive diffusion and an active efflux for 5-caffeoylquinic acid, while the ABC-efflux transporter MDR 1 and the P-gp transporter MRP 2 were identified in pig jejunal mucosa by Western blot analysis for the first time (Erk et al., 2014a). Using the same experimental model on the gastrointestinal absorption and metabolism of apple polyphenols, it was found that 1.9% 5-caffeoylquinic acid and 3.7% caffeic acid were absorbed and translocated to the basolateral side (Deußer et al., 2013).

4.3.1.2 Cellular Absorption and Metabolism

Spent coffee grounds are a potential commercial source of substantial amounts of chlorogenic acids. Bioavailability and metabolism was studied using an *in vitro* Caco-2 model of human small intestinal epithelium. During this *in vitro* digestion, lactones were partially degraded while caffeoylquinic and feruloylquinic acids were much more stable. Only 1% of the total chlorogenic acids was absorbed and transported from the apical to the basolateral side of a Caco-2 cell monolayer after 1 h. Compounds with the highest basolateral recovery were ferulic acid and dihydroferulic acid, accounting for 5.9% and 5.3% of the apical dose, respectively, indicating a higher absorption and basolateral transport than caffeic and dihydrocaffeic acids (<0.1% of the apical dose), 5-caffeoylquinic acid (0.3%), and 4,5-dicaffeoylquinic acid (0.5%). Metabolic activity was observed through isomerization of 5-caffeoylquinic acid and 4,5-dicaffeoylquinic acid, hydrolysis of chlorogenic acids and dicaffeoylquinic acid releasing caffeic acid, sulfation of caffeic acid and ferulic acid, methylation of caffeic acid yielding ferulic acid, and conversion of ferulic acid to dihydroferulic acid (Monente et al., 2015b).

Some phenolic acids appear in the blood rapidly after coffee consumption due to absorption in the small intestine. This rapid absorption could potentially be derived from free phenolic acids in instant coffee or from hydrolysis of chlorogenic acids by pancreatic or brush border enzymes. However, pharmacokinetic simulation suggests that the free phenolic acids are not sufficient to make a significant contribution to the plasma phenolic acids, even if 100% absorption is assumed. Pancreatic secretions and preparations of Caco-2 cells monolayers were used to investigate the hydrolysis of individual caffeoylquinic acids and chlorogenic acids, present in coffee. Hydrolysis of chlorogenic acids was observed with human-differentiated Caco-2 cell monolayers and with porcine pancreatin with maximal rates on 3- and 5-O-caffeoylquinic acids, respectively. The hydrolysis of chlorogenic acids into free phenolic acids is a major contributing mechanism to the early appearance of free phenolic acids in plasma (da Encarnação et al., 2015).

4.3.1.3 Microsomal and Hepatic Metabolism

Using rat microsomes, caffeic, dihydrocaffeic, and chlorogenic acid were found to be substrates for the nicotinamide adenine dinucleotide phosphate (NADPH)-supported microsomal cytochrome P450 system and resulted in *o*- and *p*-quinones, which were readily conjugated with glutathione (GSH) or formed hydroxylated adducts. They were metabolically activated by cytochrome P450 peroxygenase activity to form cytotoxic quinoid metabolites (Moridani et al., 2001). The incubation of caffeic, dihydrocaffeic, and chlorogenic acids with hepatocytes shows their metabolism by cytochrome P450, catechol-*O*-methyltransferase, and β-oxidation enzymes. Ferulic or dihydroferulic acids, formed as a result of caffeic or dihydrocaffeic-*O*-methylation by catechol-*O*-methyltransferase, were also *O*-demethylated by CYP1A1/2. Side chain dehydrogenation was also observed on dihydrocaffeic or dihydroferulic acid to form caffeic and ferulic acid, which was prevented by thioglycolic acid, an inhibitor of the β-oxidation enzyme acyl-CoA dehydrogenase. Caffeic, dihydrocaffeic, and dihydroferulic were intermetabolized to each other and to ferulic acid by isolated rat hepatocytes, while ferulic acid was metabolized only to caffeic acid but not to dihydrocaffeic and dihydroferulic acid. Evidence has been provided in this study that *O*-methylation, GSH conjugation, hydrogenation, and dehydrogenation are involved in the hepatic metabolism of caffeic and dihydrocaffeic acid (Moridani et al., 2002). As biotransformation of hydroxycinnamic acids in the human organism primarily involves Phase II conjugation reactions, the formation of these conjugates was evaluated using human liver and intestinal S9 homogenates. From the analysis of the kinetics of hydroxycinnamic acid conjugation in human S9 homogenates, it was observed that intrinsic clearance is much greater for sulfation than for glucuronidation and only isoferulic acid was significantly glucuronidated by human liver S9 homogenates. These *in vitro* data were confirmed in a human study where sulfates were detected as the main conjugates in urine, with the exception of isoferulic acid, which is mainly glucuronidated after drinking hydroxycinnamate-rich coffee (Wong et al., 2010). In another *in vitro* study, Phase II metabolism of feruloylquinic acids with human sulfotransferases and uridine 5′-diphosphoglucuronosyltransferases showed the formation of 5-*O*-feruloylquinic acid 4′-*O*-sulfate (Menozzi-Smarrito et al. 2011).

In isolated perfused rat liver, the first-pass effect of caffeic acid was not pronounced, and 93.3% appeared unchanged after one liver passage. Metabolites of caffeic acid oxidation and the methylation products, ferulic and isoferulic acid, were found in the perfusion medium as well as a cyclization product, esculetin. In the bile, mainly glucuronides as well as sulfates of caffeic acid were reported (Gumbinger et al. 1993).

4.3.2 Animal Studies

In the majority of animal and human studies on the metabolic fate of hydroxycinnamates, absorption, metabolism, and elimination have been performed on caffeic acid and its important natural depside, chlorogenic acid. In earlier studies in rats, it was suggested that chlorogenic acid is hydrolyzed in the stomach and intestine to caffeic and quinic acids (Czok et al., 1974). They did not detect chlorogenic acids in the serum or in bile after stomach or intestinal administration. It was suggested that chlorogenic acid is rapidly hydrolyzed in the gastrointestinal tract into quinic and caffeic acids and are further metabolized (Latza and Ammon, 1977).

4.3.2.1 Pharmacokinetics

In the plasma of the portal vein, free ferulic acid corresponded to 49% ± 5% of the total ferulic acid derivatives. Thus, ferulic acid is likely metabolized mainly in the liver as shown by the decline to 6.2% ± 2.7% of the fraction of free/total ferulic acid after the blood reaches the arteries (Zhao et al., 2004).

The pharmacokinetics parameters of caffeic acid and chlorogenic acid in rats have been studied after their intravenous injection. For caffeic acid, the pharmacokinetic parameter for T½, AUC0-t, and clearance were 130.91 ± 38.77 min, 4.89 ± 0.96 mg/min/L and 0.12 ± 0.02 L/min/kg, respectively. For chlorogenic acid, the pharmacokinetic parameter for T½, AUC0-t, and clearance were 49.38 ± 8.85 min, 9.54 ± 0.95 mg/min/L and 0.09 ± 0.003 L/min/kg, respectively. Caffeic acid exhibits a 2.6-fold longer half-life when compared with chlorogenic acid, a twofold lower AUC and a slightly higher value for clearance (Dai et al., 2013).

4.3.2.2 Gastrointestinal Absorption

The absorption of chlorogenic acid or caffeic acid (248 mg/kg body weight) in rats was studied after oral administration. While ingested caffeic acid was absorbed from the alimentary tract and was present in blood circulation, only traces of metabolites of caffeic and ferulic acids conjugates were detected in the plasma for 6 h after chlorogenic acid administration; most of the chlorogenic acid dose was still present in the small intestine. These results suggest that chlorogenic acid is not well absorbed from the digestive tract, unlike caffeic acid, and is subject to almost no structural changes along the gastrointestinal tract (Azuma et al., 2000).

A study was performed to evaluate whether ferulic acid is absorbed in the rat stomach. Within 25 min of stomach *in situ* perfusion, 74% ± 11% of the administered ferulic acid disappeared from the stomach, and only free ferulic acid was detected in the gastric contents and mucosa. In the plasma of the portal vein, free ferulic acid corresponded to 49% ± 5% of the total ferulic acid derivatives. Thus, ferulic acid can be rapidly absorbed from the rat stomach and found in the blood with metabolites (Zhao et al., 2004). Ferulic acid bioavailability was evaluated by measuring the urinary metabolite profiles of rats fed two different aleurone fractions of bran with high concentrations of ferulic acid and diferulic acid esters linked to arabinoxylans. Acute and chronic feeding experiments show higher increases in the excretion of phenolic metabolites/catabolites when compared with controls and ferulic acid appears to be more bioavailable in the outer part of wheat aleurone (Calani et al., 2014).

The absorption and metabolism of chlorogenic acid and caffeic acid in the small intestine were studied in rats in order to determine whether chlorogenic acid is directly absorbed or hydrolyzed in the small intestine. Chlorogenic and caffeic acids were perfused into a segment of the ileum plus jejunum during 45 min with cannulation of the biliary duct. The net absorption accounted for 19.5% and 8% of the perfused caffeic and chlorogenic acids, respectively. A minor fraction of the perfused caffeic acid was metabolized in the intestinal wall and secreted back into the gut lumen as ferulic acid. A small part of the chlorogenic acid was recovered in the gut effluent as caffeic acid, showing the presence of trace esterase activity in the gut mucosa. Although these results show that chlorogenic acid may be absorbed and hydrolyzed in the small intestine, the authors conclude that chlorogenic acid bioavailability appears to be governed largely by its uptake into the gut mucosa (Lafay et al., 2005).

Chlorogenic acid and caffeic acid appeared after 1.5 h in plasma and urine when rats were fed a diet supplemented with 0.25% weight/weight (W/W) chlorogenic acid, suggesting an absorption of chlorogenic acid into the upper part of the gastrointestinal tract. Gastric absorption of chlorogenic acid was then studied by its infusion in the ligated stomach of food-deprived rats, showing after 30 min of infusion the presence of intact chlorogenic acid in the gastric vein and aorta. These results show for the first time that chlorogenic acid is quickly absorbed in the rat stomach. Minor hydrolysis of chlorogenic acid occurred in the stomach and small intestine, whereas 15%–32% of ingested chlorogenic acid was hydrolyzed into caffeic acid in the caecum (Lafay et al., 2006).

4.3.2.3 Biliary Secretion

Radiolabeled cinnamic acids were used to study their choleretic effects and administered intraduodenally to rats. It was shown that 20% of the dose of ferulic acid, isoferulic acid, 3,4-dimethoxycinnamic acid, 3,4,5-trimethoxycinnamic acid, 8% of *p*-methoxycinnamic acid and less than 5% of caffeic acid, m-coumaric acid, and *p*-coumaric acid were recovered in biliary secretion (Westendorf and Czok, 1983).

When ferulic acid was applied *in situ* in the rat stomach, ferulic acid was also recovered in both free and conjugated forms as sulfate, glucuronide, and sulfoglucuronide conjugates in bile (Zhao et al., 2004).

From experiences of perfusion of chlorogenic and caffeic acids into a rat segment of the ileum plus jejunum, chlorogenic acid was not detected in either plasma or bile, and only low amounts of phenolic acids were secreted in the bile (Lafay et al., 2005).

4.3.2.4 Colonic Metabolism

The role of intestinal bacteria on caffeic acid metabolism was studied more than 40 years ago using germ-free (Scheline and Midtvedt, 1970) and gnotobiotic rats (Peppercorn and Goldman, 1972). Dehydroxylation was due to bacteria. The specific role of different bacteria of the flora in transforming caffeic acid into dihydrocaffeic acid, ferulic, dihydroferulic acid, 3-hydroxyphenylpropionic acid, vinyl catechol, and ethyl catechol in the host is now a major subject of research to evaluate any health benefit and risk associated with phenolic acid intake.

4.3.2.5 Urinary Excretion and Metabolic Balance

When administered intraperitoneally (i.p.) to rats, labeled cinnamic acid [3-^{14}C] and ferulic acid [2-^{14}C] were not incorporated into tissues, but most of the radioactivity was excreted in urine (48% and 68%, respectively) and feces (25% and 17%). In addition to unchanged cinnamic acid, hippuric acid was identified as the main metabolite along with benzoic acid. Unchanged ferulic acid was estimated as 25% of the administered dose, and 3-hydroxyphenylpropionic acid was also identified (Teuchy and Van Sumere, 1968). However, in contrast with others, Booth et al. (1957) were unable to show with labeled ferulic acid, the presence of dihydroferulic acid, feruloylglycine, and vanilloylglycine (Teuchy and Van Sumere, 1971).

The urinary recovery of hydroxycinnamates, ferulic acid, and chlorogenic acid was studied in the rat after oral or intravenous administration of 50 mg/kg and urine was collected over a 24 h period. For ferulic acid, 5.4% of the administered dose was orally absorbed but in contrast, neither unchanged chlorogenic acid nor the conjugated metabolites in the form of glucuronide or sulfate were detected, suggesting that renal excretion is not a major pathway of elimination for intact hydroxycinnamates in the rat (Camarasa et al., 1988).

In a rat study, four groups were fed a diet supplemented with chlorogenic, caffeic, or quinic acids or an unsupplemented diet for 8 days. The recovery of chlorogenic acid in urine 24 h after the administration was low (0.8%), and the total urinary excretion of caffeic acid liberated by the hydrolysis of chlorogenic acid and its tissue methylated metabolites (ferulic and isoferulic acids) account for 1.3% ± 0.2% of the dose ingested, while 3-coumaric acid, 3,4-dihydroxyphenylpropionic acid, 3-hydroxyphenylpropionic acid, 3-hydroxybenzoic acid, 3-hydroxyhippuric acid, and hippuric acid exhibited high urinary concentrations. These metabolites of microbial origin account for 57.4% ± 8.8% of the chlorogenic acid intake. The most abundant metabolites were hippuric acid, followed by 3-hydroxyphenylpropionic acid and 3-coumaric acid. The metabolites of microbial origin, 3-coumaric acid, 3-hydroxyphenylpropionic, benzoic, and hippuric acids, were the major compounds in both urine and plasma in rats fed chlorogenic acid. In rats fed the caffeic acid diet, the total urinary excretion of caffeic, ferulic, and isoferulic acids was 26-fold higher than that measured after the chlorogenic acid diet, and the total excretion of microbial metabolites accounted for only 28.1% ± 4.4% of caffeic acid intake. 3-Hydroxyphenylpropionic acid was also detected in the plasma of rats fed caffeic acid, in addition to caffeic acid, ferulic acid, and isoferulic acid. However, the plasma concentration of 3-hydroxyphenylpropionic acid was much lower than that of caffeic acid and its two methylated derivatives. In rats fed quinic acid, the increase in the urinary excretion of hippuric acid represented half the dose of quinic acid ingested, showing that hippuric acid largely originated from the transformation of the quinic acid moiety. The authors concluded that the bioavailability of chlorogenic acid depends largely on its metabolism by the gut microflora (Gonthier et al., 2003). A study was performed to evaluate whether ferulic acid is metabolized in the liver. In addition to free ferulic acid, three metabolites were identified after 25 min, the sulfate, glucuronide, and sulfoglucuronide conjugates were detected in the portal vein and arterial plasma (10% in the blood pool), gastric mucosa (4% ± 2%), bile (4% ± 2%), urine (3% ± 3%), and tissues (~53%) of the rats administered ferulic acid *in situ*. In the plasma of the portal vein, free ferulic acid corresponded to 49% ± 5% of the total ferulic acid derivatives. Thus, after absorption, ferulic acid is likely metabolized mainly in the liver as shown by the decline to 6.2% ± 2.7% of the fraction of free/total ferulic acid after the blood reaches the arteries (Zhao et al., 2004).

After tube feeding [3-^{14}C] caffeic acid in rats, plasma, urine, and feces were collected over 72 h and body tissues were taken at the end of the study. The recovery reached 80% of the administered dose with a major excretion in urine and an unknown metabolite was detected in feces. Nine labeled metabolites were identified, caffeic acid and its cis isomer, 3-*O*- and 4-*O*-sulfates and glucuronides of caffeic acid, 4-*O*-sulfates and glucuronides of ferulic acid, and isoferulic acid-4-*O*-sulfate; while four unidentified metabolites were also detected (Omar et al., 2012).

4.3.3 Human Studies

4.3.3.1 Pharmacokinetics

The bioavailability of polyphenols from berries was investigated in 72 volunteers consuming either a control diet or a supplement of 160 g/day berries (bilberries, lingonberries, blackcurrants, and chokeberries) for 8 weeks, providing 62.5 mg/day phenolic acids including caffeic acid (26.4 mg), 4-coumaric acid (5.5 mg), and ferulic acid (1.7 mg). In plasma, caffeic acid (+100%) and 4-coumaric acid (+40%) concentrations increased significantly in the berry compared with the control group (Koli et al., 2010). There was also a significant increase of plasma 3-hydroxyphenylpropionic acid after berry consumption, a known metabolite of caffeic and ferulic acid (Arnaud, 1993).

The plasma sample, drawn 4 h 40 min after cranberry juice intake, contained ferulic and sinapic acids, which were not detected in the samples collected at 45 min, and caffeic and coumaric acids were never found (Zhang and Zuo, 2004). The dose ingested may have been too low to get significant plasma levels or the bioavailability was low or delayed. The absorption and excretion of 20 cranberry-derived phenolics were studied after the consumption of cranberry juice and fruit by healthy volunteers. Plasma phenolics peaked between 0.5 and 2 h, and cinnamic acid, vanillic acid, and 4-coumaric acids showed second plasma concentration peaks, which was suggested by the authors to be due to the reabsorption of biliary-excreted phenolics acids (Wanga et al., 2012).

In human studies, the absorption of phenolic acids derived from coffee showed particularly rich in chlorogenic acid while free phenolic acids were undetectable. Plasma samples were collected before and 1 and 2 h after coffee administration resulting in an increased total plasma caffeic acid concentration, with absorption peak at 1 h. Caffeic acid was the only phenolic acid found in plasma samples after coffee administration while chlorogenic acid was undetectable. Most of the caffeic acid present in plasma was in bound form, mainly in the glucuronate/sulfate forms (Nardini et al., 2002).

Healthy participants were asked to randomly drink in a crossover design: instant coffee, instant coffee and 10% whole milk, or instant coffee, sugar, and nondairy creamer already premixed, with these three treatments providing 332 mg of total chlorogenic acid. Plasma pharmacokinetics showed that adding whole milk did not alter the overall bioavailability of coffee phenolic acids, whereas sugar and nondairy creamer affected the Tmax and Cmax, but not the appearance of coffee phenolics in plasma as the area under the curve (AUC) did not significantly differ between the groups (Renouf et al., 2010c).

4.3.3.2 Gastrointestinal Absorption

A low gastric pH (around 2) was suggested to facilitate the transportation of phenolic acids in an undissociated form via a passive diffusion mechanism (Tsuji and Tamai, 1996).

A dose-response study was performed in healthy subjects measuring the plasma bioavailability of phenolics after drinking three increasing doses of instant pure soluble coffee. Chlorogenic acids in their intact form were poorly absorbed, regardless of the dose. However, chlorogenic acid and phenolic acids appeared rapidly in plasma, indicating an early absorption in the gastrointestinal tract. Late-appearing metabolites were the most abundant. This study confirms that the kinetic of the appearance of coffee metabolites shows two peaks indicating that these metabolites are produced and absorbed both in the small intestine and in the colon. Late-appearing metabolites, dihydrocaffeic acid, and dihydroferulic acid have been assumed to be produced and absorbed at the level of the colon, while early-appearing metabolites, caffeic acid, and ferulic acid must be absorbed earlier in the small intestine. The overall plasma bioavailability for the three increasing doses was evaluated from the AUC of all metabolites summed and compared. A significant 2.23-fold increase in plasma appearance was observed between the low- and the medium-ingested dose, and a significant 2.38-fold increase in plasma AUC was observed between the medium- and the high-ingested dose. There was a 5.31-fold difference between the low and high dose (Renouf et al., 2014).

It is known that milk may interact with polyphenols and thus affect their bioavailability in humans. This effect was tested with the simultaneous consumption of coffee and milk, followed by the urinary excretion of chlorogenic acid and its metabolites. When subjects ingested instant coffee dissolved in water or in whole milk, excretion was significantly decreased with milk (40% ± 27%) when compared with water (68% ± 20%). This clearly shows an impairment in the bioavailability of coffee chlorogenic acids by milk in humans (Duarte and Farah, 2011) in contrast with a similar study on pharmacokinetics in coffee phenolics showing no effect of milk (Renouf et al., 2010c). Despite these advancements, a report on gastrointestinal absorption of phenolic acids has recently been published stating that the literature describing the bioavailability of chlorogenic acids is scarce and contradictory (Marín et al., 2015).

4.3.3.3 Biliary Secretion

The absorption and excretion of 20 cranberry-derived phenolics were studied after the consumption of cranberry juice and fruit by healthy volunteers. Plasma phenolics peak between 0.5 and 2 h after ingestion, and cinnamic acid, vanillic acid, and 4-coumaric acids showed second plasma concentration peaks, which may be due to the reabsorption of biliary-excreted phenolics from the jejunum (Wanga et al., 2012).

4.3.3.4 Urinary Excretion and Metabolic Balance

In 1957, it was identified that caffeic acid is the precursor of 3-hydroxyhippuric acid in human urine. In addition to unchanged caffeic acid, other acids identified are dihydrocaffeic acid, ferulic acid, dihydroferulic acid, vanillic acid, 3-coumaric acids, 3-hydroxyphenylpropionic acid, and 3-hydroxyhippuric acid as well as the glucuroconjugates, feruloylglycine, and vanilloylglycine (Booth et al., 1957).

The highest level of phenolic metabolites from dietary caffeic acid appeared in urine samples collected in the first 4 h and then decreased rapidly. In addition to caffeic acid, vanillic, ferulic, and isoferulic acids were identified and quantified. No isoferulic acid or dihydroferulic acid could be detected as metabolites of ferulic acid. As no phenolic metabolite can be detected in fecal samples, the total metabolite recovery of only 10% of the 1 g of caffeic acid dose can be questioned (Jacobson et al., 1983). The bioavailability of ferulic acid in humans has been evaluated from tomato consumption through to the monitoring of excretion in relation to intake. The results show that the peak time for maximal urinary excretion is approximately 7 h and the recovery of ferulic acid in the urine, on the basis of total free ferulic acid and feruloyl glucuronide excreted, is only 11%–25% of that ingested (Bourne and Rice-Evans, 1998).

The investigation of the absorption in humans of hydroxycinnamic acids from high-bran wheat breakfast cereal rich in ester-linked hydroxycinnamic acids, such as ferulic and diferulic acids, shows increased plasma ferulic and sinapic acid concentrations with absorption peaks between 1 and 3 h. In urine, a fourfold increase in ferulic acid and a fivefold increase in feruloylglycine were detected in 24-h urine after the consumption of the cereal. Ferulic acid detected in urine and plasma was present as conjugates, feruloylglycine and/or glucuronides, while diferulic acids were undetectable. In conclusion, ferulic and sinapic acids are absorbed in humans from dietary high-bran wheat but this absorption is limited and may originate only from the free and soluble portions present in the cereal (Kern et al., 2003).

The bioavailability of polyphenols from berries was investigated in 72 volunteers consuming a supplement of 160 g/day berries for 8 weeks, which provided 26.4 mg/day caffeic acid, 5.5 mg/day 4-coumaric acid, and 1.7 mg/day ferulic acid. In urine, with the exception of a significant increase in the excretion of 4-coumaric acid (+18%), the 24 h urinary excretions did not differ significantly between groups for any phenolic acids and their metabolites. Important individual variations in plasma and urine concentrations were observed in this study and high coffee consumption reported in Finland may explain these variations (Koli et al., 2010). After consumption of cranberry juice and fruit by healthy volunteers, all of the cranberry-derived phenolics increased significantly in urine samples after the intake of each cranberry product (Wanga et al., 2012).

Biomarkers of the bioavailability and metabolism of hydroxycinnamate derivatives from coffee through urinary elimination and the identification of the metabolites excreted were investigated. The results show a highly significant increase in the excretion of ferulic, isoferulic, dihydroferulic acid (3-(4-hydroxy-3-methoxyphenyl)-propionic acid), and vanillic acid. 3-Hydroxyhippuric acid has also been identified with a highly significant excretion increase after coffee ingestion (Rechner et al., 2001).

When human volunteers drank coffee containing 412 μmol of chlorogenic acids, 1 h after ingestion some of the components in the coffee reached nanomole peak plasma concentrations, whereas chlorogenic acid metabolites, including caffeic acid-3-O-sulfate, ferulic acid-4-O-sulfate, and sulfates of 3- and 4-caffeoylquinic acid lactones, had higher peak plasma values. The short time to reach this peak suggests their absorption by the small intestine. In contrast, dihydroferulic acid, its 4-O-sulfate, and dihydrocaffeic acid-3-O-sulfate exhibited much higher peak plasma concentrations, which was delayed 4 h after ingestion, indicating absorption in the large intestine and the probable involvement of catabolism by colonic bacteria. The volunteers of this study followed a low-polyphenol diet for 48 h before the beginning of the study and a standard lunch, containing low levels of phenolic and polyphenolic compounds, was provided after the 3 h samples were collected. Despite this control trial, ferulic acid-4-O-sulfate, dihydrocaffeic acid-3-O-sulfate, and dihydroferulic acid-4-O-sulfate were detected in the plasma of some subjects. However, the concentrations of these metabolites were 25- to 100-fold lower than the maximal values attained after coffee consumption. In urine, dihydroferulic acid, its 4-O-sulfate, dihydrocaffeic acid-3-*O*-sulfate, ferulic acid-4-*O*-sulfate, and dihydroferulic acid-4-*O*-glucuronide were major components to be excreted in urine. Although feruloylglycine is not detected in plasma, it constitutes a major urinary metabolite. Other metabolites excreted in smaller quantities included the 3-*O*-sulfate and 3-*O*-glucuronide of isoferulic acid, dihydro(iso)ferulic acid-3-*O*-glucuronide, and dihydrocaffeic acid-3-*O*-glucuronide. After 24 h metabolic balance, chlorogenic acid metabolites corresponded to 29.1% of intake, indicating that chlorogenic acids in coffee are well absorbed, and there is a need for a better recovery and further identification of two-thirds of the metabolites (Stalmach et al., 2009). For the identification of potential human metabolites of coffee polyphenols, analytical standards have been chemically prepared. Out of the 24 synthesized conjugates, 10 have been identified in human plasma and/or urine after coffee consumption. It was possible to detect hydroxycinnamic acid metabolites for the first time, such as dihydroisoferulic acid 3-*O*-glucuronide, caffeic acid 3-sulfate, as well as the sulfate and glucuronide derivatives of 3,4-dihydroxyphenylpropionic acid (Fumeaux et al., 2010). Intake of food and drink containing benzoic acid influences the urinary hippuric acid concentration, which is used to monitor toluene exposure in Japan. However, urinary hippuric acid concentration increased significantly with increasing coffee consumption in toluene-non-exposed workers despite the absence of benzoic acid in coffee. These results suggest that chlorogenic, caffeic, and quinic acids from coffee are metabolized to hippuric acid (Ogawa et al., 2011).

In a review published before 2010 on human studies looking at the bioavailability of dietary phenolic compounds, and including chlorogenic acids, the authors described the identification of metabolites and catabolites in plasma, urine, and ileal fluid (Crozier et al., 2010). When absorbed in the small intestine, they appear in the circulatory system predominantly as glucuronide, sulfate, and methylated metabolites, which are rapidly removed from the bloodstream. Up to now, the analysis of plasma provides valuable information on the identity and pharmacokinetics of circulating metabolites after acute administration but does not provide accurate quantitative assessments of uptake from the gastrointestinal tract. Urinary excretion exhibits wide variations with different classes of phenolic esters and free acids but does not allow a quantitative metabolic balance. Even when absorption occurs in the small intestine, feeding studies with ileostomy patients and control subjects reveal that substantial amounts of the parent compounds, and some of their metabolites, appear in the ileal fluid indicating that in volunteers with a functioning colon these compounds will pass to the large intestine where they are subjected to the action of the colonic microflora. Furthermore, these colonic-derived catabolites are absorbed into the bloodstream and pass through the body prior to excretion in urine. There is growing evidence that these compounds, which have only recently been investigated, are produced in the colon and form a key part of the bioavailability equation of dietary phenolic compounds (Crozier et al., 2010).

4.3.4 Role of Colonic Flora in Chlorogenic Acids Metabolism in Humans

A small part of caffeic acid administered orally to humans is excreted unchanged in the urine, but most is transformed by gut bacteria into 3-hydroxyphenylpropionic acid by a dehydroxylation process and then decarboxylated (Peppercorn and Goldman, 1971; Booth et al., 1957; Jacobson et al., 1983), and a minor part only is methylated in the liver to ferulic acid, isoferulic acid, and vanillic acids (Michaud et al., 1971). These O-methylated derivatives are excreted rapidly in the urine, while the 3-hydroxyphenyl derivatives appear later. The dehydroxylation reactions have been ascribed to the action of intestinal bacteria (Arnaud, 1988; IARC, 1993).

4.3.4.1 Ileostomy Patients

Absorption of chlorogenic acid and caffeic acid has been evaluated in healthy ileostomy patients where degradation by the colonic microflora is minimal. They ingested either 1 g of chlorogenic acid or 0.5 g of caffeic acid, and ileostomy effluent and urine were collected for 24 h. Absorption of chlorogenic acid and caffeic acid was 33% ± 17% and 95% ± 4%, respectively, of the ingested dose. Only traces of the ingested chlorogenic acid and 11% of the ingested caffeic acid were excreted in urine. These results show that one-third of chlorogenic acid and almost all of the caffeic acid were absorbed in the small intestine of humans (Olthof et al., 2001).

In a study aimed at the identification and quantitation of phenolic acid metabolites of chlorogenic acid in humans, and determination of the site of metabolism, it was shown that half of the ingested chlorogenic acid was metabolized to hippuric acid with the assumption that each molecule of chlorogenic acid can yield two molecules of hippuric acid, because the caffeic acid moiety and the quinic acid moiety of chlorogenic acid are probably metabolized to hippuric acid in humans. Of the ingested chlorogenic acid, 1.7% was recovered unchanged in urine. The most pronounced difference in the metabolic profile of chlorogenic acid between volunteers with and without a colon was the absence of hippuric acid as a metabolite of chlorogenic acid in those without a colon. These results suggest that hippuric acid arises from metabolism by micro-organisms in the colon. Subsequently, caffeic acid is dehydroxylated by bacteria in the colon and after its absorption is β-oxidized to a large extent into benzoic acid (Olthof et al., 2003).

The recovery of chlorogenic acid metabolites in 0–24 h urine sample of healthy subjects and ileostomy patients following the ingestion of 200 mL of coffee was only 29.2% and 8.0% of the intake, respectively (Del Rio et al., 2010).

Dihydroferulic acid and dihydrocaffeic acid were the major metabolites that appeared after coffee consumption, and the long time needed to reach maximum plasma concentration suggests absorption and metabolism in the colon. Phenolic acid, caffeic acid, ferulic acid, and isoferulic acid were detected earlier and they peaked at lower concentrations (Renouf et al., 2010a).

When 136 mg chlorogenic acid was ingested in a single intake of 200 mL of instant coffee by ileostomy patients to study the intestinal absorption and metabolism, 71% ± 7% of chlorogenic acid and their metabolites was present in the ileal effluent after 24 h. The metabolites including free and sulfated caffeic and ferulic acids accounted for 22% of the total ileal content, while unchanged chlorogenic acid represented 78%. In the urine, chlorogenic acid metabolites including ferulic acid-4-O-sulfate, caffeic acid-3-O-sulfate, isoferulic acid-3-O-glucuronide, and dihydrocaffeic acid-3-O-sulfate accounted for only 8% ± 1%. The main difference between ileostomy patients and healthy volunteers was a higher urine recovery (29% ± 4%) after 24 h due to the formation of dihydroferulic acid and feruloylglycine together with sulfate and glucuronide conjugates of dihydrocaffeic and dihydroferulic acids, demonstrating the importance of colonic metabolism for chlorogenic acids (Stalmach et al., 2010). In ileostomy patients, it was reported that 59%–77% of chlorogenic acids was recovered in ileal fluid after the ingestion of coffee (Erk et al., 2012; Stalmach et al., 2010). A dose-response study in ileostomy patients shows that consumption of higher chlorogenic acid content in coffee leads to faster ileal excretion, suggesting that chlorogenic acid dose might influence the gastrointestinal transit time and consequently affect chlorogenic acid absorption and metabolism. The metabolism of chlorogenic acids through glucuronidation became slightly greater with increasing dose (Erk et al., 2012).

After a caffeoylquinic acid–free diet, ileostomy volunteers consumed coffee providing 746 μmol total caffeoylquinic acid and its excretion in ileal fluid was then analyzed and quantified. Caffeoylquinic acid consumed in coffee was not influenced by interesterification reactions, while in a previous study, it was shown that interesterification of caffeoylquinic acid from cloudy apple juice and an apple smoothie was observed during gastrointestinal transit. The recovery of excreted caffeoylquinic acid varied considerably and about 26.1% of caffeoylquinic acid reached the ileal fluids after the cloudy apple juice consumption, whereas 76.2%–77.5% of caffeoylquinic acid reached the end of the small intestine after consumption of coffee and the apple smoothie. These results show that variations in food matrices as well as phenolic composition have some influence on intestinal bioavailability and interesterification of caffeoylquinic acid (Erk et al., 2014b).

4.3.4.2 Delayed Plasma Peak Absorption

Interindividual differences in excretion profiles of hydroxycinnamic acid metabolites have been observed, suggesting that the composition of the microbiota may influence the fate of dietary hydroxycinnamic acids, modifying their bioavailability (Olthof et al., 2003; Rechner et al., 2004).

Volunteers ingested instant soluble coffee (335 mg total chlorogenic acids) in water, and plasma samples were analyzed after full hydrolysis by chlorogenate esterase, glucuronidase, and sulfatase to release aglycone. Ferulic, caffeic, and isoferulic acid equivalents appeared rapidly in plasma, peaking at 1–2 h. Dihydrocaffeic and dihydroferulic acids appeared later in plasma, 6–8 h after ingestion. This study confirms that the small intestine is a significant site for absorption of some phenolic acids, but shows that the colon/microflora play a major role in absorption and metabolism of chlorogenic acids and phenolic acids from coffee (Renouf et al., 2010b). To identify coffee-derived metabolites, urine from coffee drinkers and non-coffee drinkers was screened and ferulic acid conjugates were identified as one of the major metabolites found after coffee consumption. Chlorogenic acid–derived metabolites were found to be separated into two groups showing different pharmacokinetic properties. The first group, including ferulic acid and feruloyl sulfate, appeared early in the plasma (~1 h), while the second group, containing chlorogenic acid metabolites formed by the intestinal microflora, appeared late and persisted in the plasma (>6 h). The pharmacokinetic profiles suggest that the late-appearing dihydroferulic acid, feruloylglycine, and dihydroferulic acid sulfate, formed from chlorogenic acid by the intestinal microflora, accumulated in the plasma due to their delayed colonic metabolism and absorption (Lang et al., 2013b).

4.3.4.3 Antibiotic Use and Germ-Free Studies

The role of intestinal bacteria in caffeic acid metabolism was demonstrated in humans by comparing control subjects with subjects treated with neomycin to suppress their gut flora (Shaw et al., 1963). In humans, after the oral administration of caffeic acid, the O-methylated phenolic acids (ferulic, vanillic, etc.) appeared rapidly in the urine, whereas 3-hydroxyphenyl derivatives appeared later. By suppressing the gut flora with neomycin, it was shown that the dehydroxylation reaction was due solely to the action of intestinal bacteria (Shaw et al., 1963; Daymon and Jepson, 1969).

These results were confirmed by comparing the metabolism of caffeic acid in germ-free (Scheline and Midtvedt, 1970) and various gnotobiotic (Peppercorn and Goldman, 1972) rats. However, discrepancies were observed in the ability of bacteria cultures to transform caffeic acid into ferulic acid, dihydrocaffeic acid, dihydroferulic acid, 3-hydroxypropionic acid, vinyl catechol, ethyl catechol, and the metabolites produced by these bacteria in the host.

4.3.4.4 *In Vitro* Studies with Gut Bacteria and Fecal Samples

Diferulic acids are abundant structural components of plant cell walls, especially in cereal brans. These phenolics are ester-linked to cell wall polysaccharides and cannot be absorbed in this form. However, 5–5-, 8-O-4-, and 8-5-diferulic acids were identified in the plasma of rats after their oral administration. It was shown that human and rat colonic microflora contain esterase activity able to release 5-5-, 8-O-4-, and 8-5-diferulic acids from dietary diferulates of cereal brans, followed by the absorption of the free acids (Andreasen et al., 2001a).

In the last two decades, evidence for the importance of colonic bacteria in the metabolism, absorption, and potential activity of phenolics in human health and disease has been provided. For example, it has been shown that fecal homogenates containing bacteria significantly catalyzed tea phenolics, including caffeic acid, to generate aromatic metabolites dependent on bacterial species (Lee et al., 2006).

Although caffeic acid is easily absorbed in the small intestine, its esterification with quinic acid, as in chlorogenic acid, decreases its gut absorption and increases the quantities reaching the colon and its microbiota. The effect of human fecal microbiota on the metabolism of caffeic, chlorogenic, and caftaric acids (tartaric acid ester of caffeic acid) in an *in vitro* fermentation model has been reported. These three substrates disappeared quickly and none of the free acids (caffeic, quinic, or tartaric acids) were detected after 2 h of incubation. Two major microbial metabolites were identified as 3-hydroxyphenylpropionic and benzoic acids (Gonthier et al., 2006).

4.3.4.5 Gut Bacteria and Microbial Metabolism

Due to the absence of free caffeic acid in coffee, plasma caffeic acid is likely to be derived from hydrolysis of chlorogenic acid in the gastrointestinal tract (Nardini et al., 2002). Microbial metabolism of chlorogenic acid includes the hydrolysis to quinic acid and caffeic acid, making free caffeic acid available for absorption. Free caffeic acid may be further transformed by colonic bacteria into a variety of metabolites, such as 3-coumaric acid and hydroxylated derivatives of phenylpropionic and benzoic acids (Gonthier et al., 2003, 2006; Ogawa et al., 2011; Tomás-Barberán et al., 2014). A more complex picture of the fate of chlorogenic acid has recently been described, since the colonic microbiota can hydrogenate or dehydroxylate chlorogenic acid before hydrolyzing the ester bond, or even breaking the quinic acid moiety (Tomás-Barberán et al., 2014). Bacterial biotransformation generally converges on the 3-hydroxyphenyl-propanoic acid (Rechner et al., 2004).

Like most hydroxycinnamic acids esters, most of the chlorogenic acid is not absorbed in the small intestine and reaches the colon (Stalmach et al., 2010), where it is transformed by the gut microbiota (Selma et al., 2009). It is thus well established that the majority of chlorogenic acid escapes absorption in the small intestine and reaches the colon, where the microbiota transforms it into several metabolites. The variability of bacterial metabolism on chlorogenic acid metabolism was studied in volunteers showing the formation of caffeoyl-glycerol intermediates for the first time. All the pathways converged on 3-hydroxyphenyl-propanoic acid, which was transformed to 3-hydroxyphenyl-ethanol and/or phenylacetic acid in a few subjects (Tomás-Barberán et al., 2014).

Several microbial metabolites have been identified. The main microbial metabolites of caffeic acid are 3-hydroxyphenylpropionic acid and benzoic acid, generated by the action of *Escherichia coli*, *Bifidobacterium lactis*, and *Lactobacillus gasseri*. 3-Hydroxyphenylpropionic acid is formed by de-esterification, reduction of a double bond, and dehydroxylation. Furthermore, β-oxidation shortens the side chain and forms benzoic acid. Both metabolites are also obtained from chlorogenic acid (Marín et al., 2015).

As a considerable proportion of ingested chlorogenic acids reaches the large intestine, a stirred, anaerobic, pH-controlled, batch culture fermentation model of the distal region of the colon was used to investigate the impact of coffee and chlorogenic acids on the growth of the human fecal microbiota. Incubation of coffee samples with the human fecal microbiota led to the rapid metabolism of chlorogenic acids after 4 h and the production of dihydrocaffeic acid and dihydroferulic acid. Chlorogenic acids and coffee induced a significant increase in the growth of *Bifidobacterium* spp. (Mills et al., 2015).

Bifidobacterium strains belonging to eight species occurring in the human gut were tested; among them, *Bifidobacterium animalis* were able to hydrolyze chlorogenic acid into caffeic acid and quinic acid. Only 10 out of 32 strains hydrolyzed chlorogenic acid and released caffeic acid. Both the cell-free extracts and the supernatants prepared from these strains were able to hydrolyze chlorogenic acid during growth (Raimondi et al., 2015). Bacterial species responsible for the hydrolysis by esterases of hydroxycinnamate esters in the human large intestine were identified from 35 isolates recovered after anaerobic batch culture incubation of human fecal bacteria in a chlorogenic acid–based medium were screened for cinnamoyl esterase activity. Six isolates released ferulic acid, from its ethyl ester, and were identified as *E. coli* (three isolates), *B. lactis*, and *L. gasseri* (two strains). In addition, chlorogenic acid hydrolyzing activities were essentially intracellular (Couteau et al., 2001) and a *B. bifidum* strain was able to utilize feruloyl oligosaccharides as carbon sources for removing feruloyl groups (Yuan et al., 2007). In a recent study, the genome sequences of bifidobacteria were analyzed to identify the genetic determinants that make *B. animalis* able to hydrolyze chlorogenic acid. This esterase activity was attributed to the Balat_0669 gene particular to *B. animalis* and absent in the species unable to hydrolyze chlorogenic acid (Raimondi et al., 2015).

Biotransformation of chlorogenic acid and caffeic acid in an *in vitro* mixed culture model of human intestinal microbiota was studied to determine the effects on human gut bacteria. Both chlorogenic acid and caffeic acid were metabolized rapidly, disappearing from the medium within 0.5 h and being replaced by known phenolic acid breakdown products. It was suggested that dietary polyphenol biotransformation products may have the ability to modify the gut microbial balance, rather than the original plant compounds (Parkar et al., 2013). These results agree well with previous studies, which have also shown that gut bacteria, including strains of *Lactobacillus* and *Bifidobacterium*, can metabolize chlorogenic acid to form caffeic acid and quinic acid (Couteau et al., 2001), while caffeic acid is further metabolized to form 3-coumaric acid, 3-hydroxyphenylacetic acid, and 3,4-dihydroxyphenylpropionic acid (Konishi and Kobayashi, 2004), which are then absorbed through intestinal monocarboxylate transporters.

All along the transit in the gastrointestinal tract, chlorogenic acids are metabolized and their metabolites predominate in the circulatory system rather than the ingested compounds. The catabolites produced by the colonic microflora were identified and quantified, showing that chlorogenic acids were rapidly degraded over the

6 h incubation period. Among 11 catabolites identified and quantified, caffeic and ferulic acids appeared in the first hour of incubation, and dihydrocaffeic acid, dihydroferulic acid, and 3-hydroxyphenylpropionic acid were the major end products, comprising 75%–83% of the total catabolites, whereas the remaining 17%–25% consisted of six minor catabolites. From these results, microbial and tissue metabolism can be distinguished and the authors proposed a colonic metabolic pathway and a tissue Phase I and Phase II metabolic pathway of chlorogenic acid (Ludwig et al., 2013).

4.3.5 Metabolic Pathways of Chlorogenic Acids

A number of metabolites have been identified (Table 4.3). Glucuronides of 3-coumaric acid and 3-hydroxyhippuric acid appear to be the main metabolites in humans. After oral administration of caffeic acid to human volunteers, O-methylated derivatives (ferulic, dihydroferulic, and vanillic acids) were excreted rapidly in the urine, while the 3-hydroxyphenyl derivatives appeared later. However, the dehydroxylation reactions were ascribed to the action of intestinal bacteria (Arnaud, 1988; 1993; IARC 1993).

The most frequent metabolites from ferulic acid produced by colonic microbiota are vanillic acid and 3-hydroxyphenylpropionic acid (Andreasen et al., 2001b; Couteau et al., 2001).

After 11 healthy volunteers ingested coffee beverages containing low, medium, and high amounts of chlorogenic acids, plasma and urine collected for 24 h revealed the presence of 12 metabolites in plasma and 16 metabolites in urine. They were identified as sulfates, and to a lesser extent glucuronides of caffeic, ferulic, dihydrocaffeic, and dihydroferulic acids, as well as intact feruloylquinic and caffeoylquinic acids, and sulfated caffeoylquinic acid lactones. In urine, the amounts of metabolites excreted after 24 h following consumption of the three coffees account for 24%, 25%, and 16% of the doses ingested, and these values are not significantly different, reflecting a large interindividual variability. However, peak plasma concentration and urinary excretion values showed trends toward a dose-dependent reduced bioavailability of chlorogenic acids (Stalmach et al., 2014).

4.3.6 Quinic Acid Metabolism in Animals and Humans

Quinic acid is transformed by the intestinal microflora and is excreted in the urine as catechol and hippuric acid in both rats and humans (Booth et al., 1960; Indahl and Scheline, 1973).

In 1966, it was shown that quinic acid given orally was excreted in the urine as hippuric acid in humans and some Old World monkeys but not in some New World monkeys and lemurs. Oral doses of quinic acid were aromatized to the extent of 20%–70% in humans, rhesus monkey, baboon, and green monkey, but only to 0%–10% in the other species including spider monkey, squirrel monkey, capuchin, bush baby, slow loris, tree shrew, dog, cat, ferret, rabbit, rat, mouse, guinea pig, hamster, lemming, fruit bat, hedgehog, and pigeon. No aromatization occurred in the monkey if the quinic acid was injected intraperitoneally or when they were pretreated for 4 days orally with neomycin to suppress the gut flora, and the excretion

TABLE 4.3
Clorogenic Acids and Metabolites Identified in Animals and Humans

3-Coumaric acid
4-Coumaric acid
Caffeic acid-3-*O*-sulfate
Caffeic acid-4-*O*-sulfate
3-*O*-Caffeoylquinic acid lactone-*O*-sulfate
4-*O*-Caffeoylquinic acid lactone-*O*-sulfate
Dihydroferulic acid
Dihydroferulic acid-4-*O*-sulfate
Dihydroferulic acid-4-*O*-glucuronide
Dihydro-isoferulic acid-3-*O*-glucuronide
Dihydrocaffeic acid-3-*O*-sulfate
Dihydrocaffeic acid-3-*O*-glucuronide
p-Coumaroylglucuronide
p-Coumaroylglycine
3-*O*-Feruloylquinic acid
4-*O*-Feruloylquinic acid
5-*O*-Feruloylquinic acid
Ferulic acid-4-*O*-sulfate
Feruloylglycine
Isoferulic acid (3-hydroxy-4-methoxycinnamic acid)
Isoferulic acid-3-*O*-sulfate
Isoferulic acid-3-*O*-glucuronide
Ferulic acid
3-O-Caffeoylquinic acid
5-O-Caffeoylquinic acid
4-O-Caffeoylquinic acid
Caffeic acid
Dihydrocaffeic acid
Dihydro-isoferulic acid
Vanillic acid (4-Hydroxy-3-methoxybenzoic acid)
Vanilloylglycine
3-Hydroxyphenyl-propionic acid
4-Hydroxyphenyl-propionic acid
3-Hydroxyphenyl acetic acid
3-Hydroxyphenyl ethanol
Phenyl acetate
p-Hydroxybenzoic acid
Hippuric acid (benzoylglycine)
3-Hydroxyhippuric acid (3-hydroxybenzoylglycine)
4-Hydroxyhippuric acid (4-hydroxybenzoylglycine)
Dihydrosinapic acid (3-(4-hydroxy-3,5-dimethoxyphenyl)-propionic acid)
3,5-Dihydroxyphenyl-propionic acid
3,4-Dihydroxyphenyl-propionic acid sulfate

(*Continued*)

TABLE 4.3 (CONTINUED)
Clorogenic Acids and Metabolites Identified in Animals and Humans

3,4-Dihydroxyphenyl-propionic acid glucuronide
3-Hydroxy-5-methoxycinnamic acid
3-Hydroxy-5-methoxyphenyl)-propionic acid

Source: Adapted from Booth et al., 1957, *J Biol Chem.* 229(1), 51–59; Rechner et al., 2001, *Free Rad. Biol. Med*, 30, 1213–22; Couteau et al., 2001, *J Appl Microbiol.*, 90(6), 873–81; Olthof et al., 2003, *J Nutr.*, 133(6), 1806–14; Stalmach et al., 2009, *Drug Metab Dispos.*, 37(8), 1749–58; Stalmach et al., 2010, *Arch Biochem Biophys.*, 501(1), 98–105; Fumeaux et al., 2010, *Org Biomol Chem.*, 8(22), 5199–211; Ludwig et al., 2013, *Biofactors.*, 39(6), 623–32; Tomás-Barberán et al., 2014, *Mol Nutr Food Res.*, 58(5), 1122–31; Stalmach et al., 2014, *Food Funct.*, 5(8), 1727–37; Mills et al., 2015, *Br J Nutr.*, 113(8), 1220–7.

of hippuric acid after oral doses of quinic acid was decreased to almost zero, but the ability to aromatize slowly returned over 20–30 days. These results strongly suggest that gut bacteria were responsible for the aromatization of quinic acid. When rhesus monkeys were given [^{14}C]quinic acid orally, 20%–25% of the dose was excreted in the urine as labeled hippuric acid. With this labeled quinic acid, 20%–50% of the orally administered dose was oxidized to CO_2 (Adamson et al., 1969).

The metabolic formation of an aromatic ring structure from quinic acid (1,3,4,5-tetrahydroxycyclohexane carboxylic acid) was reported more than a century ago (Arnaud, 1988). Hippuric acid was excreted in the urine after oral administration, but its formation was suppressed on parenteral injection of quinic acid in the guinea pig and after neomycin treatment in humans (Cotran et al., 1960). The fate of quinic acid was investigated in 22 species of animal including humans, where 60% of an oral dose of quinic acid was excreted as hippuric acid (Adamson et al., 1970). In the rat, the aromatization of quinic acid does not appear to be enhanced upon chronic administration and ranges from 17% to 27% and 0.7% to 2.0% of a 100 mg quinic acid dose as urinary hippuric acid and catechol, respectively. Neither protocatechuic acid nor vanillic acid was detected (Indahl and Scheline, 1973). Aromatization by the gut flora of another coffee component, shikimic acid, has also been demonstrated (Asatoor, 1965). In humans and three species of monkeys, oral quinic acid was extensively aromatized (20%–60%) and excreted in the urine as hippuric acid. When injected, quinic acid was not aromatized, but was largely excreted unchanged as well as after pretreatment with neomycin, which suppresses gut flora. The results support the view that quinic acid and shikimic acid are aromatized by the gut flora in humans and monkeys (Adamson et al., 1970).

The quinic acid moiety is dehydroxylated into cyclohexane carboxylic acid and then aromatized into benzoic acid by the colonic microflora or after absorption in body tissues. The benzoic acid formed is then conjugated with glycine and excreted in urine as hippuric acid (Olthof et al., 2003).

The metabolic pathway of phenolic acids, including chlorogenic, caffeic, and ferulic acids, is shown in Figure 4.3.

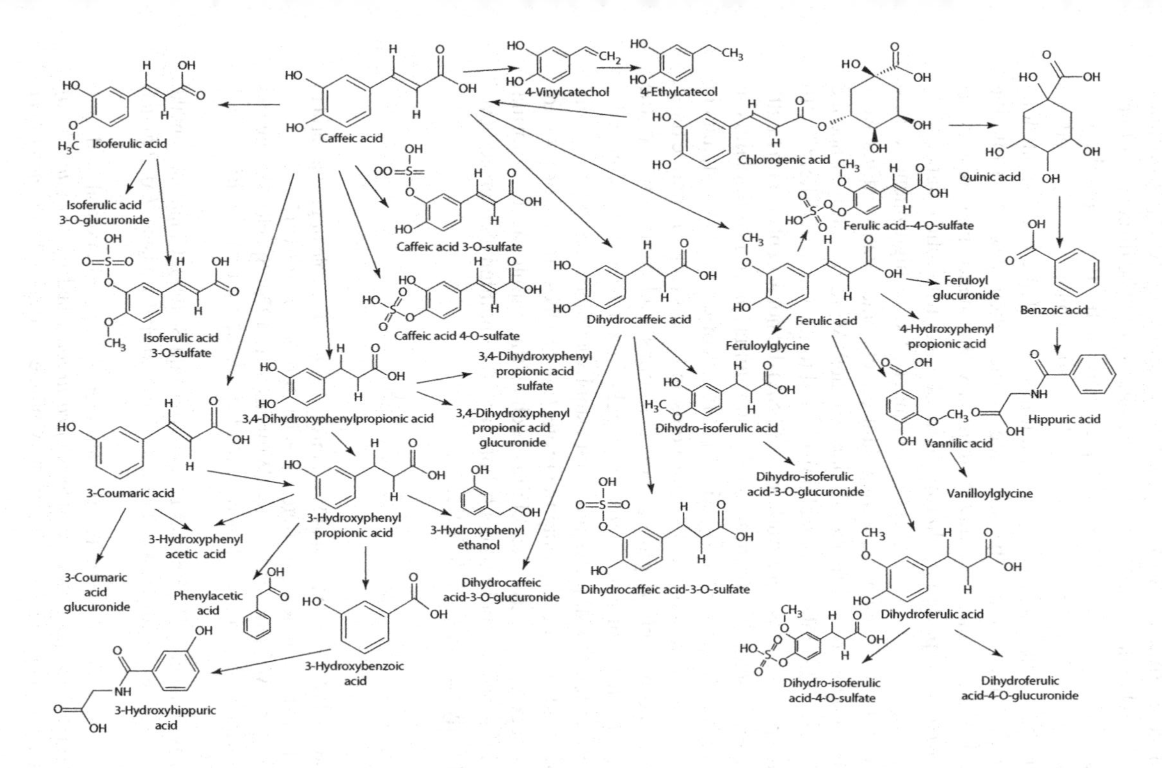

FIGURE 4.3 Metabolic pathways of chlorogenic, caffeic, and ferulic acids in animals and humans from Phase I and II enzymes as well as colonic bacteria. (Adapted from Booth et al., 1957, *J Biol Chem.* 229(1), 51–59; Arnaud, 1988, The metabolism of coffee constituents, in *Coffee, Volume 3: Physiology*, chapter 2, 33–55, eds R.J. Clarke and R. Macrae, Elsevier Applied Science, London; Arnaud, 1993, Metabolism of caffeine and other components of coffee, in *Caffeine, Coffee and Health*, ed. S. Garattini, Raven Press, New York, 43–95; Gonthier et al., 2003, *J Nutr.*, 133, 1853–9; Rechner et al., 2001, *Free Radic Biol Med.* 30, 1213–22; Couteau et al., 2001, *J Appl Microbiol.* 90(6), 873–81; Olthof et al., 2003, *J Nutr.* 133(6), 1806–14; Stalmach et al., 2009, *Drug Metab Dispos.* 37(8), 1749–58; Fumeaux et al., 2010, *Org Biomol Chem.* 8(22), 5199–211; Stalmach et al., 2010, *Arch Biochem Biophys.* 501(1), 98–105; Ludwig et al., 2013, *Biofactors.* 39(6), 623–32; Tomás-Barberán et al., 2014, *Mol Nutr Food Res.* 58(5), 1122–31; Stalmach et al., 2014, *Food Funct.* 5(8), 1727–37; Mills et al., 2015, *Br J Nutr.* 113(8), 1220–7.)

4.4 CONCLUSIONS

During the last decade, considerable effort has been put into investigating the bioavailability of phenolic acid, including its major compound, chlorogenic acid. Significant daily intakes of 0.5–1 g are reported in country surveys, stimulating industrial research to develop functional foods and helping university research institutes to evaluate the risks and benefits of these plant phenolic acids. The discovery of new compounds in plants, the study of their physiological and health effects, and the identification of metabolites in both experimental models and humans have changed our knowledge of their metabolic fate. The significant impact of colonic flora on phenolic acid bioavailability, the formation of bacterial metabolites, their absorption into the bloodstream, their hepatic metabolism, and their urinary elimination may explain the large individual variations reported in pharmacokinetics and metabolic balance.

From these studies, new food products were launched with high phenolic acid content associated with their potential antioxidant effects, and health claims were submitted with the support of published clinical studies. More research is needed to better understand the physiological mechanisms and to further prove their health benefits, as the European Food Safety Authority (EFSA) did not accept certain health claims in 2011. In their scientific opinion on the substantiation of health claims in relation to coffee, *C. arabica* L., chlorogenic acids from coffee, and antioxidants in coffee in relation to "the protection of DNA, proteins and lipids from oxidative damage, maintenance of normal blood glucose concentrations, and contribution to the maintenance or achievement of a normal body weight," the EFSA Panel concludes that a cause and effect relationship has not been established between the consumption of chlorogenic acids from coffee and the protection of DNA, lipids, or proteins from oxidative damage as well as other claims such as the maintenance of normal blood glucose concentrations and the contribution to the maintenance or achievement of a normal body weight (EFSA, 2011).

REFERENCES

Adamson R.H., Bridges J.W., Evans M.E. and Williams R.T. 1969. The role of gut bacteria in the aromatization of quinic acid in different species. *Biochem J.* 112(1):17P.

Adamson R.H., Bridges J.W., Evans M.E. and Williams R.T. 1970. Species differences in the aromatization of quinic acid *in vivo* and the role of gut bacteria. *Biochem J.* 116(3):437–43.

Ader P., Grenacher B., Langguth P., Scharrer E. and Wolffram S. 1996. Cinnamate uptake by rat small intestine: Transport kinetics and transepithelial transfer. *Exp Physiol.* 81(6):943–55.

Alonso-Salces R.M., Serra F., Reniero F. and Héberger K. 2009. Botanical and geographical characterization of green coffee (*Coffea arabica* and *Coffea canephora*): Chemometric evaluation of phenolic and methylxanthine contents. *J Agric Food Chem.* 57(10):4224–35.

Ames R.N., Profet M. and Gold L.S. 1991. Dietary carcinogens and mutagens from plants. In *Mutagens in Food: Detection and Prevention*, ed. H. Hayatsu, CRC Press, Boca Raton, FL, 29–50.

Andreasen M.F., Kroon P.A., Williamson G. and Garcia-Conesa M.T. 2001a. Intestinal release and uptake of phenolic antioxidant diferulic acids. *Free Radic Biol Med.* 31(3):304–14.

Andreasen M.F., Kroon P.A., Williamson G. and Garcia-Conesa M.T. 2001b. Esterase activity able to hydrolyze dietary antioxidant hydroxycinnamates is distributed along the intestine of mammals. *J Agric Food Chem.* 49(11):5679–84.

Andrés-Lacueva C., Medina-Remon A., Llorach R., Urpi-Sarda M., Khan N., Chiva-Blanch G., Zamora-Ros R., Rotches-Ribalta M. and Lamuela-Raventós R.M. 2009. Phenolic compounds: Chemistry and occurrence in fruits and vegetables. In *Fruit and Vegetable Phytochemicals: Chemistry, Nutritional Value, and Stability*, eds. L.A. de la Rosa, E. Alvarez-Parrilla and G.A. González-Aguilar, Wiley-Blackwell, Oxford, 53–88.

Arnaud M.J. 1988. The metabolism of coffee constituents. In *Coffee, Volume 3: Physiology*, eds. R.J. Clarke and R. Macrae, Elsevier Applied Science, London, Chapter 2, 33–55.

Arnaud M.J. 1993. Metabolism of caffeine and other components of coffee. In *Caffeine, Coffee and Health*, ed. S. Garattini, Raven Press, New York, 43–95.

Asatoor A.M. 1965. Aromatisation of quinic acid and shikimic acid by bacteria and the production of urinary hippurate. *Biochim Biophys Acta.* 100:290–2.

Azuma K., Ippoushi K., Nakayama M., Ito H., Higashio H. and Terao J. 2000. Absorption of chlorogenic acid and caffeic acid in rats after oral administration. *J Agric Food Chem.* 48(11):5496–500.

Ballistreri G., Continella A., Gentile A., Amenta M., Fabroni S. and Rapisarda P. 2013. Fruit quality and bioactive compounds relevant to human health of sweet cherry (*Prunus avium* L.) cultivars grown in Italy. *Food Chem.* 140(4):630–8.

Bastos D.H.M., Fornari A.C., Queiroz Y.S. and Torres E.A.F.S. 2006. Bioactive compounds content of chimarrão infusions related to the moisture of yerba maté (*Ilex paraguariensis*) leaves. *Braz Arch Bio Tech.* 49:399–404.

Bocco A., Cuvelier M.-E., Richard H. and Berset C. 1998. Antioxidant activity and phenolic composition of citrus peel and seed extracts. *J Agric Food Chem.* 146(6):2123–9.

Booth A.N., Emerson O.H., Jones F.T., DeEds F. 1957. Urinary metabolites of caffeic and chlorogenic acids. *J Biol Chem.* 229(1):51–9.

Booth A.N., Robbins D.J., Masri M.S. and DeEds F. 1960. Excretion of catechol after ingestion of quinic and shikimic acids. *Nature.* 187:691.

Bourne L.C. and Rice-Evans C. 1998. Bioavailability of ferulic acid. *Biochem Biophys Res Commun.* 253(2):222–7.

Brause A.R., Raterman J.M. 1982. Verification of authenticity of apple juice. *J Assoc Off Anal Chem.* 65(4):846–9.

Calani L., Ounnas F., Salen P., Demeilliers C., Bresciani L., Scazzina F., Brighenti F., Melegari C., Crozier A., de Lorgeril M. and Del Rio D. 2014. Bioavailability and metabolism of hydroxycinnamates in rats fed with durum wheat aleurone fractions. *Food Funct.* 5(8):1738–46.

Camarasa J., Escubedo E. and Adzet T. 1988. Pharmacokinetics of caffeic acid in rats by high-performance liquid chromatography method. *J Pharm Biomed Anal.* 6:503–10.

Cheng G.W. and Crisosto C.H. 1995. Browning potential, phenolic composition, and polyphenoloxidase activity of buffer extracts of peach and nectarine skin tissue. *J Am Soc Hort Sci.* 120(5):835–8.

Cilliers J.J.L., Singleton V.L. and Lamuela-Raventos R.M. 1990. Total polyphenols in apples and ciders: Correlation with chlorogenic acid. *J Food Sci.* 55:1458–9.

Clarke R.J. 1987. Coffee technology. In *Quality Control in the Food Industry*, 2nd Edition, Vol. 4, ed. S.H. Herschdoefer, Academic Press, London, 161–91.

Clifford M.N. 1985. Chlorogenic acids in coffee. In *Chemistry*, Vol. 1, eds. R.J. Clarke and R. Macrae, Elsevier Applied Science, London, 153–202.

Clifford M.N. 1999. Chlorogenic acids and other cinnamates: Nature, occurrence and dietary burden. *J Sci Food Agric.* 79:362–72.

Clifford M.N. and Knight S. 2004. The cinnamoyl-amino acid conjugates of green robusta coffee beans. *Food Chem.* 87:457–63.

Clifford M.N., Knight S., Surucu B. and Kuhnert N. 2006a. Characterization by LC-MS(n) of four new classes of chlorogenic acids in green coffee beans: Dimethoxycinnamoylquinic acids, diferuloylquinic acids, caffeoyl-dimethoxycinnamoylquinic acids, and feruloyl-dimethoxycinnamoylquinic acids. *J Agric Food Chem.* 54(6):1957–69.

Clifford M.N., Marks S., Knight S. and Kuhnert N. 2006b. Characterization by LC-MS(n) of four new classes of p-coumaric acid-containing diacyl chlorogenic acids in green coffee beans. *J Agric Food Chem.* 54(12):4095–101.

Clifford M.N. and Ramirez-Martinez J.R. 1990. Chlorogenic acids and purine alkaloid contents of mate (*Ilex paraguarensis*) leaf and beverage. *Food Chem.* 35:13–21.

Clinton W.E. 1985. The chemistry of coffee. In *Ile Colloque Scientifique International sur le Café*, Lomé, Paris, Asociation Scentifique Internationale du Café, 87–92.

Cotran R., Kendrick M.I. and Kass E.H. 1960. Role of intestinal bacteria in aromatization of quinic acid in man and guinea pig. *Proc Soc Exp Biol Med.* 104:424–6.

Couteau D., McCartney A.L., Gibson G.R., Williamson G. and Faulds C.B. 2001. Isolation and characterization of human colonic bacteria able to hydrolyse chlorogenic acid. *J Appl Microbiol.* 90(6):873–81.

Crozier A., Del Rio D. and Clifford M.N. 2010. Bioavailability of dietary flavonoids and phenolic compounds. *Mol Aspects Med.* 31(6):446–67.

Cui T., Nakamura K., Ma L., Li J.Z. and Kayahara H. 2005. Analyses of arbutin and chlorogenic acid, the major phenolic constituents in Oriental pear. *J Agric Food Chem.* 53(10):3882–7.

Czok G., Walter W., Knoche K. and Degener H. 1974. Über die Resorbierbarkeit von Chlorogensaüre durch die Ratte. *Z Ernährungswiss.* 13(3):108–12.

da Encarnação J.A., Farrell T.L., Ryder A., Kraut N.U., Williamson G. 2015. In vitro enzymic hydrolysis of chlorogenic acids in coffee. *Mol Nutr Food Res.* 59(2):231–9.

Dai G.L., Ma S.T., Liu S.J., Cheng X.G., Zang Y.X., Ju W.Z. and Tan H.S. 2013. Study on determination of caffeic acid, chlorogenic acid in rat plasma and their pharmacokinetics with LC-MS/MS. *Zhongguo Zhong Yao Za Zhi.* 38(21):3753–7.

Dayman J. and Jepson J.B. 1969. The metabolism of caffeic acid in humans: The dehydroxylating action of intestinal bacteria. *Biochem J.* 113(2):11P.

Del Rio D., Stalmach A., Calani L. and Crozier A. 2010. Bioavailability of coffee chlorogenic acids and green tea flavan-3-ols. *Nutrients.* 2(8):820–33.

Deshpande S., Jaiswal R., Matei M.F. and Kuhnert N. 2014. Investigation of acyl migration in mono- and dicaffeoylquinic acids under aqueous basic, aqueous acidic, and dry roasting conditions. *Agric Food Chem.* 62(37):9160–70.

Deußer H., Rogoll D., Scheppach W., Volk A., Melcher R. and Richling E. 2013. Gastrointestinal absorption and metabolism of apple polyphenols *ex vivo* by the pig intestinal mucosa in the Ussing chamber. *Biotechnol J.* 8(3):363–70.

Duarte G.S. and Farah A. 2011. Effect of simultaneous consumption of milk and coffee on chlorogenic acids' bioavailability in humans. *J Agric Food Chem.* 59(14):7925–31.

EFSA. 2011. Scientific opinion on the substantiation of health claims related to coffee, including chlorogenic acids from coffee. *EFSA J.* 9(4):2057.

El-Seedi H.R., El-Said A.M., Khalifa S.A., Göransson U., Bohlin L., Borg-Karlson A.K. and Verpoorte R. 2012. Biosynthesis, natural sources, dietary intake, pharmacokinetic properties, and biological activities of hydroxycinnamic acids. *J Agric Food Chem.* 60(44):10877–95.

Erk T., Hauser J., Williamson G., Renouf M., Steiling H., Dionisi F. and Richling E. 2014a. Structure- and dose-absorption relationships of coffee polyphenols. *Biofactors.* 40(1):103–12.

Erk T., Renouf M., Williamson G., Melcher R., Steiling H. and Richling E. 2014b. Absorption and isomerization of caffeoylquinic acids from different foods using ileostomist volunteers. *Eur J Nutr.* 53(1):159–66.

Erk T., Williamson G., Renouf M., Marmet C., Steiling H., Dionisi F., Barron D., Melcher R. and Richling E. 2012. Dose-dependent absorption of chlorogenic acids in the small intestine assessed by coffee consumption in ileostomists. *Mol Nutr Food Res.* 56:1488–500.

Farah A. 2012. Coffee constituents. In *Coffee: Emerging Health Effects and Disease Prevention*, ed. Y.-F. Chu, Wiley-Blackwell, Oxford, and the Institute of Food Technologists, 21–58.

Farah A., de Paulis T., Moreira D.P., Trugo L.C. and Martin P.R. 2006. Chlorogenic acids and lactones in regular and water-decaffeinated arabica coffees. *J Agric Food Chem.* 54(2):374–81.

Farah A., de Paulis T., Trugo L.C. and Martin P.R. 2005. Effect of roasting on the formation of chlorogenic acid lactones in coffee. *J Agric Food Chem.* 53(5):1505–13.

Farrell T.L., Dew T.P., Poquet L., Hanson P. and Williamson G. 2011. Absorption and metabolism of chlorogenic acids in cultured gastric epithelial monolayers. *Drug Metab Dispos.* 39(12):2338–46.

Ferreres F., Valentão P., Llorach R., Pinheiro C., Cardoso L., Pereira J.A., Sousa C., Seabra R.M. and Andrade P.B. 2005. Phenolic compounds in external leaves of tronchuda cabbage (*Brassica oleracea* L. var. costata DC). *J Agric Food Chem.* 53(8):2901–7.

Fineli. 2007. The Finnish food composition database (homepage on the Internet) (Release 7). KTL (National Public Health Institute), Nutrition Unit, Helsinki. Available from: http://www.fineli.fi.

Fumeaux R., Menozzi-Smarrito C., Stalmach A., Munari C., Kraehenbuehl K., Steiling H., Crozier A., Williamson G. and Barron D. 2010. First synthesis, characterization, and evidence for the presence of hydroxycinnamic acid sulfate and glucuronide conjugates in human biological fluids as a result of coffee consumption. *Org Biomol Chem.* 8(22):5199–211.

Gonthier M.P., Remesy C., Scalbert A., Cheynier V., Souquet J.M., Poutanen K. and Aura A.M. 2006. Microbial metabolism of caffeic acid and its esters chlorogenic and caftaric acids by human faecal microbiota *in vitro. Biomed Pharmacother.* 60(9):536–40.

Gonthier M.P., Verny M.A., Besson C., Rémésy C. and Scalbert A. 2003. Chlorogenic acid bioavailability largely depends on its metabolism by the gut microflora in rats. *J Nutr.* 133:1853–9.

Grosso G., Stepaniak U., Topor-Mądry R., Szafraniec K. and Pająk A. 2014. Estimated dietary intake and major food sources of polyphenols in the Polish arm of the HAPIEE study. *Nutrition.* 30(11–12):1398–403.

Gumbinger H.G., Vahlensieck U. and Winterhoff H. 1993. Metabolism of caffeic acid in the isolated perfused rat liver. *Planta Medica.* 59:491–3.

Hatcher D.W. and Kruger J.E. 1997. Simple phenolic acids in flours prepared from Canadian wheat: Relationship to ash content, color, and polyphenol oxidase activity. *Cereal Chem.* 74:337–43.

Heck C.I., Schmalko M. and Gonzalez de Mejia E. 2008. Effect of growing and drying conditions on the phenolic composition of mate teas (*Ilex paraguariensis*). *J Agric Food Chem.* 56(18):8394–403.

IARC. 1991. Monographs on the evaluation of the carcinogenic risk to humans. Coffee, tea, mate, methylxanthines and methylglyoxal, Vol. 51: Chemical composition. World Health Organization, International Agency for Research on Cancer, Geneva, 61–81.

IARC. 1993. Monograph on the evaluation of the carcinogenic risk to humans. Some naturally occurring substances: Food items and constituents, heterocyclic aromatic amines and mycotoxins, Vol. 56: Caffeic acid. World Health Organization, International Agency for Research on Cancer, Geneva, 115–34.

Im H.W., Suh B.S., Lee S.U., Kozukue N., Ohnisi-Kameyama M., Levin C.E. and Friedman M. 2008. Analysis of phenolic compounds by high-performance liquid chromatography and liquid chromatography/mass spectrometry in potato plant flowers, leaves, stems, and tubers and in home-processed potatoes. *J Agric Food Chem.* 56(9):3341–9.

Indahl, S.R. and Scheline R.R. 1973. Quinic acid aromatization in the rat. Urinary hippuric acid and catechol excretion following the singular or repeated administration of quinic acid. *Xenobiotica.* 3(8):549–56.

IUPAC Commission on the Nomenclature of Organic Chemistry (CNOC) and IUPAC-IUB Commission on Biochemical Nomenclature. 1976. Nomenclature of cyclitols, recommendations 1973. *Biochem J.* 153:23–31.

Jacobson E.A., Newmark H., Baptista J. and Bruce W.R. 1983. A preliminary investigation of the metabolism of dietary phenolics in humans. *Nutr Rep Int.* 28:1409–17.

Jaiswal R. 2011. Synthesis and analysis of the dietary relevant isomers of chlorogenic acids, their derivatives and hydroxycinnamates. PhD Thesis, Jacobs University, School of Engineering and Science, Bremen, Germany.

Jaiswal R., Matei M.F., Golon A., Witt M. and Kuhnert N. 2012. Understanding the fate of chlorogenic acids in coffee roasting using mass spectrometry based targeted and non-targeted analytical strategies. *Food Funct.* 3(9):976–84.

Jaiswal R., Patras M.A., Eravuchira P.J. and Kuhnert N. 2010. Profile and characterization of the chlorogenic acids in green Robusta coffee beans by LC-MS(n): Identification of seven new classes of compounds. *J Agric Food Chem.* 58(15):8722–37.

Kammerer D., Carle R. and Schieber A. 2004. Characterization of phenolic acids in black carrots (*Daucus carota* ssp. sativus var. atrorubens Alef.) by high-performance liquid chromatography/electrospray ionization mass spectrometry. *Rapid Commun Mass Spectrom.* 18(12):1331–40.

Kern S.M., Bennett R.N., Mellon F.A., Kroon P.A. and Garcia-Conesa M.-T. 2003. Absorption of hydroxycinnamates in humans after high-bran cereal consumption. *J Agric Food Chem.* 51(20) 6050–5.

Koli R., Erlund I., Jula A., Marniemi J., Mattila P. and Alfthan G. 2010. Bioavailability of various polyphenols from a diet containing moderate amounts of berries. *J Agric Food Chem.* 58(7):3927–32.

Konishi Y. and Kobayashi S. 2004. Transepithelial transport of chlorogenic acid, caffeic acid, and their colonic metabolites in intestinal Caco-2 cell monolayers. *J Agric Food Chem.* 52:2518–26.

Kuhnert N., Jaiswal R., Eravuchira P., El-Abassy R.M., von der Kammerb B. and Materny A. 2011. Scope and limitations of principal component analysis of high resolution LC-TOF-MS data: The analysis of the chlorogenic acid fraction in green coffee beans as a case study. *Anal Methods.* 3:144–55.

Kusnawidjaja K., Thomas H. and Dirscherl W. 1969. Uber das Vorkommen von Vanillinsäure, Ferulasäure und Kaffeesäure in pflanzlichen Nahrungsmitteln. *Z Ernahrungswiss.* 9(4):290–300.

Lafay S., Gil-Izquierdo A., Manach C., Morand C., Besson C. and Scalbert A. 2006. Chlorogenic acid is absorbed in its intact form in the stomach of rats. *J Nutr.* 136(5):1192–7.

Lafay S., Morand C., Manach C., Besson C. and Scalbert A. 2005. Absorption and metabolism of caffeic acid and chlorogenic acid in the small intestine of rats. *Br J Nutr.* 96:39–46.

Lang R., Dieminger N., Beusch A., Lee Y.M., Dunkel A., Suess B., Skurk T., Wahl A., Hauner H. and Hofmann T. 2013b. Bioappearance and pharmacokinetics of bioactives upon coffee consumption. *Anal Bioanal Chem.* 405(26):8487–503.

Lang R., Yagar E.F., Wahl A., Beusch A., Dunkel A., Dieminger N., Eggers R., Bytof G., Stiebitz H., Lantz I. and Hofmann T. 2013a. Quantitative studies on roast kinetics for bioactives in coffee. *J Agric Food Chem.* 61(49):12123–8.

Latza R. and Ammon R. 1977. Gaschromatographischer Nachweis von Stoffwechselprodukten der Chlorogensaure. *Ernährung-Umsch.* 24:169–71.

Lautemann, E. 1863. Ueber die Reduction der Chinasäure zu Benzoësäure und die Verwandlung derselben in Hippursäure im thierischen Organismus, *Justus Liebigs Ann Chem.* 125:9–13.

Lempereur I., Rouau X. and Abecassis J. 1997. Genetic and agronomic variation in arabinoxylan and ferulic acid contents of durum wheat (*Triticum durum* L.) grain and its milling fractions. *J Cereal Sci* 25:103–10.

Llorach R., Martínez-Sánchez A., Tomás-Barberán F.A., Gil M.I. and Ferreres F. 2008. Characterisation of polyphenols and antioxidant properties of five lettuce varieties and escarole. *Food Chem.* 108(3):1028–38.

Ludwig I.A., Mena P., Calani L., Cid C., Del Rio D., Lean M.E. and Crozier A. 2014. Variations in caffeine and chlorogenic acid contents of coffees: What are we drinking? *Food Funct.* 5(8):1718–26.

Ludwig I.A., Paz de Peña M., Concepción C. and Crozier A. 2013. Catabolism of coffee chlorogenic acids by human colonic microbiota. *Biofactors.* 39(6):623–32.

Maier H.G. and Grimsehl A. 1982. Die Säuren des Kaffees III. Chlorogensäuren im Röstkaffee. *Kaffee Tee Markt.* 32(23):3–6.

Manach C., Scalbert A., Morand C., Rémésy C. and Jiménez L. 2004. Polyphenols: Food sources and bioavailability. *Am J Clin Nutr.* 79(5):727–47.

Mattila P., Hellström J. and Törrönen R. 2006. Phenolic acids in berries, fruits, and beverages. *J Agric Food Chem.* 54(19):7193–9.

Menozzi-Smarrito C., Wong C.C., Meinl W., Glatt H., Fumeaux R., Munari C., Robert F., Williamson G. and Barron D. 2011. First chemical synthesis and in vitro characterization of the potential human metabolites 5-o-feruloylquinic acid 4′-sulfate and 4′-O-glucuronide. *J Agric Food Chem.* 59(10):5671–6.

Michaud J., Lesca M.F. and Roudge A.M. 1971. Métabolisme hépatique de dérivés caféiques. *Bull Soc Pharm Bordeaux.* 110:65–72.

Mills C.E., Oruna-Concha M.J., Mottram D.S., Gibson G.R. and Spencer J.P. 2013. The effect of processing on chlorogenic acid content of commercially available coffee. *Food Chem.* 141(4):3335–40.

Mills C.E., Tzounis X., Oruna-Concha M.J., Mottram D.S., Gibson G.R. and Spencer J.P. 2015. *In vitro* colonic metabolism of coffee and chlorogenic acid results in selective changes in human faecal microbiota growth. *Br J Nutr.* 113(8):1220–7.

Monente C., Ludwig I.A., Irigoyen A., De Peña M.P. and Cid C. 2015a. Assessment of total (free and bound) phenolic compounds in spent coffee extracts. *J Agric Food Chem.* 63(17):4327–34.

Monente C., Ludwig I.A., Stalmach A., de Peña M.P., Cid C. and Crozier A. 2015b. *In vitro* studies on the stability in the proximal gastrointestinal tract and bioaccessibility in Caco-2 cells of chlorogenic acids from spent coffee grounds. *Int J Food Sci Nutr.* 66(6):657–64.

Monteiro M.C. and Farah A. 2012. Chlorogenic acids in Brazilian *Coffea arabica* cultivars from various consecutive crops. *Food Chem.* 134:611–4.

Moon J.K., Yoo H.S. and Shibamoto T. 2009. Role of roasting conditions in the level of chlorogenic acid content in coffee beans: correlation with coffee acidity. *J Agric Food Chem.* 57(12):5365–9.

Moreira A.S., Coimbra M.A., Nunes F.M., Passos C.P., Santos S.A., Silvestre A.J., Silva A.M., Rangel M. and Domingues M.R. 2015. Chlorogenic acid-arabinose hybrid domains in coffee melanoidins: Evidences from a model system. *Food Chem.* 185:135–44.

Moridani M.Y., Scobie H., Jamshidzadeh A., Salehi P. and O'Brien P.J. 2001. Caffeic acid, chlorogenic acid, and dihydrocaffeic acid metabolism: Glutathione conjugate formation. *Drug Metab Dispos.* 29(11):1432–9.

Moridani M.Y., Scobie H. and O'Brien P.J. 2002. Metabolism of caffeic acid by isolated rat hepatocytes and subcellular fractions. *Toxicol Lett.* 133(2–3):141–51.

Nardini M., Cirillo E., Natella F. and Scaccini C. 2002. Absorption of phenolic acids in humans after coffee consumption. *J Agric Food Chem.* 50(20):5735–41.

Ogawa M., Suzuki Y., Endo Y., Kawamoto T. and Kayama F. 2011. Influence of coffee intake on urinary hippuric acid concentration. *Ind Health.* 49(2):195–202.

Okamura S. and Watanabe M. 1981. Determination of phenolic cinnamates in white wine and their effect on wine quality. *Agric Biol Chem.* 45(9):2063–70.

Olthof M.R., Hollman P.C., Buijsman M.N., van Amelsvoort J.M. and Katan M.B. 2003. Chlorogenic acid, quercetin-3-rutinoside and black tea phenols are extensively metabolized in humans. *J Nutr.* 133(6):1806–14.

Olthof M.R., Hollman P.C. and Katan M.B. 2001. Chlorogenic acid and caffeic acid are absorbed in humans. *J Nutr.* 131(1):66–71.

Omar M.H., Mullen W., Stalmach A., Auger C., Rouanet J.M., Teissedre P.L., Caldwell S.T., Hartley R.C. and Crozier A. 2012. Absorption, disposition, metabolism, and excretion of [3-(14)C]caffeic acid in rats. *J Agric Food Chem.* 60(20):5205–14.

Ovaskainen M.L., Törrönen R., Koponen J.M., Sinkko H., Hellström J., Reinivuo H. and Mattila P. 2008. Dietary intake and major food sources of polyphenols in Finnish adults. *J Nutr.* 138(3):562–6.

Parkar S.G., Trower T.M. and Stevenson D.E. 2013. Fecal microbial metabolism of polyphenols and its effects on human gut microbiota. *Anaerobe.* 23:12–9.

Peppercorn M.A. and Goldman P. 1971. Caffeic acid metabolism by bacteria of the human gastrointestinal tract. *J Bacteriol.* 108:996–1000.

Peppercorn M.A. and Goldman P. 1972. Caffeic acid metabolism by gnotobiotic rats and their intestinal bacteria. *Proc Natl Acad Sci USA.* 69(6):1413–5.

Radtke J., Linseisen J. and Wolfram G. 1998. Phenolsäurezufuhr Erwachsener in einem bayerischen Teilkollektiv der Nationalen Verzehrsstudie. *Z Ernahrungswiss.* 37:190–7.

Raimondi S., Anighoro A., Quartieri A., Amaretti A., Tomás-Barberán F.A., Rastelli G. and Rossi M. 2015. Role of bifidobacteria in the hydrolysis of chlorogenic acid. *Microbiologyopen.* 4(1):41–52.

Rapisarda P., Bellomo S.E. and Intelisano S. 2001. Storage temperature effects on blood orange fruit quality. *J Agric Food Chem.* 49(7):3230–5.

Rapisarda P., Carollo G., Fallico B., Tomaselli F. and Maccarone E. 1998. Hydroxycinnamic acids as markers of Italian blood orange juices. *J Agric Food Chem.* 46(2):464–70.

Rechner A.R., Smith M.A., Kuhnle G., Gibson G.R., Debnam E.S., Srai S.K., Moore K.P. and Rice-Evans C.A. 2004. Colonic metabolism of dietary polyphenols: Influence of structure on microbial fermentation products. *Free Radic Biol Med.* 36(2):212–25.

Rechner A.R., Spencer J.P.E., Kuhnle G., Hahn U. and Rice-Evans C.A. 2001. Novel biomarkers of the metabolism of caffeic acid derivatives *in vivo*. *Free Radic Biol Med.* 30:1213–22.

Renouf M., Guy P.A., Marmet C., Fraering A.L., Longet K., Moulin J., Enslen M., Barron D., Dionisi F., Cavin C., Williamson G. and Steiling H. 2010b. Measurement of caffeic and ferulic acid equivalents in plasma after coffee consumption: small intestine and colon are key sites for coffee metabolism. *Mol Nutr Food Res.* 54(6):760–6.

Renouf M., Guy P., Marmet C., Longet K., Fraering A.L., Moulin J., Barron D., Dionisi F., Cavin C., Steiling H. and Williamson G. 2010a. Plasma appearance and correlation between coffee and green tea metabolites in human subjects. *Br J Nutr.* 104(11):1635–40.

Renouf M., Marmet C., Giuffrida F., Lepage M., Barron D., Beaumont M., Williamson G. and Dionisi F. 2014. Dose-response plasma appearance of coffee chlorogenic and phenolic acids in adults. *Mol Nutr Food Res.* 58(2):301–9.

Renouf M., Marmet C., Guy P., Fraering A.L., Longet K., Moulin J., Enslen M., Barron D., Cavin C., Dionisi F., Rezzi S., Kochhar S., Steiling H. and Williamson G. 2010c. Nondairy creamer, but not milk, delays the appearance of coffee phenolic acid equivalents in human plasma. *J Nutr.* 140(2):259–63.

Rodrigues N.P., Salva T.J.C. and Bragagnolo N. 2015. Influence of coffee genotype on bioactive compounds and the *in vitro* capacity to scavenge reactive oxygen and nitrogen species. *J Agric Food Chem.* 63(19):4815–26.

Rodríguez-Arcos R.C., Smith A.C. and Waldron K.W. 2004. Ferulic acid crosslinks in asparagus cell walls in relation to texture. *J Agric Food Chem.* 52(15):4740–50.

Scheline R.R. and Midtvedt T. 1970. Absence of dehydroxylation of caffeic acid in germ-free rats. *Experientia.* 26(10):1068–9.

Schütz K., Kammerer D., Carle R. and Schieber A. 2004. Identification and quantification of caffeoylquinic acids and flavonoids from artichoke (*Cynara scolymus* L.) heads, juice, and pomace (pulpe) by HPLC-DAD-ESI/MS(n). *J Agric Food Chem.* 52(13):4090–6.

Selma M.V., Espín J.C. and Tomás-Barberán F.A. 2009. Interaction between phenolics and gut microbiota: Role in human health. *J Agric Food Chem.* 57(15):6485–501.

Shaw K.N.F., Gutenstein M. and Jepson J.B. 1963. Intestinal flora and diet in relation to m-hydroxyphenyl acids of human urine. In *Proc. 5th Int. Cong. Biochem.*, 1961, Moscow, N.M. Sissakian, Vol. 9, Pergamon Press, Oxford, 427.

Smrke S., Kroslakova I., Gloess A.N. and Yeretzian C. 2015. Differentiation of degrees of ripeness of Catuai and Tipica green coffee by chromatographical and statistical techniques. *Food Chem.* 174:637–42.

Sosulski F., Krygier K. and Hogge L. 1982. Free, esterified, and insoluble-bound phenolic acids. 3. Composition of phenolic acids in cereal and potato flours. *J Agric Food Chem.* 30:337–40.

Spencer J.P., Chowrimootoo G., Choudhury R., Debnam E.S., Srai S.K. and Rice-Evans C. 1999. The small intestine can both absorb and glucuronidate luminal flavonoids. *FEBS Lett.* 458(2):224–30.

Spiller, M.A. 1984. The chemical components of coffee. In *The Methylxanthine Beverages and Foods: Chemistry, Consumption, and Health Effects*, eds. G.A. Spiller, Alan R. Liss, New York, 91–147.

Stalmach A., Mullen W., Barron D., Uchida K., Yokota T., Cavin C., Steiling H., Williamson G. and Crozier A. 2009. Metabolite profiling of hydroxycinnamate derivatives in plasma and urine after the ingestion of coffee by humans: Identification of biomarkers of coffee consumption. *Drug Metab Dispos.* 37(8):1749–58.

Stalmach A., Steiling H., Williamson G. and Crozier A. 2010. Bioavailability of chlorogenic acids following acute ingestion of coffee by humans with an ileostomy. *Arch Biochem Biophys.* 501(1):98–105.

Stalmach A., Williamson G. and Crozier A. 2014. Impact of dose on the bioavailability of coffee chlorogenic acids in humans. *Food Funct.* 5(8):1727–37.

Sulaiman S.F., Moon J.K. and Shibamoto T. 2011. Investigation of optimum roasting conditions to obtain possible health benefit supplement, antioxidants from coffee beans. *J Diet Suppl.* 8(3):293–310.

Teuchy H. and Van Sumere C.F. 1971. The metabolism of (1-^{14}C) phenylalanine, (3-^{14}C) cinnamic acid and (2-^{14}C) ferulic acid in the rat. *Arch Int Physiol Biochim.* 79(3):589–618.

Tomás-Barberán F., García-Villalba R., Quartieri A., Raimondi S., Amaretti A., Leonardi A. and Rossi M. 2014. *In vitro* transformation of chlorogenic acid by human gut microbiota. *Mol Nutr Food Res.* 58(5):1122–31.

Trugo L.C. and Macrae R. 1984. Chlorogenic acid composition of instant coffees. *Analyst.* 109(3):263–6.

Truong V.D., McFeeters R.F., Thompson R.T., Dean L.L. and Shofran B. 2007. Phenolic acid content and composition in leaves and roots of common commercial sweet potato (*Ipomea batatas* L.) cultivars in the United States. *J Food Sci.* 72(6):C343–9.

Tsuji A. and Tamai I. 1996. Carrier-mediated intestinal transport of drugs. *Pharm Res.* 13(7):963–77.

Tudela J.A., Cantos E., Espín J.C., Tomás-Barberán F.A. and Gil M.I. 2002. Induction of antioxidant flavonol biosynthesis in fresh-cut potatoes. Effect of domestic cooking. *J Agric Food Chem.* 50(21):5925–31.

Viani R. 1988. Physiologically active substances in Coffee. In *Coffee*, vol. 3, Physiology, eds. R.J. Clarke and R. Macrae, Elsevier Applied Science, London and New York, 1–31.

Viani R. 1993. The composition of coffee. In *Caffeine, Coffee, and Health*, ed. S Garattini, Raven Press, New York, 17–41.

Wakabayashi K., Soga K., Hoson T., Kotake T., Yamazaki T., Higashibata A., Ishioka N., Shimazu T., Fukui K., Osada I., Kasahara H. and Kamada M. 2015. Suppression of hydroxycinnamate network formation in cell walls of rice shoots grown under microgravity conditions in space. *PLoS One.* 10(9):e0137992.

Wang C. and Zuo Y. 2011. Ultrasound-assisted hydrolysis and gas chromatography-mass spectrometric determination of phenolic compounds in cranberry products. *Food Chem.* 128(2):562–8.

Wanga C., Zuo Y., Vinson J.A. and Deng Y. 2012. Absorption and excretion of cranberry-derived phenolics in humans. *Food Chem.* 132:1420–8.

Westendorf J. and Czok G. 1983. Die biliäre Ausscheidung choleretisch aktiver Zimtsäure-Derivate durch die RatteZ. *Ernahrungswiss.* 22(4):255–70.

Willeman H., Hance P., Fertin A., Voedts N., Duhal N., Goossens J.F. and Hilbert J.L. 2014. A method for the simultaneous determination of chlorogenic acid and sesquiterpene lactone content in industrial chicory root foodstuffs. *Scientific World J.* 2014:583180.

Wojdyło A., Nowicka P., Laskowski P. and Oszmiański J. 2014. Evaluation of sour cherry (*Prunus cerasus* L.) fruits for their polyphenol content, antioxidant properties, and nutritional components. *J Agric Food Chem.* 62(51):12332–45.

Wolffram S., Weber T., Grenacher B. and Scharrer E. 1995. A Na(+)-dependent mechanism is involved in mucosal uptake of cinnamic acid across the jejunal brush border in rats. *J Nutr.* 125(5):1300–8.

Wong C.C., Meinl W., Glatt H.R., Barron D., Stalmach A., Steiling H., Crozier A. and Williamson G. 2010. *In vitro* and *in vivo* conjugation of dietary hydroxycinnamic acids by UDP-glucuronosyltransferases and sulfotransferases in humans. *J Nutr Biochem.* 21(11):1060–8.

Yuan J.P., Wang J.H. and Liu X. 2007. Metabolism of dietary soy isoflavones to equol by human intestinal microflora: Implications for health. *Mol Nutr Food Res.* 51:765–81.

Zhang K. and Zuo Y. 2004. GC-MS determination of flavonoids and phenolic and benzoic acids in human plasma after consumption of cranberry juice. *J Agric Food Chem.* 52(2):222–7.

Zhao Z., Egashira Y. and Sanada H. 2004. Ferulic acid is quickly absorbed from rat stomach as the free form and then conjugated mainly in liver. *J Nutr.* 134:3083–8.

5 Mechanism of the Inhibition by Chlorogenic Acids against Postprandial Increase in Blood Glucose Level

Yusaku Narita and Kuniyo Inouye

CONTENTS

5.1 CHLOROGENIC ACIDS

Chlorogenic acids (CGAs) are a family of esters that are structural analogs of quinic acid (QA) that carry either one or multiple cinnamate derivatives such as caffeic (CA), ferulic (FA), and *p*-coumaric acids. CGAs are widely distributed among plants such as apple, prune, yacon, blueberry, broccoli, burdock, and sweet potato,[1–5] and are one of the most commonly consumed polyphenols in diets worldwide. QA has a chemical structure with an equatorial hydroxyl group at the 4- and 5-positions and an axial hydroxyl group at the 1- and 3-positions (Figure 5.1).[6–8] The nomenclature of CGAs follows the preferred IUPAC numbering system with QA as the parent structure.[6–8] In general, 5-caffeoylquinic acid (5-CQA) is called chlorogenic acid (CGA). The UV-visible absorption spectra of CGA in distilled water at room temperature shows two absorption peaks at 324 and 217 nm, two shoulders at 296 and 240 nm, and one trough at 262 nm.[9] Commonly, quantitative and qualitative analysis of CGAs from coffee is performed using reverse-phase high-performance liquid chromatography (HPLC) with a UV or photodiode array detector.[10–13] Green coffee beans have nine main CGA isomers: three mono-caffeoylquinic acids (CQAs) (3-, 4-, and 5-CQAs), three di-caffeoylquinic acids (diCQAs) (3,4-, 3,5-, and 4,5-diCQAs), and three mono-feruloylquinic acid (FQAs) (3-, 4-, and 5-FQAs) (Figure 5.1).[8,13] The two species of coffee in world trade are *Coffea arabica* (arabica coffee) and *Coffea canephora* "Robusta" (robusta coffee), and they account for approximately 75% and 24% of the market, respectively. Robusta coffee [3.92–11.32% (w/w) dry matter] contains more CGAs than arabica coffee does [3.02–7.49% (w/w) dry matter] (Table 5.1).[8,14–18] Although CGAs in green coffee beans and brewed coffee are conventionally analyzed using HPLC, analysis of trace amounts of CGAs using liquid chromatography–mass spectrometry (LC–MS) has recently been reported.[19–23] Eighty-two CGAs have been detected in green coffee beans by LC–MS analysis.[19–22]

5.2 COFFEE DRINKING AND RISK OF TYPE 2 DIABETES

Diabetes is a common chronic disease. According to the International Diabetes Federation (IDF), there were 387 million people with diabetes in 2014, and the prevalence of diabetes in people in the age range of 20–79 years was 8.3%, with 1/12 of the human population estimated to be diabetic.[24] The IDF predicted that if effective measures to reduce the number of diabetic patients were not taken, the number would become 592 million by 2035. As of 2014, the country with the largest number of diabetes patients was China (96.29 million people), the second largest rate is India (66.85 million), followed by the United States (25.78 million). The number of diabetic patients in Japan was 7.21 million, ranking in 10th place. The number of people dying of diabetes was 4.9 million per year, meaning that every 7 s, one person dies of diabetes somewhere in the world.

Diabetes is an autoinflammatory syndrome that is a collection of many disorders such as hyperglycemia, dyslipidemia, and insulin resistance.[25] Diabetes has been divided into type 1 diabetes (T1D) and type 2 diabetes (T2D). T1D is a congenital autoimmune disease with an absolute deficiency in insulin secretion resulting from destruction of pancreatic β-cells. In contrast, T2D is an acquired disease with a combination of insulin resistance and inadequate insulin secretion caused by interacting genetic, diet, and lifestyle factors. Currently, measures to prevent T2D on a global scale are considered urgent because the prevalence of the condition is increasing rapidly in developed and developing countries, and it is becoming a worldwide health problem. Hypertension is common in patients with T2D, affecting up to 60% of diabetic patients.[26] Epidemiological studies have indicated that subjects with hypertension are more likely to develop T2D.[27] Thus, diabetes and hypertension have many common risk factors and elements such as sedentary lifestyle, lack of exercise, obesity, insulin resistance, mental stress, and aging. Several dietary factors have also been associated with insulin sensitivity, glucose metabolism, and risk of hypertension and T2D.[28,29]

There have been many epidemiologic studies of coffee drinking aimed at investigating its effect on the risk of cancer and chronic diseases. Coffee drinking may reduce the risk of liver cancer.[30–33] As to its effect on diabetes, Van Dam and Hu selected for meta-analysis 7 case–control and 8 cohort studies, Huxley et al. selected 18 cohort studies, and Ding et al. selected 1 case–control and 27 cohort studies.[34–36]

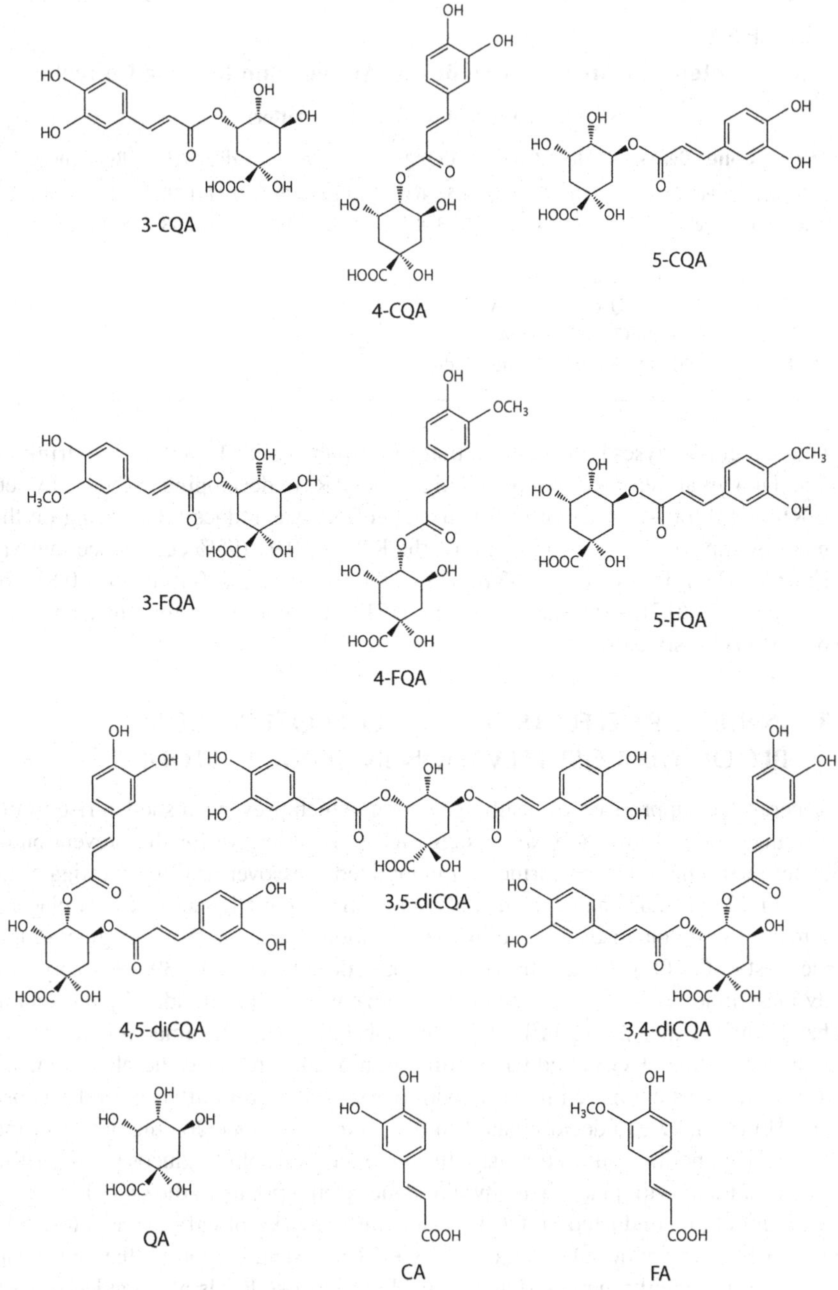

3-CQA

4-CQA

5-CQA

3-FQA

4-FQA

5-FQA

3,5-diCQA

4,5-diCQA

3,4-diCQA

QA

CA

FA

FIGURE 5.1 Chemical structures of nine CGAs, QA, CA, and FA.

TABLE 5.1
CGA Contents in Green Coffee Beans (Arabica and Robusta Coffee)

	Content (w/w %, Dry Matter)				
Green Coffee Beans	Total CGA[a]	CQA[b]	FQA[c]	diCQA[d]	References
Arabica coffee	3.02–7.49	2.58–6.63	0.12–0.79	0.27–1.39	8, 15–18
Robusta coffee	3.92–11.32	2.79–8.33	0.47–1.19	0.61–1.98	8, 14, 15, 18

[a] Total of CQA, FQA, and diCQA.
[b] Total of 3-CQA, 4-CQA, and 5-CQA.
[c] Total of 3-FQA, 4-FQA, and 5-FQA.
[d] Total of 3,4-diCQA, 3,5-diCQA, and 4,5-diCQA.

All these meta-analyses indicated that the risk of diabetes can be reduced by drinking coffee. Ding et al. reported that the relative risk (RR) in developing diabetes, by setting RR = 1.0 for the case without drinking coffee, was reduced depending on the number of cups of coffee drunk per day; the RR was 0.92 (95% confidence interval [CI]: 0.90 – 0.94) for one cup, 0.85 (0.82 – 0.88) for two cups, 0.79 (0.75 – 0.83) for three cups, 0.75 (0.71 – 0.80) for four cups, 0.71 (0.65 – 0.76) for five cups, and 0.67 (0.61 – 0.74) for six cups.[36]

5.3 INHIBITORY EFFECTS OF CGAs ON POSTPRANDIAL BLOOD GLUCOSE ELEVATION IN CLINICAL STUDIES

In general, the suppression of insulin secretion, which prevents a sudden rise in the blood glucose level after a meal, is suggested to be effective for the prevention of diabetes. Van Dijk et al. performed a randomized crossover trial to investigate the effects of 12 g decaffeinated coffee, 500 mg CGAs, 1 g trigonelline, or a placebo (1 g mannitol) on glucose and insulin concentrations during a 75-g oral glucose tolerance test (OGTT) in 15 healthy, overweight male subjects [age, 39.9 ± 16.5 years; body mass index (BMI) which means a person's weight (kg) divided by the square of height (m^2), 27.6 ± 2.2 kg/m^2].[37] Each test substance was consumed 30 min before the glucose uptake. CGAs and trigonelline significantly reduced the blood glucose and insulin levels compared to those with placebo at 15 min after an oral glucose load.[37] However, 12 g of decaffeinated coffee, which contained 264 mg of CGAs and 72 mg of trigonelline, showed no significant changes in blood glucose and insulin levels from those with placebo at any of the measuring points in the OGTT.[37]

Graham et al. conducted an OGTT test using 5 mg/kg of caffeine as a test substance in 18 young male subjects (age, 23.3 ± 1.1 years) and reported that their insulin levels significantly increased and their blood glucose levels also tended to rise, with no significant difference between 15 and 120 min after an oral glucose load.[38] The test substance was consumed 60 min before the oral glucose load. It is noteworthy from this test that the results showed that the caffeine intake group had a 60% greater area under the curve (AUC) for insulin during the OGTT than that of the placebo group, but a corresponding rise in blood glucose levels was not seen with the AUC for blood glucose of the caffeine intake group showed only 37% greater than that of the placebo group. Graham et al. proposed that caffeine inhibited the action of insulin by promoting glucose uptake in skeletal muscle, given that caffeine is a nonselective adenosine receptor antagonist, and that such antagonists reduce cell-surface GLUT-4 and glucose uptake *in vitro* in resting rat muscles exposed to insulin.[38]

Moisey et al. investigated the influence of drinking 5 mg/kg of caffeinated coffee or 5 mg/kg of decaffeinated coffee as a test substance for insulin and blood glucose levels after ingestion of low- or high-glycemic index (GI) cereals with nonfat milk on 10 young male subjects (age, 23.3 ± 1.1 years; BMI, 25.3 ± 1.1 kg/m^2).[39] Here, the GI values of the low- or high-GI cereals with nonfat milk were 41 and 81, respectively. The cereal and nonfat milk contained 75 g of carbohydrate and the test substance was consumed 60 min before ingestion of the cereal with nonfat milk. The blood glucose levels after ingestion of caffeinated coffee and the high-GI cereal with nonfat milk were significantly greater than those after ingestion of decaffeinated coffee at the times of 30, 45, 60, 90, and 120 min. The blood glucose levels after ingestion of the low-GI cereal and nonfat milk with caffeinated coffee was significantly greater than those after the ingestion with decaffeinated coffee at the times of 15, 45, 60, 90, and 120 min. The AUCs for blood glucose in the groups consuming low- or high-GI cereals and nonfat milk with caffeinated coffee were approximately 3 and 2.5 times higher, respectively, than those of the groups consuming them with decaffeinated coffee. The insulin level after ingestion of high-GI cereal and nonfat milk with caffeinated coffee was significantly greater than that after the ingestion with decaffeinated coffee at 120 min. The blood glucose levels after the ingestions of low-GI cereal and nonfat milk with caffeinated coffee were significantly greater than those with decaffeinated coffee at the times of 60, 90, and 120 min. The insulin levels in the group consuming low- or high-GI cereals and nonfat milk with caffeinated coffee were approximately 1.3—1.4 times higher, respectively, than those of the group consuming them with decaffeinated coffee. From these results, Moisey et al. suggested that the intake of caffeinated coffee markedly reduced the insulin sensitivity in comparison with that with decaffeinated coffee.[39]

Iwai et al. reported that the influence of decaffeinated green coffee bean extract, after extraction with 56% ethanol from green coffee beans decaffeinated by the supercritical CO_2 process, filtered, concentrated, and spray-dried, on blood glucose levels rose after rice ball ingestion in 41 healthy subjects (age, 34.8 ± 8.0 years; BMI, 22.0 ± 3.1 kg/m^2).[40] This test was performed as a randomized, double-blind, placebo-controlled, single-ingestion crossover clinical trial, and water or water containing 100 or 300 mg of decaffeinated green coffee bean extracts were consumed simultaneously with 200 g of rice balls, with all being consumed in 10 min. The blood glucose level at 30 min after the ingestion of 300 mg of the extract was significantly lower than that of the placebo (Figure 5.2). Moreover, the blood glucose levels were slightly lower at 30-min after ingestion of 100 mg of the extract than those of the ingestion of the placebo. However, a significant reduction in postprandial blood glucose levels after the ingestion of 100 mg of the extract was observed only to the high-glycemic-response group (n = 18; age, 35.1 ± 8.5 years; BMI, 21.4 ± 3.0 kg/m^2) (Figure 5.2). In other analyses, the insulin levels were not different from those with

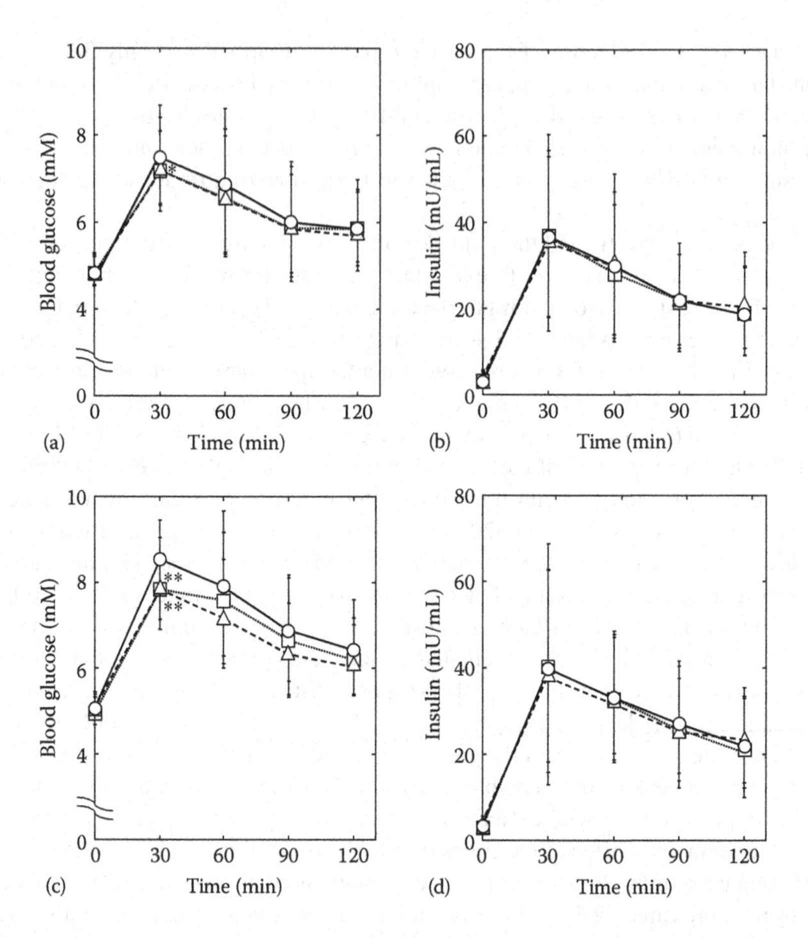

FIGURE 5.2 Changes in postprandial blood glucose and insulin response after ingestion of decaffeinated green coffee bean extract. Data are expressed as means ± SD. Significant difference was shown with repeated analysis of variance followed by Dunnett's multiple comparison. $^*p < 0.05$, $^{**}p < 0.01$ vs. control. Symbols are as follows: placebo group (open circles), 100 mg decaffeinated green coffee bean extract ingestion group (open triangles), 300 mg decaffeinated green coffee bean extract ingestion group (open squares). (a) Blood glucose levels in all subjects ($n = 41$), (b) insulin response in all subjects, (c) blood glucose levels in high-glycemic-response subjects ($n = 18$), (d) insulin response in high-glycemic subjects. (From Iwai et al., 2012, *Food Sci. Technol. Res.* 18, 849–860.)

the placebo (Figure 5.2). The decaffeinated green coffee bean extract contained approximately 40% CGAs, 0.003% caffeine, and 3.2% trigonelline. Iwai et al. considered that the main ingredients contributing to the inhibitory effect on the rise in postprandial blood glucose levels might be CGAs, given that CGAs inhibit glucose transport and enzyme inhibition.

These reports together suggest that the ingestion of up to 264 mg CGAs does not but that of 500 mg CGAs may significantly affect the insulin sensitivity.[37,40] They also suggest that the amounts of CGAs required to control the blood glucose levels after carbohydrate intake may be dependent on the intake timings, such as before the meals or during the meals.[37,40]

Caffeine is contained not only in roasted but also in green coffee beans. Caffeine intake may increase insulin resistance and raise the postprandial blood glucose levels. Accordingly, it may be undesirable in the treatment and prevention of diabetes. Many clinical trials have been performed to determine the effects of intake of caffeinated and decaffeinated coffee on insulin sensitivity and postprandial blood sugar levels. However, reports often do not describe the amount of caffeine in the decaffeinated coffee. The caffeine content in decaffeinated coffee is less than that of caffeinated coffee but is not zero. In future studies, it should be considered whether caffeine intake may increase the insulin sensitivity and postprandial blood glucose level with the parallel clinical trials with decaffeinated coffee and decaffeinated green coffee beans. In the previous studies investigating the effects of intake of coffee and coffee components (such as caffeine, trigonelline, and CGAs) on postprandial blood glucose and insulin levels, the timing of administration of these test samples in many cases has been assumed according to the previous studies to be before or during a meal. However, in general, coffee is drunk after a meal. For this reason, studies in which coffee or coffee components are administered after carbohydrate intake will remain important in the future.

5.4 INHIBITION OF α-AMYLASE AND α-GLUCOSIDASE BY CGAs

Dietary carbohydrate is not absorbed directly from the intestine unless it has been subjected to the action of α-glycosidases (EC 3.2.1) such as α-amylase and α-glucosidase in saliva and the small intestine. Inhibition of α-glycosidase activity would be an effective approach to controlling hyperglycemia. Specific pancreatic α-glycosidase inhibitors such as acarbose, voglibose, and miglitol are used clinically to prevent hyperglycemia.[41,42] Recently, interest in diabetes prevention employing components derived from natural products instead of these chemical compounds has increased.

α-Amylases (1,4-α-D-glucan-glucanohydrolase, EC 3.2.1.1) are endoglucanases that catalyze the hydrolysis of the α-1,4-glucosidic linkages in starch and related polysaccharides, and they are secretory products of the pancreas and salivary glands in mammals. α-Amylase inhibitors assist in the cure and prevention of diabetes and obesity by controlling the increase of postprandial blood glucose levels by delaying and blocking postprandial carbohydrate digestion and absorption. Rohn et al. reported that the hydrolysis of starch by crude porcine pancreas α-amylase (PPA) was inhibited by 5-CQA, CA, FA, and QA, and that the inhibitory potencies were in the order 5-CQA > CA > FA > QA.[43] Narita and Inouye reported that purified PPA isozyme (PPA-I) catalyzed the hydrolysis of *p*-nitrophenyl-α-D-maltoside (G_2-*p*NP) as a substrate (Table 5.2).[44–46] The strongest inhibitory effect of the nine main CGAs contained in green coffee beans and structural components of the CGAs against PPA-I hydrolysis of G_2-*p*NP was from 3,4-diCQA and 4,5-diCQA, followed, in descending order, by 3,5-diCQA, 5-CQA, 4-CQA, 3-CQA, CA, 5-FQA, 4-FQA, 3-FQA, FA, and QA (Table 5.2).[44–46] The authors described the mechanism of inhibition of PPA-I by CGAs and their architectural components. The inhibition modes

TABLE 5.2
Kinetic Parameters of Inhibitors of PPA-I Activity with G^2-*p*NP and Thermodynamic Binding Parameters for Interactions of Inhibitors with PPA-I

Inhibitor	IC_{50} (mM)	K_i (mM)	K_i' (mM)	K_m (mM)	ΔG°_{Ki} (kJ/mol)	$\Delta G^\circ_{Ki'}$ (kJ/mol)	ΔH°_{Ki} (kJ/mol)	$\Delta H^\circ_{Ki'}$ (kJ/mol)	$T\Delta S^\circ_{Ki}$ (kJ/mol)	$T\Delta S^\circ_{Ki'}$ (kJ/mol)	References
3-CQA	0.23	0.61	0.13	2.37	N. A.	N. A.	N. A.	N. A.	N. A.	N. A.	45
4-CQA	0.12	0.24	0.10	3.77	N. A.	N. A.	N. A.	N. A.	N. A.	N. A.	45
5-CQA	0.08	0.23	0.05	3.04	–21.7	–25.5	–70.3	–59.0	–48.5	–33.4	44
3-FQA	2.55	6.14	1.74	2.34	N. A.	N. A.	N. A.	N. A.	N. A.	N. A.	45
4-FQA	2.02	4.34	1.40	2.97	N. A.	N. A.	N. A.	N. A.	N. A.	N. A.	45
5-FQA	1.09	1.95	0.99	4.51	–16.2	–17.3	–40.5	–36.9	–24.3	–19.6	45
3,4-diCQA	0.02	0.01	0.02	7.70	N. A.	N. A.	N. A.	N. A.	N. A.	N. A.	45
3,5-diCQA	0.03	0.10	0.01	1.18	–23.6	–28.9	–47.8	–74.8	–24.2	–43.8	45
4,5-diCQA	0.02	0.01	0.03	9.02	–27.9	–25.9	–47.4	–53.0	–19.5	–27.1	45
CA	0.40	1.12	0.27	3.04	–17.9	–18.0	–78.9	–58.3	–61.0	–40.3	44
FA	5.45	11.17	4.87	3.15	N. A.	N. A.	N. A.	N. A.	N. A.	N. A.	45
QA	26.5	N. A.[a]	N. A.	N. A.	N. A.	N. A.	N. A.	N. A.	N. A.	N. A.	44

[a] N.A., not analyzed.

of the nine CGAs, CA, and FA against the PPA-I-catalyzed hydrolysis of G_2-*p*NP were determined to be of mixed type.[44–46] Narita and Inouye proposed a hypothetical model for the inhibitor-binding site (I site), which was separated into two subsites: namely, the CA or FA subsite and the QA subsite, on the enzyme surface. CA (or FA) and QA sub-structures connected via an ester bond in CQA (or FQA) were proposed to bind to corresponding subsites in the I site.[44–46] 3-CQA, 4-CQA, 5-CQA, 3-FQA, 4-FQA, 5-FQA, 3,5-diCQA, CA, and FA were proposed to bind to the enzyme–substrate (ES) complex more strongly than to free enzyme (E) because the modes of their inhibition of PPA-1 with G_2-*p*NP were demonstrated to be of mixed type with $K_i > K_i'$ (K_i and K_i' are inhibitor constants for the free enzyme and enzyme–substrate complex, respectively) (Table 5.2). In contrast, 3,4-diCQA and 4,5-diCQA bind to free E more strongly than to ES complex because their inhibition modes were of mixed type, with $K_i < K_i'$ (Table 5.2). The K_i and K_i' values of CQAs were one-half, one-third, and one-fifth of the respective values of CA, and these values of FQAs were also one-half, one-third, and one-fifth of the respective values of FA (Table 5.2). These results support the above hypothetical model for the I site, meaning that CQA and FQA bind to the same I site separated into two subsites. It has been suggested that the interactions of 5-CQA, 5-FQA, 3,5-diCQA, 3,4-diCQA, or CA with PPA-I are enthalpy driven, given that the interactions were exothermic with a large increase in $\Delta H°$ (Table 5.2).[44–46]

CGAs have also an inhibitory effect on α-glucosidases with maltase and sucrose.[47] The inhibitory activity of 3-CQA against rat intestine crude α-glucosidase using maltose as substrate is lower than that of 5-CQA, in agreement with the inhibitory effects of PPA-I.[45,47] However, the inhibition modes of 5-CQA and 3-CQA against the crude α-glucosidase with maltose are of the noncompetitive type and are different from the mixed-type inhibition shown against PPA-1 with G_2-*p*NP.[47] CGAs inhibit enzymes other than α-amylase and α-glucosidase, such as lipase and glucose-6-phosphatase.[48,49]

Type 2 diabetes causes postprandial hyperglycemia via a decrease and/or a delay in the timing of insulin secretion corresponding to the rise of postprandial blood glucose levels and insulin resistance in the liver and skeletal muscle. The insulin action is more effective on postprandial hyperglycemia when inhibitors against α-glucosidase and α-amylase are present because the insulin secretion and the rise of the blood glucose value occur by gradual absorption and decomposition of carbohydrate under the action of the inhibitors. We propose that CGAs have a potential role in the prevention and treatment of diabetes, given their inhibitory effects on α-amylase and α-glucosidase similar to those of acarbose, a diabetes drug.

5.5 INHIBITION OF GLUCOSE ABSORPTION IN SMALL INTESTINE BY CGAs

Glucose is absorbed into enterocytes mainly through the sodium-dependent glucose transporter (SGLT-1). SGLT-1 transports 1 mol of glucose and 2 mol of sodium ions into the cell using a high extracellular sodium ion concentration generated by a sodium-potassium pump (Na^+/K^+-ATPase). Welsch et al. reported that glucose uptake by brush border membrane vesicles, which are spherical membrane vesicles on which SGLT1 is expressed, isolated from the small intestine in rat was inhibited by 80%, 35%, and 38% by 1 mM of 5-CQA, CA, and FA, respectively.[50] Green tea polyphenols such as epicatechin and epigallocatechin gallate have been shown to inhibit glucose transport by brush border membrane vesicles isolated from small intestine in rabbit.[51] CGAs, CA, and FA inhibit SGLT1 as well as other polyphenols.[52]

5.6 CONCLUSION

There have been many epidemiologic studies indicating that drinking coffee correlates to a decrease in the risk of diabetes. Reduction in the relative risk of developing diabetes was suggested to depend on the number of cups of coffee drunk per day in the range between 1 and 6 cups/day based on a study reported by Ding et al. However, insulin levels increased significantly and blood glucose levels also tended to rise, though non-significantly, with consumption of caffeinated coffee in an OGTT in humans. Insulin sensitivity decreased with consumption of caffeinated coffee.[39], and this appears to contradict the results of this clinical study, and the previously mentioned epidemiological study. Although insulin resistance is transiently increased by caffeine intake, insulin sensitivity is suggested to improve with chronic caffeine intake via the reduction of inflammatory adipocytokine expression.[53] In any case, further studies are needed to establish the relationship of consumption of caffeinated coffee or caffeine with diabetes.

CGAs are major components of coffee and have inhibitory effects on α-glucosidase and α-amylase and on glucose transport through SGLT1. Their consumption contributes to moderate postprandial blood glucose level increases. CGA ingestion led to significantly lower blood glucose concentrations in an OGTT. Intake of decaffeinated green coffee bean extract containing 40% CGAs suppressed a blood glucose increase observed with a placebo in a clinical trial involving simultaneous consumption of rice balls and extract. It is concluded that consumption of CGAs and decaffeinated green coffee bean extract is effective for the prevention of diabetes.

REFERENCES

1. Takenaka, M., Yan, X., Ono, H., Yoshida, M., Nagata, T., and Nakanishi, T. 2003. Caffeic acid derivatives in the roots of yacon (*Smallanthus sonchifolius*). *J. Agric. Food Chem.* 51:793–796.
2. Maruta, Y., Kawabata, J., and Niki, R. 1995. Antioxidative caffeoylquinic acid derivatives in the roots of burdock (*Arctium lappa* L.). *J. Agric. Food Chem.* 43:2592–2595.
3. Islam, M. S., Yoshimoto, M., Yahara, S., Okuno, S., Ishiguro, K., and Yamakawa, O. 2002. Identification and characterization of foliar polyphenolic composition in sweetpotato (*Ipomoea batatas* L.) genotypes. *J. Agric. Food Chem.* 50:3718–3722.
4. Nakatani, N., Kayano, S., Kikuzaki, H., Sumino, K., Katagiri, K., and Mitani, T. 2000. Identification, quantitative determination, and antioxidative activities of chlorogenic acid isomers in Prune (*Prunus domestica* L.). *J. Agric. Food Chem.* 48:5512–5516.
5. Clifford, M. N. 1999. Chlorogenic acids and other cinnamates–nature, occurrence and dietary burden. *J. Sci. Food Agric.* 79:362–372.
6. Clifford, M. N. 1987. Chlorogenic acids. In *Coffee*, Vol. 1, ed. R. J. Clarke and R. Macrae, 153–202. Elsevier Applied Science, London.

7. IUPAC. 1976. Nomenclature of cyclitos. *Biochem. J.* 153:23–31.
8. Farah, A., and Donangelo, C. M. 2006. Phenolic compounds in coffee. *Braz. J. Plant Physiol.* 18:23–36.
9. Belay, A., and Gholap, A. V. 2009. Characterization and determination of chlorogenic acids (CGA) in coffee beans by UV-Vis spectroscopy. *Afr. J. Pure Appl. Chem.* 3:234–240.
10. Clifford, M. N., Shutler, S., Thomas, G. A., and Ohiokpehai, O. 1987. The chlorogenic acids content of coffee substitutes. *Food Chem.* 24:99–107.
11. Ky, C.-L., Noirot, M., and Hamon, S. 1997. Comparison of five purification methods for chlorogenic acids in green coffee beans (*Coffea* sp.). *J. Agric. Food Chem.* 45:786–790.
12. Fujioka, K., and Shibamoto, T. 2008. Chlorogenic acid and caffeine contents in various commercial brewed coffees. *Food Chem.* 106:217–221.
13. Narita, Y., and Inouye, K. 2013. Degradation kinetics of chlorogenic acid at various pH values and effects of ascorbic acid and epigallocatechin gallate on its stability under alkaline conditions. *J. Agric. Food Chem.* 61:966–972.
14. Clifford, M. N., and Jarvis, T. 1988. The chlorogenic acids content of green robusta coffee beans as a possible index of geographic origin. *Food Chem.* 29:291–298.
15. Anthony, F., Clifford, M. N., and Noirot, M. 1993. Biochemical diversity in the genus *Coffea* L.: Chlorogenic acids, caffeine and mozambioside contents. *Genet. Resour. Crop Evol.* 40:61–70.
16. Farah, A., de Paulis, T., Moreira, D. P., Trugo, L. C., and Martin, P. R. 2006. Chlorogenic acids and lactones in regular and water-decaffeinated arabica coffees. *J. Agric. Food Chem.* 54:374–381.
17. Ky, C.-L., Louarn, J., Dussert, S., Guyot, B., Hamon, S., and Noirot, M. 2001. Caffeine, trigonelline, chlorogenic acids and sucrose diversity in wild *Coffea arabica* L. and *C. canephora* P. accessions. *Food Chem.* 75:223–230.
18. Alonso-Salces, R. M., Serra, F., Reniero, F., and Héberger, K. 2009. Botanical and geographical characterization of green coffee (*Coffea arabica* and *Coffea canephora*): Chemometric evaluation of phenolic and methylxanthine contents. *J. Agric. Food Chem.* 57:4224–4235.
19. Clifford, M. N., Johnston, K. L., Knight, S., and Kuhnert, N. 2003. Hierarchical scheme for LC-MS^n identification of chlorogenic acids. *J. Agric. Food Chem.* 51:2900–2911.
20. Clifford, M. N., Knight, S., Surucu, B., and Kuhnert, N. 2006. Characterization by LC-MS^n of four new classes of chlorogenic acids in green coffee beans: dimethoxycinnamoylquinic acids, diferuloylquinic acids, caffeoyl-dimethoxycinnamoylquinic acids, and feruloyl-dimethoxycinnamoylquinic acids. *J. Agric. Food Chem.* 54:1957–1969.
21. Clifford, M. N., Marks, S., Knight, S., and Kuhnert, N. 2006. Characterization by LC-MS^n of four new classes of *p*-coumaric acid-containing diacyl chlorogenic acids in green coffee beans. *J. Agric. Food Chem.* 54:4095–4101.
22. Jaiswal, R., Patras, M. A., Eravuchira, P. J., and Kuhnert, N. 2010. Profile and characterization of the chlorogenic acids in green robusta coffee beans by LC-MS^n: Identification of seven new classes of compounds. *J. Agric. Food Chem.* 58:8722–8737.
23. Narita, Y., and Inouye, K. 2014. Chlorogenic acids from coffee. In *Coffee in Health and Disease Prevention*, ed. V. R. Pready, 189–199, Elsevier, Amsterdam.
24. International Diabetes Federation. 2014. *Diabetes Atlas*, 6th ed., International Diabetes Federation, Brussels, Belgium.
25. Akash, M. S. H., Rehman, K., and Chen, S. 2014. Effects of coffee on type 2 diabetes mellitus. *Nutrition* 30:755–763.
26. American Diabetes Association. 2003. Treatment of hypertension in adults with diabetes. *Diabetes Care* 26:S80–S82.

27. Meisinger, C., Thorand, B., Schneider, A., Stieber, J., Doring, A., and Lowel, H. 2002. Sex differences in risk factors for incident type 2 diabetes mellitus: The MONICA Augsburg cohort study. *Arch. Intern. Med.* 162:82–89.
28. Reddy, K. S., and Katan, M. B. 2004. Diet, nutrition and the prevention of hypertension and cardiovascular diseases. *Public Health Nutr.* 7:167–186.
29. Steyn, N. P., Mann, J., Bennett, P. H., Temple, N., Zimmet, P., Tuomilehto, J., and Louheranta, A. 2004. Diet, nutrition and the prevention of type 2 diabetes. *Public Health Nutr.* 7:147–165.
30. Larsson, S. C., and Wolk, A. 2007. Coffee consumption and risk of liver cancer: A meta-analysis. *Gastroenterology* 132:1740–1745.
31. Bravi, F., Bosetti, C., Tavani, A., Bagnardi, V., Gallus, S., Negri, E., Franceschi, S., and La Vecchia, C. 2007. Coffee drinking and hepatocellular carcinoma risk: A meta-analysis. *Hepatology* 46:430–435.
32. Masterton, G. S., and Haves, P. C. 2010. Coffee and the liver: a potential treatment for liver disease? *Eur. J. Gastroenterol. Hepatol.* 22:1277–1283.
33. Sang, L.-X., Chang, B., Li, X.-H., and Jiang, M. 2013. Consumption of coffee associated with reduced risk of liver cancer: a meta-analysis. *BMC Gastroenterolo.* 13:34.
34. van Dam, R. M., and Hu, F. B. 2005. Coffee consumption and risk of type 2 diabetes: a systematic review. *J. Am. Med. Assoc.* 294:97–104.
35. Huxley, R., Lee, C. M. Y., Barzi, F., Timmermeister, L., Czernichow, S., Perkovic, V., Grobbee, D. E., Batty, D., and Woodward, M. 2009. Coffee, decaffeinated coffee, and tea consumption in relation to incident type 2 diabetes mellitus: A systematic review with meta-analysis. *Arch. Intern. Med.* 169:2053–2063.
36. Ding, M., Bhupathiraju, S. N., Chen, M., van Dam, R. M., and Hu, F. B. 2014. Caffeinated and decaffeinated coffee consumption and risk of type 2 diabetes: A systematic review and a dose-response meta-analysis. *Diabetes Care* 37:569–586.
37. van Dijk, A. E., Olthof, M. R., Meeuse, J. C., Seebus, E., Heine, R. J., and van Dam, R. M. 2009. Acute effects of decaffeinated coffee and the major coffee components chlorogenic acid and trigonelline on glucose tolerance. *Diabetes Care* 32:1023–1025.
38. Graham, T. E., Sathasivam, P., Rowland, M., Marko, N., Greer, F., and Battram, D. 2001. Caffeine ingestion elevates plasma insulin response in humans during an oral glucose tolerance test. *Can. J. Physiol. Pharmacol.* 79:559–565.
39. Moisey, L. L., Kacker, S., Bickerton, A. C., Robinson, L. E., and Graham, T. E. 2008. Caffeinated coffee consumption impairs blood glucose homeostasis in response to high and low glycemic index meals in healthy men. *Am. J. Clin. Nutr.* 87:1254–1261.
40. Iwai, K., Narita, Y., Fukunaga, T., Nakagiri, O., Kamiya, T., Ikeguchi, M., and Kikuchi, Y. 2012. Study on the postprandial glucose responses to a chlorogenic acid-rich extract of decaffeinated green coffee beans in rats and healthy human subjects. *Food Sci. Technol. Res.* 18:849–860.
41. van de Laar, F. A., Lucassen, P. L., Akkermans, R. P., van de Lisdonk, E. H., Rutten, G. E., and van Weel, C. 2005. α-Glucosidase inhibitors for patients with type 2 diabetes. *Diabetes Care* 28:166–175.
42. Olokoba, A. B., Obateru, O. A., and Olokoba, L. B. 2012. Type 2 diabetes mellitus: A review of current trends. *Oman Med. J.* 27:269–273.
43. Rohn, S., Rawel, H. M., and Kroll, J. 2002. Inhibitory effects of plant phenols on the activity of selected enzymes. *J. Agric. Food Chem.* 50:3566–3571.
44. Narita, Y., and Inouye, K. 2009. Kinetic analysis and mechanism on the inhibition of chlorogenic acid and its components against porcine pancreas α-amylase isozymes I and II. *J. Agric. Food Chem.* 57:9218–9225.
45. Narita, Y., and Inouye, K. 2011. Inhibitory effects of chlorogenic acids from green coffee beans and cinnamate derivatives on the activity of porcine pancreas α-amylase isozyme I. *Food Chem.* 127:1532–1539.

46. Narita, Y., and Inouye, K. 2014. Inhibition of porcine pancreas α-amylase by chlorogenic acids from green coffee beans and cinnamic acid derivatives: A focus on kinetic. In *Coffee in Health and Disease Prevention*, ed. V. R. Pready, 757–763, Elsevier, Amsterdam.
47. Ishikawa, A., Yamashita, H., Hiemori, M., Inagaki, E., Kimoto, M., Okamoto, M., Tsuji, H., Memon, A. N., Mohammadi, A., and Natori, Y. 2007. Characterization of inhibitors of postprandial hyperglycemia from the leaves of *Nerium indicum*. *J. Nutr. Sci. Vitaminol.* 53:166–173.
48. Narita, Y., Iwai, K., Fukunaga, T., and Nakagiri, O. 2012. Inhibitory activity of chlorogenic acids in decaffeinated green coffee beans against porcine pancreas lipase and effect of a decaffeinated green coffee bean extract on an emulsion of olive oil. *Biosci. Biotechnol. Biochem.* 76:2329–2331.
49. Henry-Vitrac, C, Ibarra, A., Roller, M., Merillon, J.-M., and Vitrac, X. 2010. Contribution of chlorogenic acids to the inhibition of human hepatic glucose-6-phosphatase activity in vitro by svetol, a standardized decaffeinated green coffee extract. *J. Agric. Food Chem.* 58:4141–4144.
50. Welsch, C. A., Lachance, P. A., and Wasserman, B. P. 1989. Dietary phenolic compounds: inhibition of Na^+-dependent D-glucose uptake in rat intestinal brush border membrane vesicles. *J. Nutr.* 119:1698–1704.
51. Kobayashi, Y., Suzuki, M., Satsu, H., Arai, S., Hara, Y., Suzuki, K., Miyamoto, Y., and Shimizu, M. 2000. Green tea polyphenols inhibit the sodium-dependent glucose transporter of intestinal epithelial cells by a competitive mechanism. *J. Agric. Food Chem.* 48:5618–5623.
52. Tunnicliffe, J. M., Cowan, T., and Shearer, J. 2014. Chlorogenic acids in whole body and tissue-specific glucose regulation. In *Coffee in Health and Disease Prevention*, ed. V. R. Pready, 777–785, Elsevier, Amsterdam.
53. Matsuda, Y., Kobayashi, M., Yamauchi, R., Ojika, M., Hiramitsu, M., Inoue, T., Katagiri, T., Murai, A., and Horio, F. 2011. Coffee and caffeine improve insulin sensitivity and glucose tolerance in C57BL/6J mice fed a high-fat diet. *Biosci. Biotechnol. Biochem.* 75:2309–2315.

6 Beneficial Effects of Green Coffee Bean Extract and Coffee Polyphenols on Metabolic Syndrome

Ichiro Tokimitsu and Takatoshi Murase

CONTENTS

6.1 INTRODUCTION

Metabolic syndrome (MetS) is defined as a cluster of multiple risk factors, including central obesity, hyperglycemia, hyperlipidemia, and hypertension, which together are associated with greater cardiovascular disease risk [1,2]. The prevalence of MetS has increased over recent decades, reaching alarming rates worldwide [3,4].

Because coffee is one of the most widely consumed beverages in the world [5], even potentially small health benefits associated with coffee intake may have important implications for public health. Although some epidemiological studies had previously investigated the relationship between coffee consumption and MetS, the results of these studies have not been conclusive.

From a cross-section study of Japanese civil servants, Matsuura et al. [6] reported that moderate coffee consumption was significantly associated with a lower prevalence of MetS. In this study, MetS was diagnosed in 374 of 2335 men or 16.0%, and 32 of 948 women or 3.4%. Multiple logistic regression analyses show that the odds ratio in men for the presence of MetS was 0.61 (0.39–0.95) among moderate coffee drinkers who drank >4 cups of coffee per day when compared with non-coffee drinkers. Among all the components of MetS, high blood pressure and high triglyceride levels were inversely associated with moderate coffee consumption in men, whereas in women, there was no significant association between moderate coffee consumption and the prevalence of MetS or its components. Other studies conducted in Japan [7,8] and the Mediterranean [9] have also demonstrated a significant inverse correlation between coffee consumption and MetS.

On the other hand, Driessen et al. [10] reported that there was no association between coffee consumption and the development of MetS in a longitudinal study. They investigated the association of long-term coffee consumption between the ages of 27 and 36 years, and the prevalence of MetS at the age of 36. Data on coffee consumption and MetS components were obtained from a healthy cohort of 174 men and 194 women when followed up from the age of 27 years onward. At the age of 36 years, the prevalence of MetS was 10.1%, and coffee consumption did not differ significantly between subjects with or without MetS or its components. Other studies [11,12] conducted in Europe also failed to demonstrate any association between coffee consumption and MetS prevalence.

As coffee is a complex beverage containing hundreds of biologically active components [13], it remains unknown what components may have an effect on the prevalence of MetS. In this chapter, we introduce the anti-MetS effects (antiobesity, antihyperglycemia, and antihyperlipidemia) of green coffee bean extract (GCBE) and coffee polyphenols (CPP), such as caffeoylquinic acids, feruloylquinic acids, and dicaffeoylquinic acids, and we discuss their possible mechanisms of action. The effects of GCBE on hypertension are reviewed in Chapter 8.

6.2 EFFECTS OF GREEN COFFEE BEAN EXTRACT AND COFFEE POLYPHENOLS ON OBESITY, HYPERGLYCEMIA, AND HYPERLIPIDEMIA (ANIMAL STUDIES)

Murase et al. [14] investigated the effect of CPP on diet-induced body fat accumulation. C57BL/6J mice, prone to develop high-fat/high-sucrose diet–dependent obesity, were administered high purity CPP after the removal of caffeine, which is just as abundant in coffee. The administration of CPP inhibited the high-fat diet–dependent increase in abdominal fat (mesenteric, perirenal, retroperitoneal, and periepididymal fat) in a dose-dependent manner, and also inhibited body weight gain, demonstrating that CPP are effective in inhibiting obesity (Figure 6.1). Additionally, triglyceride and cholesterol accumulation in the liver was also significantly inhibited (Figure 6.1). Inflammatory changes in adipose tissue in obesity, including macrophage infiltration, have recently been attracting attention as a possible underlying mechanism of MetS [15]. In adipocytes enlarged due to a high-fat diet, the marked macrophage infiltration and increase in mRNA expression of monocyte chemoattractant protein-l (MCP-1) were shown to be inhibited by CPP ingestion.

Expired gas analysis demonstrated CPP ingestion significantly increased oxygen utilization or energy utilization, without influencing the respiratory quotient, suggesting that energy utilization increased due to the promoted utilization of both lipids and sugars as energy sources. CPP-induced changes in the expression of energy metabolism–related molecules in animals fed a high-fat diet were analyzed using reverse transcription polymerase chain reaction (RT-PCR) (Figure 6.2).

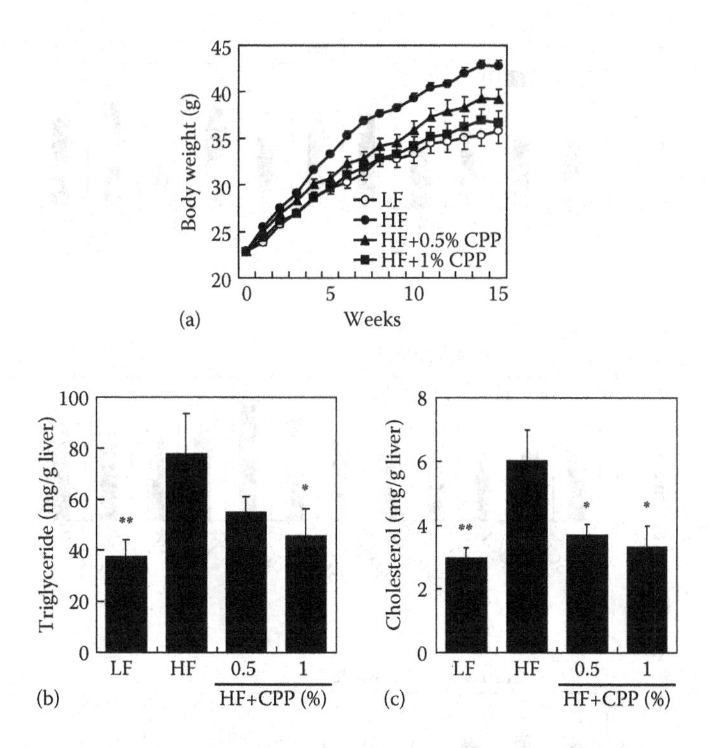

FIGURE 6.1 Effects of coffee polyphenols (CPP) on body fat accumulation (a); mean body weight of 10 mice at each time point (b, c); hepatic lipids were extracted from the liver and quantified. Values are means ± SE of 10 mice, $*p < .05$, $**p < .01$ vs. high-fat control group. (Modified from Murase T. et al., *Am. J. Endocrinol. Metab.*, 2011, 300, E122–E133.)

No significant changes were noted in the mRNA expression of PPARα and acyl-CoA oxidase (ACO), which are important for fatty acid and energy metabolism in the liver, or in monoacylglycerol acyltransferase (MGAT) and diacylglycerol acyltransferase (DGAT), which are important for triglyceride synthesis. On the other hand, CPP ingestion significantly reduced the mRNA expression levels of sterol regulatory element–binding protein-lc (SREBP-lc), a key regulator of fatty acid metabolism, as well as fatty acid synthase (FAS), stearoyl-CoA desaturase 1 (SCDl), acetyl-CoA carboxylase 1 (ACCl), and ACC2, which are regulated by SREBP-lc. CPP also significantly decreased the mRNA expression levels of SREBP-lc, FAS, SCDl, ACCl, and ACC2 in perirenal adipose tissue. No significant changes were noted in energy metabolism–related gene expression in brown adipose or muscle tissue, suggesting that the liver and white adipose tissue are involved in the CPP-induced promotion of energy utilization and antiobesity effects. FAS and ACCl are enzymes involved in the fatty acid synthesis pathway, and the inhibition of their expression has been reported to result in an increase in energy utilization and a reduction in body fat [16–19]. A reduction of ACC2 expression is thought to enhance fatty acid oxidation in mitochondria via the production of malonyl-CoA, by inhibiting carnitine palmitoyl transferase (CPT-I) [20]. After CPP ingestion, ACC activity in the liver decreased

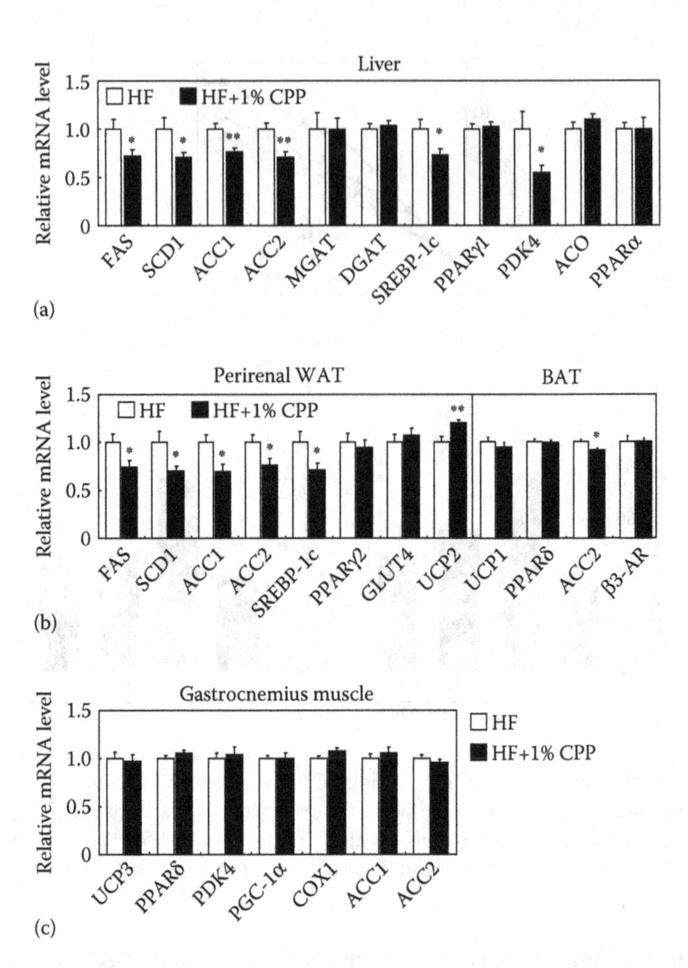

FIGURE 6.2 Effects of coffee polyphenols (CPP) on mRNA levels in the liver (a), dipose tissue (b), and skeletal muscle (c). Values are means ± SE of 10 mice, $*p < .05$, $**p < .01$ vs. high-fat control group. (Modified from Murase T. et al., *Am. J. Endocrinol. Metab.*, 2011, 300, E122–E133.)

with a reduction of its mRNA expression, leading to a significant decrease in its metabolite, malonyl-CoA. Pyruvate dehydrogenase kinase-4 (PDK4) switches the energy source from sugars to fatty acids via phosphorylation of pyruvate dehydrogenase complex (PDC), which is important for glucose homeostasis [21]. CPP ingestion reduced PDK4 expression in the liver. It is hypothesized that reduced PDK4 expression promotes glucose metabolism.

Furthermore, Murase et al. [14] also investigated CPP-induced changes in energy metabolism–related gene expression using cultured hepatocytes. As observed in mice, mRNA expression of SREBP-lc and its associated proteins significantly decreased with exposure to CPP. The main polyphenols found in coffee, caffeoylquinic acids (3-/4-/5-caffeoylquinic acid [CQA]), feruloylquinic acids (3-/4-/5-feruloylquinic acid

[FQA]), and dicaffeoylquinic acids (3,4-/3,5-/4,5-dicaffeoylquinic acid [diCQA]), were individually purified, isolated, and assessed for their effects on gene expression *in vitro*. The expression of SREBP-lc and its associated proteins was strongly inhibited by CQA and diCQA. Because total CPP, CQA, FQA, and diCQA did not activate AMP-activated protein kinase (AMPK) or peroxisome proliferator–activated receptor PPARα, PPARδ, or PPARγ, the CPP effects observed may not be mediated via these pathways.

Murase et al. [14] proposed CPP's mechanism of action based on these findings as follows: when CPP is ingested, ACC1, FAS, and SCDl expression decreases in the liver due to the inhibition of SREBP-lc expression, and fatty acid synthesis is inhibited. It is also known that the inhibition of SCDl increases energy utilization [19]. Reduced ACC2 expression decreases malonyl-CoA production, which enhances CPT-I activity and promotes fatty acid oxidation. On the other hand, glucose utilization increases due to the inhibition of PDK4 expression. CPP-induced inhibition of fat synthesis and an increase in energy utilization may prevent body fat accumulation.

Several animal studies have reported the effects of GCBE and CPP on obesity (Table 6.1). Mubarak et al. [25] reported that supplementation of chlorogenic acid in a high-fat diet did not reduce body weight when compared with mice fed a high-fat diet alone. Moreover, Li Kwok Cheong et al. [27] also reported that GCE, rich in chlorogenic acid, did not attenuate high-fat diet–induced obesity. Although explanations for these discrepancies had not been presented, one explanation may be that the dosage of the CPP varied due to the difference in sources. Significant differences in CPP composition have been described between roasted and unroasted coffee beans [30]. The use of different strains of mice may have also contributed to these differences. Further work using CPP with varying composition and in various strains of experimental animals is required to determine the effects of GCE and CPP on obesity.

Medium- to long-term CPP ingestion increases energy utilization via changes in gene expression, whereas a single ingestion of CPP induces changes in the blood hormone levels and the ratios of utilized energy substrates by inhibiting digestive enzymes. [31]. CPP were not observed to influence oxygen consumption when they were administered orally as an emulsion of corn oil and either starch or sucrose; however, significant inhibition of the elevation of the respiratory quotient, suggesting an increase in the ratio of lipid utilization, was observed with the ingestion of CPP. Postprandial energy metabolism is markedly influenced by ingested energy substrates, and hormones secreted in response to these. Murase et al. [31] reported that increases in the blood levels of glucose, insulin, glucose-dependent insulinotropic polypeptide (GIP), and triglycerides were inhibited after the administration of a carbohydrate (starch or sucrose), lipid, and CPP mixture. Insulin secreted in response to carbohydrate-derived glucose promotes the incorporation of blood glucose into peripheral tissue via the glucose transporter (GLUT). Insulin also promotes fatty acid synthesis by activating ACCl, and inhibits lipolysis by inhibiting hormone-sensitive lipase (HSL) and fatty acid oxidation via ACC2 activation and malonyl-CoA production [32–34]. GIP secreted by upper

TABLE 6.1
Effects of Green Coffee Bean Extract and Chlorogenic Acids on Metabolic Syndrome (Animal Studies)

Authors, Year	Experimental Design and Treatments	Results
Shimoda et al., 2006 [22]	Male ddy mice, 14 day • Active group supplemented with 0.5% and 1% green coffee bean extract • Control groupstandard diet	Green coffee bean extract is possibly effective against weight gain and fat accumulation by inhibition of fat absorption and activation of fat metabolism in the liver
Tanaka et al., 2009 [23]	Male Sprague–Dawley rats, 4 w • Active group supplemented with 1% green coffee bean extract extract; 10% caffeine, 27% chlorogenic acid • Control group supplemented with 0% green coffee extract	Green coffee extract has potent antiobesity and hypotriglyceridemic properties, and there is a possibility that these effects are exerted at least in part by the suppression of lipogenesis and the acceleration of lipolysis
Cho et al., 2010 [24]	Male Sprague–Dawley rats, 8 w • Active group high-fat diet supplemented with 0.02% (wt/wt) caffeic acid or chlorogenic acid • Control group normal diet, high-fat diet	Both caffeic acid and chlorogenic acid significantly lowered body weight, visceral fat mass and plasma leptin and insulin levels compared with the high-fat control group. Chlorogenic acid seem to be more potent for body weight reduction and the regulation of lipid metabolism than caffeic acid.
Murase et al., 2011 [14]	C57BL/6 J mice, 2–15 w • Active group high-fat diet supplemented with 0.5, 1.0% coffee polyphenol • Control group normal diet, high-fat diet	Supplementation with coffee polyphenol significantly reduced body weight gain, abdominal and liver fat accumulation, and infiltration of macrophages into adipose tissue. Energy expenditure evaluated by indirect calorimetric was significantly increased in coffee polyphenol-fed mice
Mubarak et al., 2013 [25]	C57BL/6 male mice, 12 w • Active group high-fat diet supplemented with chlorogenic acid (1 g/kg of diet) • Control group normal diet, high-fat diet	Supplementation of chlorogenic acid in the high-fat diet did not reduce body weight compared with mice fed the high-fat diet alone. Chlorogenic acid resulted in increases insulin resistance compared with mice fed a high-fat diet only.

Song et al., 2014 [26]	C57BL/6 N male mice, 11 w • Active group high-fat diet supplemented with 0.1%, 0.3%, and 0.9% decaffeinated green coffee bean extract, and 0.15% 5-caffeoylqunic acid • Control coffee chow diet, high-fat diet	Based on the reduction in high-fat diet–induced body weight gain and increments in plasma lipids, glucose, and insulin levels, the minimum effective dose of green coffee extract appears to be 0.3%.
Li Kwok Cheong et al., 2014 [27]	C57BL6 mice, 12 w • Active group high-fat diet supplemented with 0.5% green coffee bean extract rich in chlorogenic acid • Control group normal diet, high-fat diet	Green coffee extract did not attenuate high-fat diet–induced obesity, glucose intolerance, insulin resistance, or systemic oxidative stress. Furthermore, green coffee extract did not protect against ex vivo oxidant (hypochlorous acid)-induced endothelial dysfunction.
Huang et al., 2014 [28]	Male Sprague–Dawley rats, 12 w • Active group high-fat diet supplemented with 20 and 90 mg/kg 5-caffeoylquinic acid • Control group normal diet, high-fat diet	5-Caffeoylquinic acid suppressed high-fat diet–induced increases in body weight and visceral fat pad weight, serum lipid levels, and serum and hepatic free fatty acids in a dose-dependent manner.
Ma et al., 2015 [29]	C57BL/6 male mice, 15 w • Active group regular chow diet or high-fat diet with intraperitoneal injection of chlorogenic acid (100 mg/kg) twice weekly • Control group regular chow diet or high-fat diet with intraperitoneal injection of DMSO (carrier solution) twice per weekly Obese C57BL/6 male mice, 6 w • Active group intraperitoneal injection of chlorogenic acid (100 mg/kg) twice weekly • Control group intraperitoneal injection of DMSO (carrier solution) twice weekly	Chlorogenic acid significantly blocked the development of diet-induced obesity but did not affect body weight in obese mice. Chlorogenic acid treatment curbed high-fat diet–induced hepatic steatosis and insulin resistance.

gastrointestinal K-cells in response to glucose and lipid ingestion has an indirect effect on the promotion of fat accumulation by promoting insulin secretion and acting on adipocytes. Accordingly, CPP-induced inhibition of insulin and GIP elevation may influence the metabolic energy balance via glucose utilization and fatty acid metabolism.

CPP-induced reduction of blood glucose and hormone levels may also involve the inhibition of glycosidase. In an *in vitro* study [31] investigating the influence of CPP on carbohydrate digestive enzymes, CPP was shown to inhibit maltase and sucrase. Murase et al. [31] investigated nine individual polyphenols found in CPP and observed that diCQA strongly inhibited maltase, whereas CQA and diCQA strongly inhibited sucrase, suggesting that CQA and diCQA are significant contributors to the changes in energy metabolism induced after a single ingestion of CPP.

As described above, continuous CPP ingestion may inhibit body fat accumulation by inhibiting SREBP-lc expression. Because SREBP-lc expression is enhanced by glucose and insulin, it is also possible that the inhibition of the postprandial elevation of insulin by CPP via the inhibition of glycosidase also contributes to the CPP-induced inhibition of SREBP-lc expression, thus resulting in the inhibition of body fat accumulation. Because GIP has been reported to be involved in fat synthesis and the development of obesity, the inhibition of its secretion by CPP may also contribute to the antiobesity effect of continuous CPP ingestion.

Recently, many studies have explored CPP involvement in lipid and glucose metabolism. Tanaka et al. [23] reported that GCBE significantly reduced serum and liver triglyceride concentration in male Sprague–Dawley rats after 4 weeks. Cho et al. [24] also reported that chlorogenic acid lowered triglyceride (in the plasma, liver, and heart) and cholesterol levels (in the plasma, adipose tissue, and heart) in high-fat diet–induced obese mice. Huang et al. [28] investigated the effect of 5-CAQ on liver lipid metabolism of Sprague–Dawley rats fed a high-fat diet. They showed that 5-CQA may reduce serum lipid levels by altering the expression PPARα and LXRα. Several studies [29] suggested that CPP is a novel insulin sensitizer and capable of maintaining glucose homeostasis. Mechanistic studies [35,36] have shown that CPP may delay intestinal glucose absorption and inhibit gluconeogenesis. Moreover, other studies [37] have shown that CPP may enhance glucose uptake in skeletal muscle. Murase et al. [14] reported that the ingestion of CPP significantly reduced the high-fat diet–induced elevation of plasma glucose levels in C57BL/6J mice. Recently, Ong et al. [38] investigated the effect of chlorogenic acid on glucose tolerance, insulin sensitivity, hepatic gluconeogenesis, lipid metabolism, and skeletal muscle glucose uptake in $Lepr^{db/db}$ mice. They demonstrated that chronic administration of chlorogenic acid improved fasting glucose level, glucose tolerance, insulin sensitivity, and dyslipidemia. Moreover, they showed that chlorogenic acid activated AMPK, subsequently leading to beneficial metabolic outcomes, such as the suppression of hepatic glucose production and fatty acid synthesis. Further work is required to clarify the mechanisms of these observation at the molecular level, particularly to identify the first target molecules of CPP after ingestion. It is also of interest to identify what components in coffee may synergistically contribute to the anti-MetS effect in collaboration with CPP.

6.3 EFFECTS OF GREEN COFFEE BEAN EXTRACT AND COFFEE POLYPHENOLS ON OBESITY, HYPERGLYCEMIA, AND HYPERLIPIDEMIA (HUMAN STUDIES)

The antiobesity action of CPP has also been confirmed in humans [39]. When male subjects, with a body mass index (BMI) of 25–30 kg/m^2 and a visceral fat area of 80–170 cm^2, ingested a coffee beverage containing 297 mg CPP/can or a placebo beverage containing 2 mg CPP/can for 12 weeks, body weight significantly decreased after 4 weeks in the CPP group, and body weight changes by 12 weeks were −0.3 and −1.5 kg in the placebo and CPP groups, respectively, showing a significantly greater decrease in the CPP group (Figure 6.3). CT analysis of the abdominal, visceral, and subcutaneous fat areas showed a significant decrease by 12 weeks in the CPP group. These findings confirm that CPP are also effective in reducing abdominal fat and body weight in humans.

Some human studies have reported the effects of GCBE and CPP on obesity (Table 6.2). Recently, Vinson et al. [41] conducted a 22 week crossover study to examine the efficacy and safety of GCBE at reducing weight and body mass in 16 overweight adults. They reported that GCBE may be an effective nutraceutical in reducing weight in borderline obese adults, and may be an inexpensive means of preventing obesity in overweight adults. These findings warrant future large-scale studies to determine if CPP are able to protect against obesity, as well as to investigate modulating factors, such as genetic predisposition, sex, age, and CPP composition and dose.

To clarify the mechanism of the antiobesity effect of CPP, Ota et al. [42] investigated the effect of daily consumption of CPP on energy metabolism in humans. Subjects consumed 185 g of a test beverage with or without CPP (359 mg) daily for 1 week. Energy metabolism was evaluated by indirect calorimetry before and after the test period after fasting and up to 3.5 h postprandially, and during cycle ergometry. Indirect calorimetry showed that, compared with the control beverage, 1-week ingestion of the CPP beverage led to a higher fat utilization in the sedentary period and a higher anaerobic threshold during exercise. Moreover, Soga et al. [43]

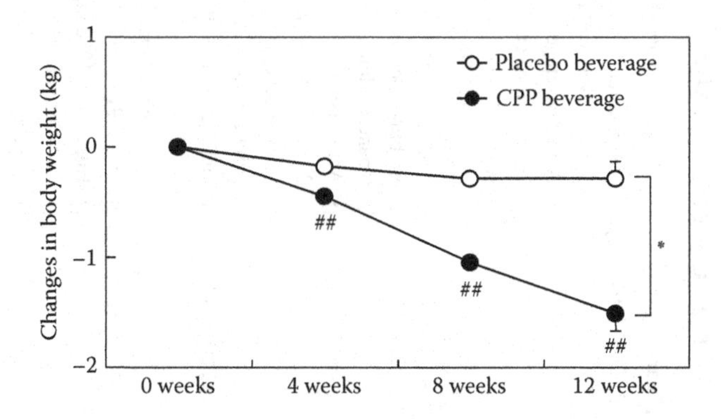

FIGURE 6.3 Effect of CPP on changes in body weight. Average ± SE, *$p < .05$, ##$p < .01$ vs. 0w. (Modified from Nagao et al., *Jpn. Pharmacol. Ther.*, 2009, 37, 333–344.)

TABLE 6.2
Effects of Green Coffee Bean Extract and Chlorogenic Acids on Metabolic Syndrome (Human Studies)

Authors, Year	Experimental Design and Treatments	Results
Thorn et al., 2007 [40]	Comparative, randomized, double-blind study, 12 w 30 slightly to moderately overweight (BMI 27.5–32.0 kg/m^2) nonsmokers • Active beverage instant coffee enriched with chlorogenic acid (a total of 200 mg per 2200 mg of the coffee comprises an extract of green coffee) • Control beverage commercial instant coffee	Results from the weight study show the mean ± SD weight reductions for active beverage and control beverage drinkers were 5.4 ± 0.6 and 1.7 ± 0.9 kg, respectively. The difference in weight loss between the two groups was statistically significant and the weight loss in the active beverage group by the end of study was also statistically significant compared with the start.
Nagao et al., 2009 [39]	Double-blind, randomized, placebo-controlled intervention study, 12 w 109 Japanese adults with a BMI of 25 to < 30 kg/m^2 • Active beverage 297 mg chlorogenic acid per 185 g coffee • Control beverage 2 mg chlorogenic acid per 185 g coffee	After 12 weeks of beverage consumption, changes from week-0 values (active vs. control, mean ± SE) in visceral fat area (−4.4 ± 2.1 vs. 3.6 ± 2.3 cm^2), waist circumference (1–8 ± 0.2 vs. 0.0 ± 0.2 cm^2), and BMI (−0.6 ± 0.1 vs. −0.1 ± 0.1 kg/cm^2) were greater in the active group than in the control group.
Vinson et al., 2012 [41]	Randomized, double-blind, placebo-controlled, linear dose, crossover study, 22 w 16 Overweight adults; average BMI at the start of the study was 28.22 ± 0.91 kg/m^2 • High-dose (1050 mg) green coffee extract • Low-dose (700 mg) green coffee extract • Placebo green coffee extract; 45.9% chlorogenic acids	Significant reduction was observed in body weight, body mass index, and percent body fat; as well as a small decrease in heart rate, but with no significant changes to diet over the course of the study.

reported a similar effect of CPP on energy metabolism in humans, suggesting that these effects may be important for the antiobesity effect of CPP.

Epidemiologic surveys have shown high coffee consumption is associated with lower incidence of type 2 diabetes [44–49]. These beneficial effects of coffee are also observed with decaffeinated coffee, indicating that components in coffee other than caffeine may play a role in this observation. There has recently been increased interest in CPP after several animal studies reported that CPP may prevent insulin resistance induced by a high-fat diet [35–37]. In a human study, van Dijk et al. [50] evaluated the acute effects of chlorogenic acid on glucose tolerance. They reported that chlorogenic acid ingestion significantly reduced glucose and insulin concentration 15 min following a 2 h oral glucose tolerance test when compared with a placebo. Iwai et al. [51] investigated the antihyperglycemic effects of GCBE, showing that GCBE significantly reduced plasma glucose levels after carbohydrate ingestion, particularly in subjects with a high-glycemic response. However, little is known about the effects of GCBE and CPP on fasting plasma glucose and triglyceride levels in humans. Further long-term studies are necessary to clarify these effects in hyperglycemic and hyperlipidemic subjects.

6.4 CONCLUSIONS

The increase in patients with MetS due to changes in dietary habits and lifestyles has become a serious social problem worldwide. Lifestyle improvements, such as undertaking an exercise regimen and developing healthy eating habits, are important for the prevention of MetS, but adoption of these practices is often difficult. In animal studies, GCBE or CPP have been shown to have anti-MetS effects, and their possible mechanisms of action have been presented at the molecular level. Although the evidence for GCBE and CPP to prevent or improve MetS in humans requires further investigation, as a potential lifestyle modification, GCBE or CPP may hold promise in the pursuit of healthier body condition.

REFERENCES

1. Eckel RH, Drundy SM, Zimmet PZ. The metabolic syndrome. *Lancet*, 2005, 365, 1415–1428.
2. Grundy SM, Cleeman JI, Daniels SR, Donato KA, Eckel RH, Franklin BA, Gordon DJ, Krauss RM, Savage PJ, Smith SC Jr, Spertus JA, Costa F. Diagnosis and management of the metabolic syndrome: An American/National Heart, Lung, and Blood Institute scientific statement. *Circulation*, 2005, 112, 2735–2752.
3. Ford ES, Giles WH, Dietz WH. Prevalence of the metabolic syndrome among US adults: Findings from the third National Health and Nutrition Examination Survey. *JAMA*, 2002, 287, 356–359.
4. Hu G, Qiao Q, Tuomilehto J, Balkau B, Borch-Johnsen K, Pyorala K. Prevalence of the metabolic syndrome and its relation to all-cause and cardiovascular mortality in nondiabetic European men and women. *Arch. Intern. Med.*, 164, 1066–1076.
5. Schaefer B. Coffee consumption and type 2 diabetes mellitus. *Ann. Intern. Med.*, 2004, 141, 321–324.

6. Matsuura H, Mure K, Nishio N, Kitano N, Nagai N, Takeshita T. Relationship between coffee consumption and prevalence of metabolic syndrome among Japanese civil servants. *J. Epidemiol.*, 2012, 22, 160–166.
7. Hino A, Adachi H, Enomoto M, Furuki K, Shigetoh Y, Ohtska M, Kumagae S, Hirai Y, Jalaldin A, Satoh A, Imaizumi T. Habitual coffee but not green tea consumption is inversely associated with metabolic syndrome: An epidemiological study in a general Japanese population. *Diabetes Res. Clin. Pract.*, 2007, 76, 383–389.
8. Takami H, Nakamoto M, Uemura H, Katsuura S, Yamaguchi M, Hiyoshi M, Sawachika F, Juta T, Arisawa K. Inverse correlation between coffee consumption and prevalence of metabolic syndrome: Baseline survey of the Japan Multi-Institutional Collaborative Cohort (J-MICC) Study in Tokushima, Japan. *J. Epidemiol.*, 2013, 23, 12–20.
9. Grosso G, Marventano S, Galvano F, Pajak A, Mistretta A. Factors associated with metabolic syndrome in a Mediterranean population: Role of caffeinated beverages. *J. Epidemiol.*, 2014, 24, 327–333.
10. Driessen MT, Koppes LLJ, Veldhuis L, Samoocha D, Twisk JWR. Coffee consumption is not related to the metabolic syndrome at the age of 36 years: The Amsterdam Growth and Health Longitudinal Study. *Eur. J. Clin. Nutr.*, 2009, 63, 536–542.
11. Balk L, Hoekstra T, Twisk J. Relationship between long-term coffee consumption and components of the metabolic syndrome: The Amsterdam Growth and Health Longitudinal Study. *Eur. J. Epidemiol.*, 2009, 24, 203–209.
12. Hosmark AT. The Oslo Health Study: Soft drink intake is associated with the metabolic syndrome. *Appl. Physiol. Nutr. Metab.*, 2010, 35, 635–642.
13. Yesil A, Yilmaz, Y. Review article: Coffee consumption, the metabolic syndrome and non-alcoholic fatty liver disease. *Aliment. Pharmacol. Thr.*, 2013, 38, 1038–1044.
14. Murase T, Misawa K, Minegishi Y, Aoki M, Ominami H, Suzuki Y, Shibuya Y, Hase T. Coffee polyphenols suppress diet-induced body fat accumulation by downregulating SREBP-1c and related molecules in C57/6J mice. *Am. J. Endocrinol. Metab.*, 2011, 300, E122–E133.
15. Hotamisligil GS. Inflammation and metabolic disorder. *Nature*, 2006, 444, 860–867.
16. Dobryn A, Ntambi JM. The role of stearoyl-CoA desaturase in body weight regulation. *Trends Cardovasc. Med.*, 2004, 14, 77–81.
17. Mao J, DeMayo FJ, Li H, Abu-Elheiga L, Gu Z, Shaikenov TE, Kordari P, Chirala SS, Heird WC, Wakil SJ. Liver-specific deletion of acetyl-CoA carboxylase 1 reduces hepatic triglyceride accumulation without affecting glucose homeostasis. *Proc. Natl. Acad. Sci. USA*, 2006, 103, 8552–8557.
18. Savage DB, Choi CS, Samuel VT, Liu ZX, Zhang D, Wang A, Zhang XM, Cline GW, Yu XX, Geisler JG, Bhnot S, Monia BP, Shulman GI. Reversal of diet-induced hepatic steatosis and hepatic insulin resistance by antisense oligonucleotide inhibitors of acetyl-CoA carboxylase 1 and 2. *J. Clin. Invest.*, 2006, 116, 817–824.
19. Ntambi JM, Miyazaki M, Stoehr JP, Lan H, Kendziorski CM, Yandell BS, Song Y, Cohen P, Friedman JM, Attie AD. Loss of stearoyl-CoA desaturase-1 function protects mice against adiposity. *Proc. Natl. Acad. Sci. USA*, 2002, 99, 11482–11486.
20. McGarry JD, Brown NF. The mitochondrial carnitine palmitoyltransferase system. From concept to molecular analysis. *Eur. J. Biochem.*, 1997, 244, 1–14.
21. Sugden MC, Holness MJ. Recent advances in mechanisms regulating glucose oxidation at the level of the pyruvate dehydrogenase complex by PDKs. *Am. J. Physiol. Endocrinol. Metab.*, 2003, 284, E855–E862.
22. Shimoda H, Seki E, Aitani M. Inhibitory effect of green coffee bean extract on fat accumulation and body weight gain in mice. *BMC Complement. Altern. Med.*, 2006, 6, 1–9.

23. Tanaka K, Nishizono S, Tamura S, Kondo M, Shimoda H, Tanaka J, Okada T. Anti-obesity and hypotriglyceridemic properties of coffee bean extract in SD rats. *Food Technol. Res.*, 2009, 15, 147–152.
24. Cho A-S, Jeon S-M, Kim M-J, Yeo J, Seo K-I, Choi M-S, Lee M-K. Chlorogenic acid exhibits anti-obesity property and improves lipid metabolism in high-fat diet-induced obese mice. *Food Chem. Toxicol.*, 2010, 48, 937–943.
25. Mubarak A, Hodgson JM, Considine MJ, Croft KD, Matthews VB. Supplementation of a high-fat diet with chlorogenic acid is associated with insulin resistance and hepatic lipid accumulation in mice. *J. Agri. Food Chem.*, 2013, 61, 4371–4378.
26. Song SJ, Choi S, Park T. Decaffeinated green coffee bean extract attenuates diet-induced obesity and insulin resistance in mice. *Evid. Based Complement. Alternat. Med.*, 2014, 2014, 718379.
27. Li Kwok Cheong JD, Croft KD, Henry PD, Matthews V, Hodgson JM, Ward NC. Green coffee polyphenols do not attenuate features of the metabolic syndrome and improve endothelial function in mice fed a high fat diet. *Arch. Biochem. Biophys.*, 2014, 559, 46–52.
28. Huang K, Liang X-C, Zhong Y-I, He W-Y, Wang Z. 5-Caffeoylquinic acid decreases diet-induced obesity in rats by modulating PPARα and LXRα transcription. *J. Sci. Food Aglic.*, 2015, 95, 1903–1910.
29. Ma Y, Gao M, Liu D. Chlorogenic acid improves high fat diet-induced hepatic steatosis and insulin resistance in mice. *Pharm. Res.*, 2015, 32, 1200–1209.
30. Jaiswal R, Matei MF, Golon A, Witt M, Kuhnert N. Understanding the fate of chlorogenic acids in coffee roasting using mass spectrometry based targeted and non-targeted analytical strategies. *Food Funct.*, 2012, 3, 976–984.
31. Murase T, Yokoi Y, Misawa K, Ominami H, Suzuki Y, Sgibuya Y, Hase T. Coffee polyphenols modulates whole-body substrate oxidation and suppress postprandial hyperglycaemia, hyperinsulinaemia and hyperlipidaemia. *Br. J. Nutr.*, 2012, 107, 1757–1765.
32. Brownsey RW, Boone AN, Elliott JE, Kulpa JE, Lee WM. Regulation of acetyl-CoA carboxylase. *Biochem. Soc. Trans.*, 2006, 34, 223–227.
33. Holm C. Molecular mechanisms regulating hormone-sensitive lipase and lipolysis. *Biochem. Soc. Trans.*, 2003, 31, 1120–1124.
34. Bandyopadhyay GK, Yu JG, Ofrecio J, Olefsky JM. Increased malonyl-CoA levels in muscle from obese and type 2 diabetic subjects lead to decreased fatty acid oxidation and increased lipogenesis; thiazolidinedione treatment reverses these defects. *Diabetes*, 2006, 55, 2277–2285.
35. Hemmerle H, Burger H-J, Below P, Schubert G, Rippel R, Schindler PW, Paulus E, Herling AW. Chlorogenic acid and synthetic chlorogenic acid derivatives: Novel inhibitors of hepatic glucose-6-phosphatase translocase. *J. Med. Chem.*, 1997, 40, 137–140.
36. Bassoli BK, Cassolla P, Borba-Murad GR, Constantin J, Salgueiro-Pagadigorria CL, Bazotte RB, da Silva RSSF, de Souza HM. Chlorogenic acid reduces the plasma glucose peak in the oral glucose tolerance test: Effects on hepatic glucose release and glycaemia. *Cell Biochem. Funt.*, 2008, 26, 320–328.
37. Prabhakar PK, Doble M. Synergistic effects of phytochemicals in combination with hypoglycemic drugs on glucose uptake in myotubes. *Phytomedicine*, 2009, 16, 1119–1126.
38. Ong KW, Hsu A, Tan BKH. Anti-diabetic and anti-lipidemic effects of chlorogenic acid are mediated by ampk activation. *Biochem. Pharmacol.*, 2013, 85, 1341–1351.
39. Nagao T, Ochiai R, Watanabe T, Kataoka K, Komikado M, Tokimitsu I, Tsuchida T. Visceral fat-reducing effect of continuous coffee beverage consumption in obese subjects. *Jpn. Pharmacol. Ther.*, 2009, 37, 333–344.

40. Thom E. The effect of chlorogenic acid enriched coffee on glucose absorption in healthy volunteers and its effect on body mass when used long-term in overweight and obese people. *J. Int. Med. Res.*, 2007, 35, 900–908.
41. Vinson JA, Burnham BR, Nagendran MV. Randomized, double-blind, placebo-controlled, linear dose, crossover study to evaluate the efficacy and safety of a green coffee bean extract in overweight subjects. *Diabetes Metab. Syndr. Obes.*, 2012, 5, 21–27.
42. Ota N, Soga S, Murase T, Shimotoyodome A, Hase T. Consumption of coffee polyphenols increases fat utilization in humans. *J. Health Sci.*, 2010, 56, 745–751.
43. Soga S, Ota N, Shimotoyodome A. Stimulation of postprandial fat utilization in healthy humans by daily consumption of chlorogenic acids. *Biosci. Biotechnol. Biochem.*, 2013, 77, 1633–1636.
44. Bhupathiraju SN, Pan A, Malik VS, Manson JE, Willett WC, van Dam RM, Hu FB. Caffeinated and caffeine-free beverages and risk of type 2 diabetes. *Am. J. Clin. Nutr.*, 2013, 97, 155–166.
45. Pereira MA, Parker ED, Folson AR. Coffee consumption and risk of type 2 diabetes mellitus: An 11-year prospective study of 28812 postmenopausal women. *Arch. Intern Med.*, 2006, 166, 1311–1316.
46. Satorelli DS, Fagherazzi G, Balkau B, Touillaud MS, Boutron-Ruault MC, de Lauzon-Guillan B, Clavel-Chapelon F. Differential effects of coffee on the risk of type 2 diabetes according to meal consumption in a French cohort of women: The E3N/EPIC cohort study. *Am. J. Clin. Nutr.*, 2010, 91, 1002–1012.
47. Van Dam RM, Hu FB. Coffee consumption and risk of type 2 diabetes: A systematic review. *JAMA*, 2005, 294, 97–104.
48. Salazar-Martinez E, Willett WC, Ascherio A, Manson JE, Leitzmann MF, Stampfer MJ, Hu FB. *Ann. Intern. Med.*, 2004, 140, 1–8.
49. Van Dam RM, Feskens EJ. Coffee consumption and risk of type 2 diabetes mellitus. *Lancet*, 2002, 360, 1477–1478.
50. van Dijk AE, Olthof MR, Meeuse JC, Seebus E, Heine RJ, van Dam RM. Acute effects of decaffeinated coffee and the major coffee components chlorogenic acid and trigonelline on glucose tolerance. *Diabetes Care*, 2009, 32, 1023–1025.
51. Iwai K, Narita Y, Fukunaga T, Nakagiri O, Kamiya T, Ikeguchi M, Kikuchi Y. Study on the postprandial responses to a chlorogenic acid-rich extract of decaffeinated green coffee beans in rats and healthy human subjects. *Food Sci. Technol. Res.*, 2012, 18, 849–860.

7 Antiobesity Profile of Green Coffee Extract

Hiroshi Shimoda

CONTENTS

ABSTRACT

Green coffee bean extract (GCBE) contains chlorogenic acid derivatives including caffeoylquinic acids and feruloylquinic acids, and has been in focus as a weight loss ingredient. In mice fed a high-fat diet (HFD), GCBE suppresses body weight gain and fat accumulation in a range of 0.3%–2.0% in an HFD. The antiobese mechanism of GCBE causes suppression of adipogenesis and proinflammatory pathways in the adipocytes, and leads to an improvement of insulin responsiveness in the muscles. On the other hand, lipid metabolism is enhanced by GCBE in the liver. GCBE especially enhances the activity of carnitine palmitoyltransferase (CPT), which is a rate-limiting enzyme for β-oxidation. 3-Mono caffeoylquinic acid and feruloylquinic acids are active ingredients on activation of CPT. While the expression of enzymes synthesizing hepatic lipids is downregulated by monocaffeoylquinic acids and dicaffeoylquinic acids, those mechanisms in the liver and skeletal muscles are regulated by AMP-activated protein kinase (AMPK). Regarding the clinical studies of GCBE, five trials were performed in mildly obese subjects. The dosage of GCBE was in the range of 100–1000 mg/day and subjects consumed GCBE for 4–12 weeks. A systematic review of the studies showed more than 400 mg/day of GCBE (180 mg of chlorogenic acids equivalent) was required to reduce body weight gain and BMI. However, more well-designed trials performed on a larger scale will be required to confirm the antiobese effect of GCBE.

7.1 INTRODUCTION

For the past decade, green coffee bean extract (GCBE) has been in focus as a weight loss ingredient. GCBE has a high content of chlorogenic acid derivatives (CGA), including 3-, 4-, and 5-caffeoylquinic acids; 3,4-, 3,5-, and 4,5-dicaffeoylquinic acids; and monoferuloylquinic acids. Among these derivatives, there is a particularly high content of 5-caffeoylquinic acid, which possesses antioxidant activity. Meng et al. [1] reviewed the antiobesity effect of chlorogenic acid in rodents, revealing that it improves various types of obesity and diabetic states. The primary antiobesity mechanism of chlorogenic acid is activation of the AMP-activated protein kinase (AMPK), which regulates energy balance. AMPK activation enhances fatty acid oxidation in the liver and skeletal muscles. In addition, chlorogenic acid upregulates hepatic expression of PPARα, which enhances β-oxidation. Thus, chlorogenic acid is thought to reduce body fat accumulation by increasing the consumption of fatty acids.

Although many preclinical studies of GCBE have been performed, there are few clinical studies. Some reviews have pointed out inadequacies in the design of previous clinical studies on GCBE [2,3] and one report was retracted by the authors [4]. However, an antiobesity effect is claimed for a canned coffee beverage containing GCBE (Kao Co. Ltd., Japan) marketed in Japan as a food for specified health use (FORSHU), because its fat utilization [5] and safety [6] have been confirmed and accepted by the Japanese government. In addition, we have been providing standardized GCBE for 12 years as a weight loss ingredient.

In this chapter, as a manufacturer of GCBE, we introduce the antiobesity effects of GCBE demonstrated in our animal studies and describe the clinical efficacy of GCBE for weight loss.

7.2 ANTIOBESITY EFFECTS OF GCBE IN RODENTS

GCBE has been reported to reduce fat accumulation in mice and rats. For evaluating GCBE, C57BL/6 mice fed a high-fat diet (HFD mice) have frequently been used. Song et al. [7] fed an HFD containing 0.3% decaffeinated GCBE (Svetol, Naturex Inc., France) to C57BL/6 mice and found that it suppressed body weight gain and reduced visceral fat accumulation. They also confirmed downregulation of genes related to WNT10b- and galanin-mediated adipogenesis, and to the TLR4-mediated proinflammatory pathways in adipose tissue. On the other hand, Ghadieh et al. [8] studied the effect of oral administration of Svetol in HFD mice, instead of adding it to the diet. They administered 5.25 mg/kg of Svetol orally for 3 weeks and found that weight gain was suppressed. They concluded that maintenance of glucose metabolism and insulin responsiveness were involved in the mechanism of weight loss. Jia et al. [9] evaluated changes of gene expression in skeletal muscle when C57BL/6 mice were fed an HFD containing 2% GCBE. While visceral fat accumulation was not suppressed by GCBE, it suppressed weight gain and hepatic fat accumulation, as well as upregulating gene expression related to the insulin receptor pathway in skeletal muscle. These reports demonstrated that GCBE contributes to weight loss, improvement of insulin resistance, and suppression of fat accumulation in mice. However, several investigators have obtained different results in HFD mice. Li et al. [10] reported that an HFD containing 0.5% GCBE did not improve fat accumulation or glucose intolerance in C57BL/6 mice, while Mubarak et al. [11] reported that adding chlorogenic acid (0.1%) to an HFD did not suppress weight gain, fat accumulation, or insulin resistance. Thus, the reported antiobesity effects of GCBE have varied. Therefore, we conducted a study of GCBE (Green coffee bean extract-P, Oryza Oil & Fat Chemical. Co. Ltd.) in HFD mice to further evaluate its influence on fat accumulation. The GCBE used in our study contained 15% caffeine and 49% chlorogenic acid derivatives, including 24% chlorogenic acid. We found that adding 0.5% GCBE to the diet strongly suppressed weight gain (Figure 7.1), as well as liver and epididymal fat weight (Table 7.1). Activation of lipid oxidation in the liver was involved in the mechanism by which GCBE suppressed fat accumulation. GCBE and its constituents, 3-chlorogenic acid and feruloyl quinic acids, were confirmed to enhance the activity of carnitine palmitoyltransferase (CPT), which is a rate-limiting enzyme for β-oxidation [12]. We also confirmed that adding 1% GCBE to an HFD suppressed weight gain and fat accumulation in the liver and adipose tissue in rats [13]. Hepatic CPT activity was increased, while the activity of some lipogenic enzymes, including fatty acid synthase (FAS), was suppressed.

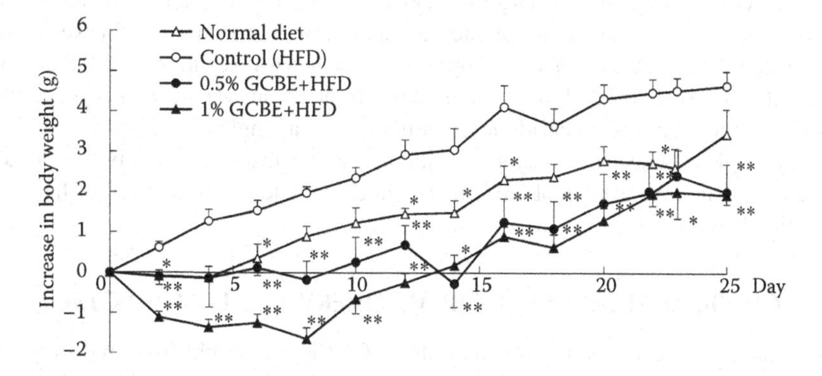

FIGURE 7.1 Effect of GCBE on weight gain in mice fed an HFD. C57BL/6J mice (male, 9 weeks old) were fed an HFD [20% corn oil, 10% lard, 13% sucrose, 20% casein, 4% cellulose, 3.5% mineral mixture (Harpers mixture), 1% vitamin mixture (Harpers mixture), and 28.5% corn starch] or a normal diet (5% corn oil, 20% casein, 4% cellulose, 3.5% mineral mixture [Harpers mixture], 1% vitamin mixture [Harpers mixture], and 66.5% corn starch). GCBE was mixed with the HFD and given for 25 days. Each point represents the mean ± SE ($n=6$). Asterisks denote significant differences from the control: * $p<.05$ and ** $p<.01$.

TABLE 7.1
Effects of GCBE in HFD-fed C57BL/6 Mice

	Increase of Body Weight (g)	Food Consumption (g)	Liver Weight (g)	Epididymal Fat (g)
Normal diet	3.5 ± 0.6	95.3	1.22 ± 0.04	0.30 ± 0.04**
Control (HFD)	4.6 ± 0.4	65.5	1.13 ± 0.04	0.52 ± 0.05
0.5% GCBE+HFD	2.0 ± 0.7**	67.4	0.95 ± 0.07**	0.36 ± 0.07*
1% GCBE+HFD	1.9 ± 0.2**	57.9	1.00 ± 0.02*	0.26 ± 0.02**

Note: Each value represents the mean ± SE ($n=6$). Asterisks denote significant differences from the control: *$p<.05$ and **$p<.01$.

Other researchers have also focused on the metabolism of liver fat by GCBE. Murase et al. [14] reported that the caffeoylquinic acids and dicaffeoylquinic acids in GCBE downregulate the expression of enzymes synthesizing hepatic lipids, such as sterol regulatory element–binding protein (SREBP)-1c and acetyl-CoA carboxylases (ACC)-1 and 2. As suppression of ACC2 induces the activation of CPT-1, the findings of Murase et al. [14] support the effects of GCBE that we observed [12]. Based on this evidence, GCBE enhances hepatic lipid oxidation, leading to consumption of fat.

We also confirmed that the weight loss effect of GCBE required both chlorogenic acid and caffeine in mice fed a normal diet. As shown in Figure 7.2, weight loss due to caffeine or chlorogenic acid alone was smaller than that caused by GCBE. The suppressive effect of both compounds on visceral fat accumulation was weaker than that of GCBE (Table 7.2). Zheng et al. [15] reported similar results and explained that the combination of chlorogenic acid and caffeine is required to reduce fat accumulation. They gave chlorogenic acid and caffeine to mice for 24 weeks and found that fat accumulation was suppressed, along with elevation of CPT activity and reduction of fatty acid synthase activity. In addition, we showed that caffeine decreases the serum triglyceride level in mice after a single oral dose (Figure 7.3), while a single oral dose of caffeine also suppressed fat absorption in olive oil–loaded mice [12]. Thus, the effects of caffeine might contribute to suppression of fat accumulation by GCBE.

7.3 CLINICAL TRIALS OF GCBE IN OVERWEIGHT SUBJECTS

There have not been many clinical trials of GCBE for weight loss, and only two systematic reviews on the antiobesity effects of GCBE have been published [16,17]. However, one review [16] was based solely on the reduction of body weight as the primary outcome, and the other review [17] contained a study that was retracted in 2014. Therefore, we conducted a new systematic review and meta-analysis to assess the influence of GCBE on weight loss. We searched the Cochrane Library, PubMed, Google, JAMA, and Japanese (JAPICDOC and JMEDPlus) databases in July 2015 (Figure 7.4) using the following search terms: green coffee bean, chlorogenic acid, quinic acid, caffeic acid, and obesity. Two additional references were included and 139 references were identified as targets for initial screening. Finally, five articles were identified that described placebo-controlled randomized clinical trials of GCBE for weight loss. The characteristics of those five trials are summarized in Table 7.3 and the risk of bias is evaluated in Table 7.4. A high level of indirectness was observed in the studies using Svetol as GCBE [18–20], and the risk of bias was high in all reports. Dellalibera et al. [18] conducted a clinical trial of Svetol, which is a caffeine-free GCBE containing 45% chlorogenic acid derivatives including chlorogenic acid. Subjects with a BMI > 25 kg/m^2 ingested 400 mg/day of Svetol (180 mg of chlorogenic acids) for 60 days, resulting in significant improvement of body weight and BMI (Table 7.5). Two additional clinical studies of Svetol have been performed in the EU. Thom [19] performed a clinical trial using instant coffee containing Svetol and subjects with a BMI range of 27.5 to 32 kg/m^2 were given coffee containing 200 mg of Svetol 5 times a day for 12 weeks. The change of BMI was not

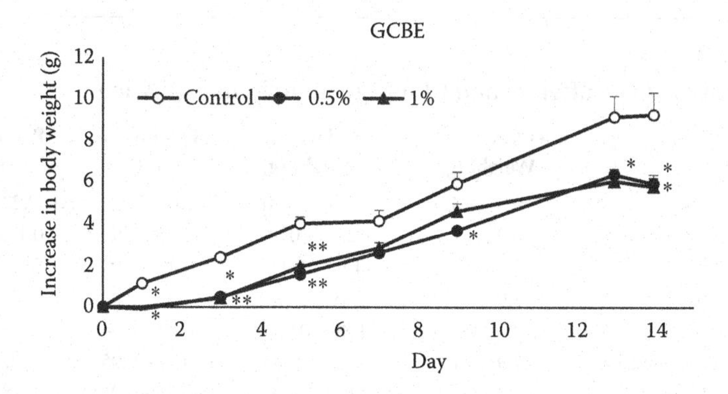

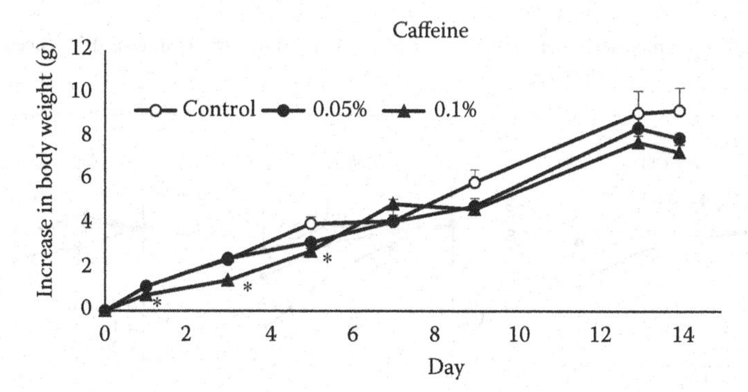

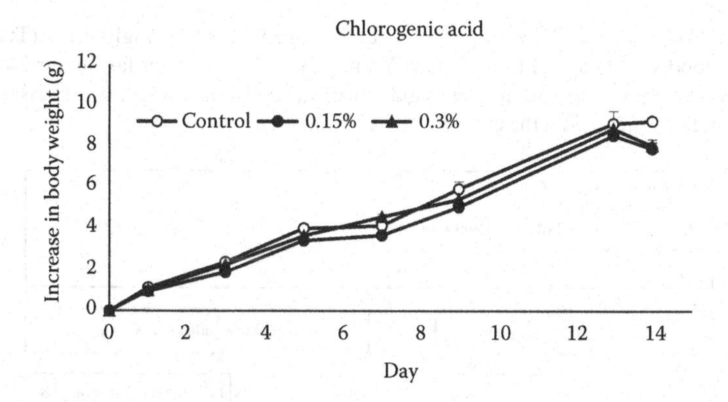

FIGURE 7.2 Effect of GCBE, caffeine, and chlorogenic acid on weight gain in mice fed a normal diet. Male ddY mice (6 weeks old) were fed a normal diet (CE-2, Clea Japan) containing GCBE, caffeine, and chlorogenic acid for 14 days. Each point represents the mean ± SE ($n = 7$). Asterisks denote significant differences from the control: * $p < .05$ and ** $p < .01$.

TABLE 7.2
Effects of GCBE, Caffeine, and Chlorogenic Acid in ddY Mice

	Increase of Body Weight (g)	Liver Weight (g)	Epididymal Fat (g)	Perinephric Fat (g)
Control	9.3±0.4	2.31±0.10	0.61±0.07	0.22±0.04
0.5% GCBE	6.0±0.1	2.13±0.08	0.39±0.06	0.11±0.02*
1% GCBE	5.8±0.2	1.93±0.11*	0.45±0.07	0.12±0.02*
0.05% Caffeine	8.0±0.2	1.88±0.06**	0.54±0.06	0.15±0.03
0.1% Caffeine	7.3±0.2	1.88±0.05**	0.49±0.04	0.15±0.02
0.15% Chlorogenic acid	7.9±0.1	1.95±0.03	0.57±0.05	0.17±0.02
0.3% Chlorogenic acid	8.1±0.2	1.88±0.05	0.61±0.08	0.18±0.03

Note: Each value represents the mean ± SE (n=7). Asterisks denote significant differences from the control: *p<.05 and **p<.01.

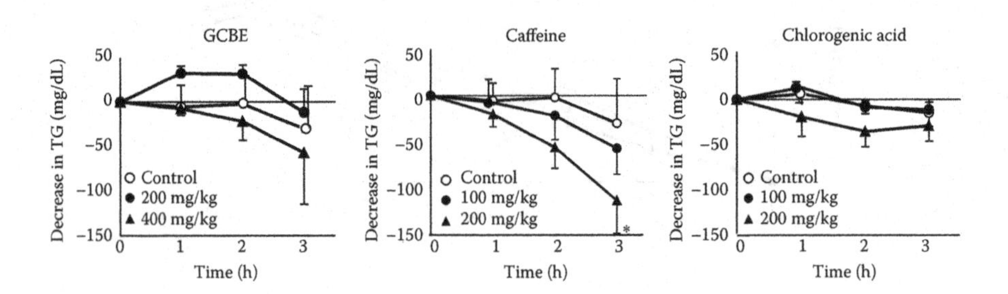

FIGURE 7.3 Effect of GCBE, caffeine, and chlorogenic acid on triglyceride (TG) levels in mice. Blood was collected from male ddY mice (6 weeks old) after fasting for 24 h. Each test agent was given orally 30 min later and blood was collected every 1 h. Asterisks denote significant differences from the control: * p<.05 and ** p<.01.

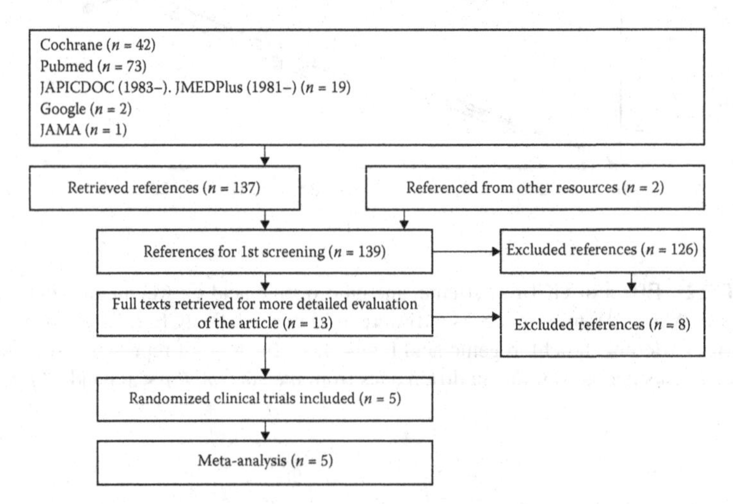

FIGURE 7.4 Flow chart showing selection of the randomized clinical trials.

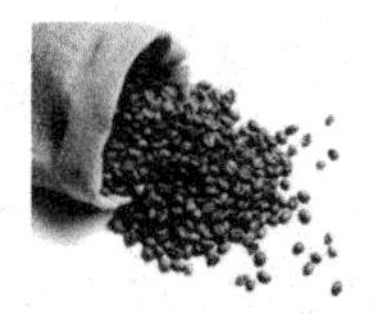

FIGURE 1.1 Green coffee bean fruit.

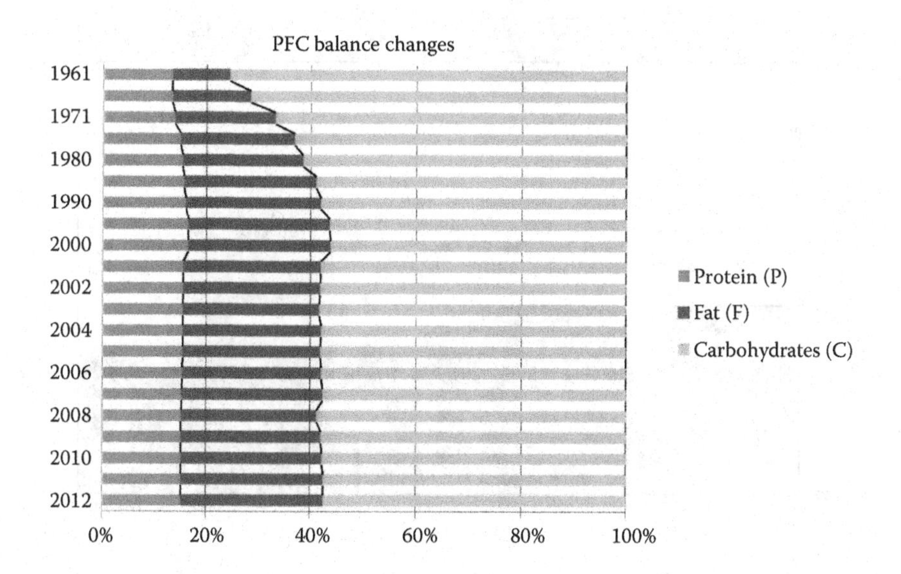

FIGURE 2.1 The changing dietary structure of the Japanese. (From MHLW (Ministry of Health, Labor, and Welfare), National health and nutrition survey, MHLW, Tokyo, 2012, sections 44, 45 and 46 [35].)

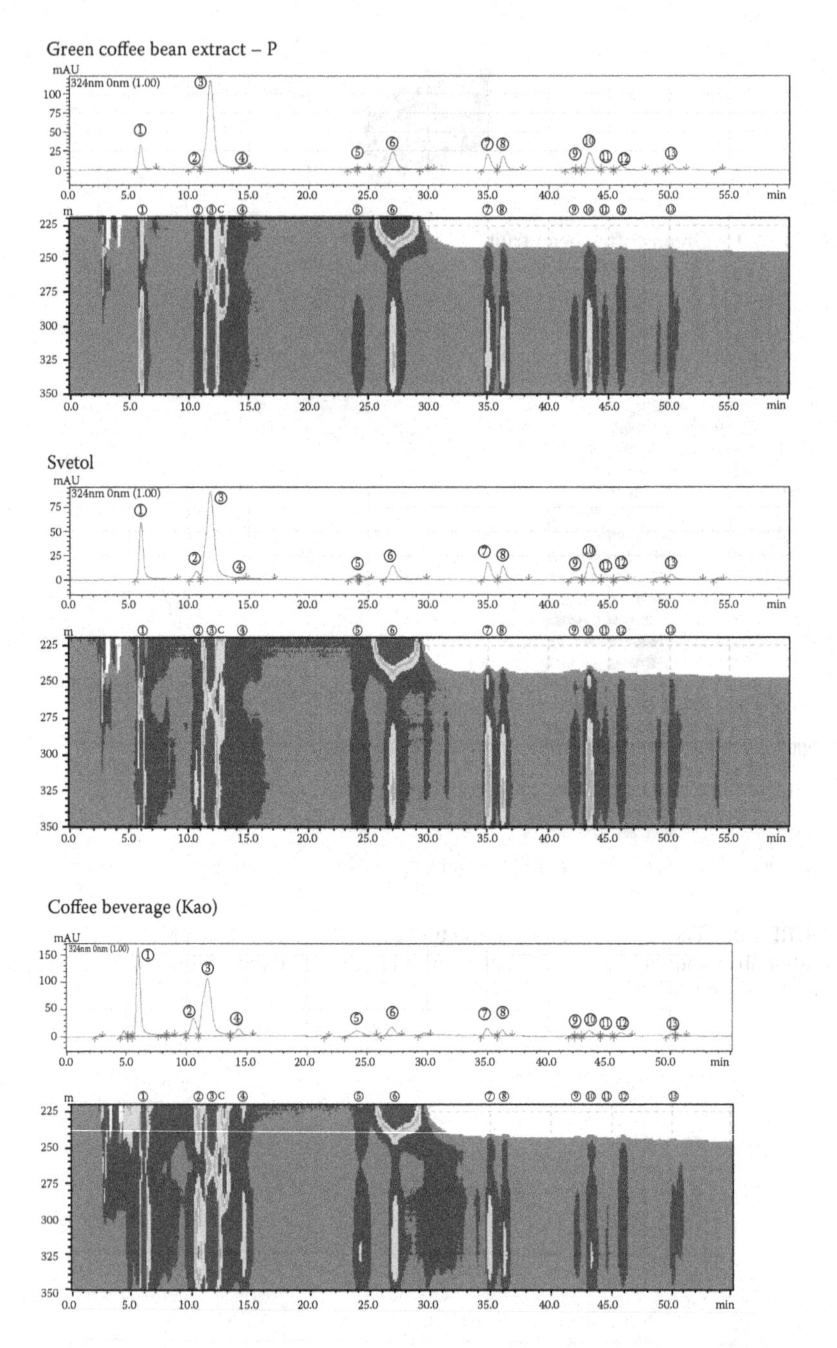

FIGURE 7.6 Comparison of HPLC chromatograms of GCBE products used for the clinical trials. Peak 1: 3-caffeoylquinic acid; 2: 4-caffeoylquinic acid; 3: chlorogenic acid; 4: 3-feruloylquinic acid; 5: 4-feruloylquinic acid; 6: 5-feruloylquinic acid; 7: 3,4-dicaffeoylquinic acid; 8: 3,5-dicaffeoylquinic acid; 10: 4,5-dicaffeoylquinic acid; C: caffeine; Peaks 9, 11–13: unknown peaks.

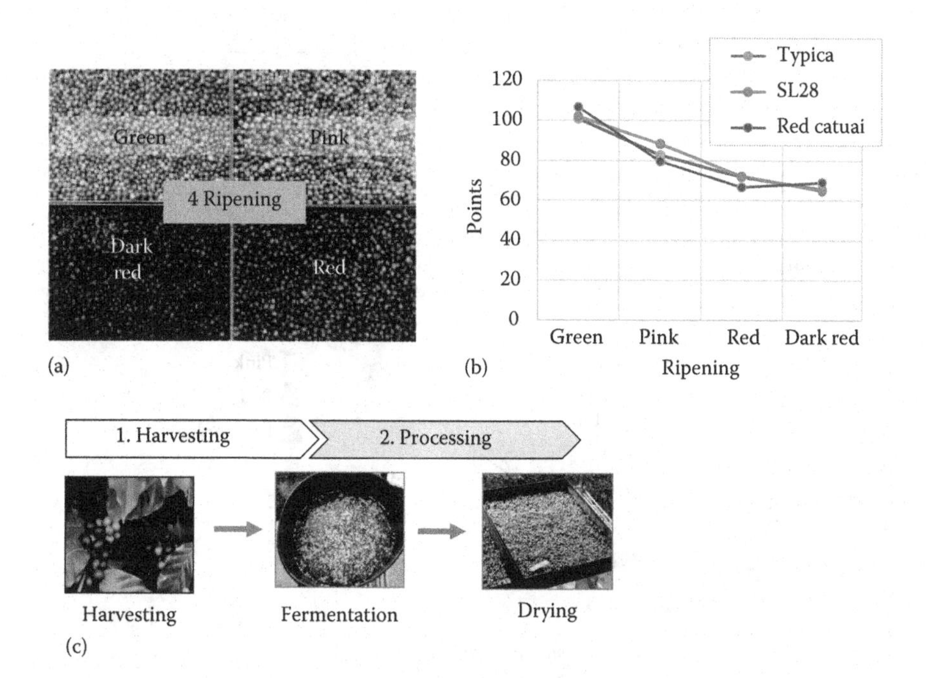

FIGURE 12.2 Green *C. arabica* beans at four stages of ripening. (a) Coffee cherries of four ripening stages. (b) Hardness values of the coffee cherries. (c) The process from harvesting of coffee cherries to green beans.

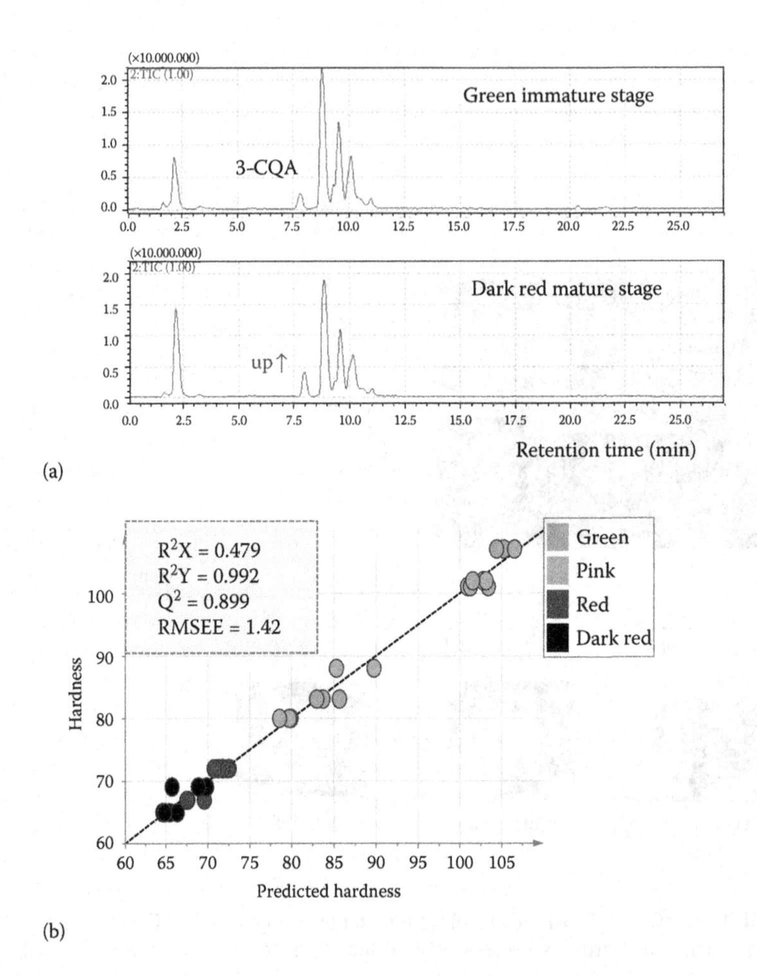

FIGURE 12.3 Multivariate analyses. (a) Total ion chromatogram of bean extracts of Typica at green immature stage (upper) and dark red mature stage (lower) in negative ion mode by LC–MS measurements. The peak (3-CQA), which is more abundant in the bean extract (at dark red stage), is shown. (b) OPLS regression model. Hardness values (the ripening stages) were predicted by the metabolite information in the green beans.

(*Continued*)

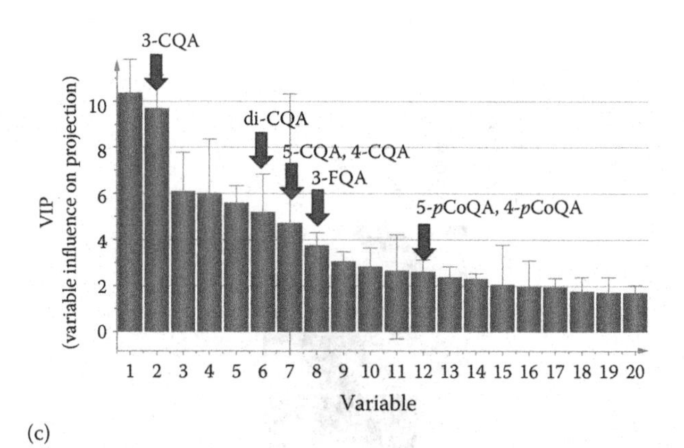

(c)

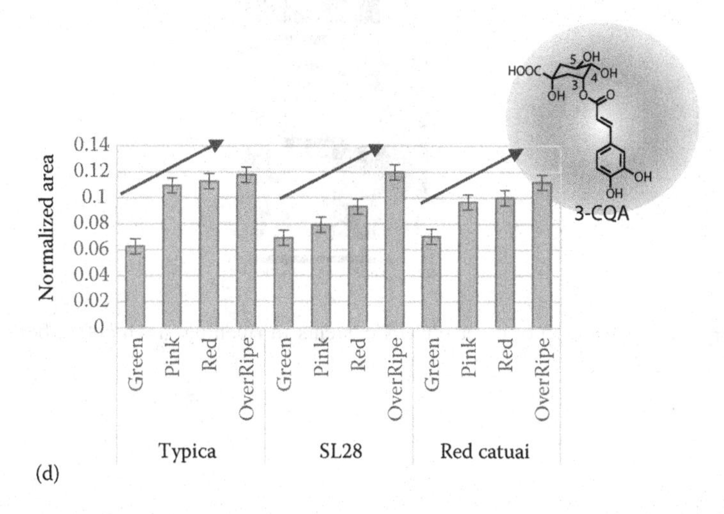

(d)

FIGURE 12.3 (Continued) Multivariate analyses. (c) The variable influence on projection (VIP) plots. The top 20 variables are shown. The arrowheads indicate CGA in the lists. (d) 3-CQA exists in greater amounts in riper beans.

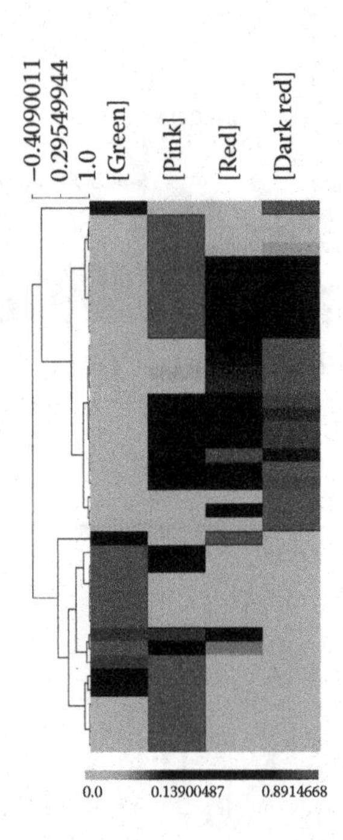

FIGURE 12.4 Heat map of diverse CGA contents in ripening green coffee beans of Red Catuai.

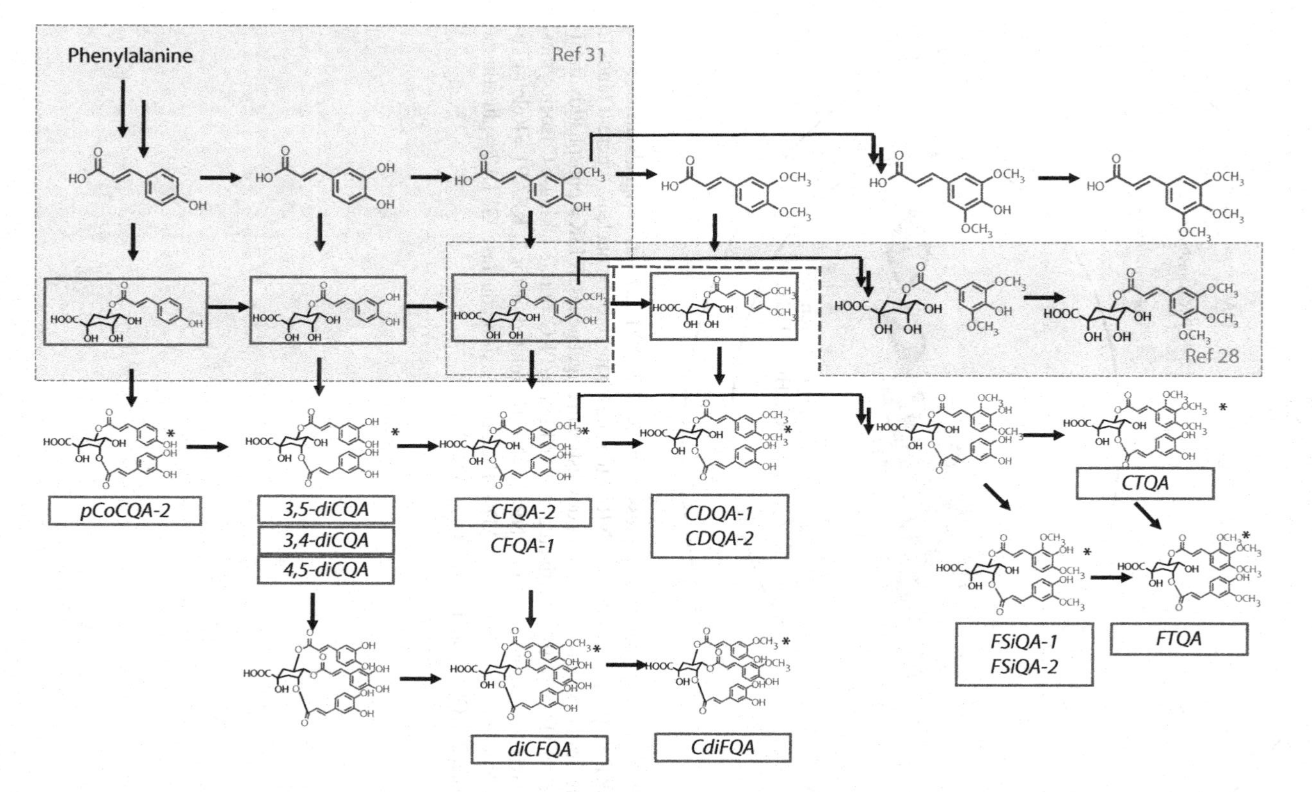

FIGURE 12.6 Proposed CGA metabolic pathway and changes of diverse CGA contents in ripening. CGA isomers circled with a green line are present in higher amounts in the immature beans, and those circled with a red line are present in higher amounts in the mature beans. Isomer structures with an asterisk (*) are unknown and one possibility of regioisomers are presented. The pathways with gray circles were described in a previous report. (From Jaiswal et al., *J. Agric. Food Chem.* 2010, 58, 8722–8737; Koshiro et al., *Z Naturforsch C.*, 2007, 62, 731–742.)

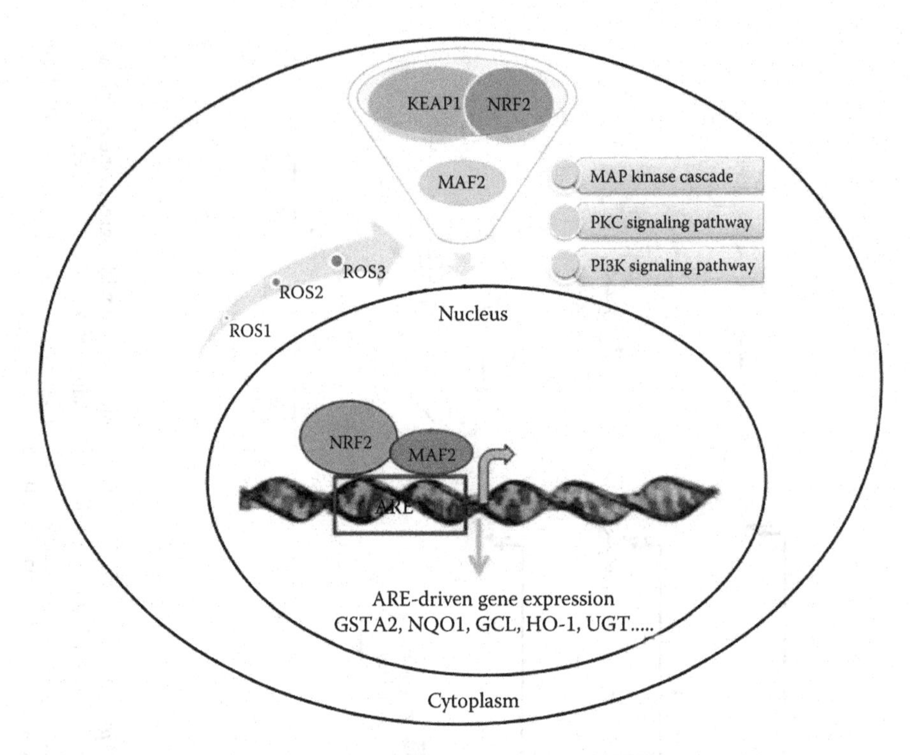

FIGURE 13.2 ARE-driven gene expression by NRF2. ARE activation signals disassociate the NRF2-KEAP1 complex allowing NRF2 to translocate into the nucleus, where it binds to the ARE and transcriptionally activates downstream target genes. (PI3K = phosphatidylinositol 3-kinase, MAPK = mitogen activated protein kinase, PKC = protein kinase C isoenzymes, ARE = antioxidant response element, NRF2 = NF-E2-related factor 2, KEAP1 = Kelch-like-ECH-associated protein 1, NQO1 = NAD(P)H:quinone oxidoreductase, GSTA2 = glutathione S-transferases 2, ROS = reactive oxygen species.)

TABLE 7.3
Methodological Characteristics of the Studies Analyzed

Author and Country	Journal	Study Design	PICO or PECO	Setting	Specification of Subjects	Intervention	Control	Analytical Method	Primary Outcome	Secondary Outcome	Abnormality Detected	Peer Review
Dellalibera O., Lemaire B., Lafai S., Italy and France	*Phytotherapie* 4, 1–4 (2006).	RCT Parallel 60 days	Can GCBE suppress overweight in subjects with BMI >25 compared to placebo capsule?	ND	BMI >25, males and females aged 19–75	GCBE (Svetol, 200 mg) capsule, twice a day (n=30)	Placebo (Dextrin 200 mg) capsule twice a day (n=20)	PPS	Body weight, BMI, muscle/fat ratio	Subjective symptoms	NO	+
Thom E., Norway	*J. Int. Med. Res.* 35, 900–8 (2007).	RCT Parallel 12 weeks	Can coffee beverage containing GCBE suppress overweight in subjects with BMI of 27.5–32.0 compared to placebo coffee beverage?	ND	BMI 27.5–32.0, non-smoker, no medication	Coffee beverage containing GCBE (Svetol, 200 mg), 5 times a day (n=15)	Placebo coffee beverage, 5 times a day (n=15)	PPS	Body weight, body fat ratio	ND	ND	+
Yeon P.J., Young K.J., Pyo L.S., Ho L.J., South Korea	*Korean J. Nutr.* 43, 374–81 (2010).	RCT Parallel 8 weeks	Can GCBE containing chlorogenic acids suppress overweight in subjects with BMI >23 or 27% body fat ratio compared to placebo capsule?	South Korea	BMI >23 or body fat ratio >27%, females aged 19 to 55[a]	GCBE (50 mg) and dextrin (150 mg) Two capsules, twice a day (n=23)	Placebo (Dextrin 200 mg) One capsule, twice a day (n=20)	PPS	Body weight, BMI, waist, waist/hip ratio, body fat ratio, abdominal fat area by CT	Blood pressure, energy expenditure, blood parameters	NO	+

(Continued)

TABLE 7.3 (CONTINUED)
Methodological Characteristics of the Studies Analyzed

Author and Country	Journal	Study Design	PICO or PECO	Setting	Specification of Subjects	Intervention	Control	Analytical Method	Primary Outcome	Secondary Outcome	Abnormality Detected	Peer Review
Nagao T., Ochiai T., Watanabe T., Kataoka K., Komikado M., Tokimitsu I., Tsuchida T., Japan	*Jpn. Pharmacol. Ther.* 37, 333–44 (2009)	RCT Parallel 12 weeks	Can coffee beverage containing GCBE with high concentration of chlorogenic acids affect visceral fat in subjects with BMI of 25–30 compared to placebo coffee beverage?	Japan	BMI 25 to 30, Visceral fat area >80–170 cm^2, males and females[b]	Coffee beverage containing 297 mg of chlorogenic acids, once a day ($n=53$)	Coffee beverage containing 2 mg of chlorogenic acids, once a day ($n=56$)	PPS	Visceral and subcutaneous fat areas in abdomen, BMI, body weight, body fat ratio, waist/hip ratio	Blood pressure, blood parameters, urine parameters, energy intake	NO	+
Ayton global research, England	Independent market study on the effect of coffee shape on weight loss 2009, June, 1–7	RCT Parallel 4 weeks	Can coffee beverage containing GCBE suppress overweight in subjects with BMI of 25–30 compared to placebo coffee beverage?	ND	BMI 25–30, non-smoker, no medication	Coffee beverage containing GCBE (Svetol, 200 mg), ($n=30$)	Placebo coffee beverage (Nescafe Expresso Pure Arabica Original blend), ($n=32$)	PPS	Body weight, waist, hip, bust, ratio of subjects losing weight	ND	ND	–

[a] Maintained body weight for 3 months.
[b] Excluded heavy smokers, heavy drinkers, and serious diseases at diagnosis.
ND: not described, NO; not observed.

TABLE 7.4
Evaluation of Bias Risk in the Studies Analyzed

	Risk of Bias								
	Selection Bias		Blind Bias		Reduce Number Bias				
References	Randomization Appropriate	Allocation Concealed	Subjects Blinded	Outcome Assessor Blinded	ITT, FAS, PPS	Incomplete Outcome Data	Reported Selective Outcome	Other Bias	Conclusion
Dellalibera (2006)	−2	−2	−1	−2	−2	−2	−2	−2	−2
Thom (2007)	−2	−2	−1	−2	−2	0	0	0	−2
Yeon (2010)	0	−2	−1	0	−2	−2	0	−2	−2
Nagao (2009)	−1	−1	0	0	−2	0	0	−2	−1
Ayton (2009)	−2	−2	−1	0	−2	0	0	0	−2

Note: High, −2; middle, −1; low, 0.

TABLE 7.5
Evaluation of Indirectness, BMI, and Body Weight in the Studies Analyzed

	Indirectness					Dosage of GCBE and Chlorogenic Acids (mg/day)	Values Before and After Ingestion									Difference of Changed Average Value between Active and Placebo	p Value
	Group	Active	Placebo	Outcome	Conclusion		Outcome	Placebo (Before)	Placebo (After)	Difference of Average	p Value	Active (Before)	Active (After)	Difference of average	p Value		
Dellalibera (2006)	−2	0	0	−2	−2	400	BMI (kg/m²)	ND	ND	−1.9	ND	ND	ND	−0.9	ND	−1	<0.001
						180	BW (kg)	ND	ND	−2.45	ND	ND	ND	−4.97	ND	−2.52	<0.001
Thom (2007)	−2	−2	−1	0	−2	1000	BMI (kg/m²)	29.9	ND	ND	–	29.2	ND	ND	–	ND	–
						450	BW (kg)	84.3	82.6	−1.7	NS	85.2	79.8	−5.4	0.003	−3.7	<0.05
Yeon (2010)	−1	0	0	0	−1	200	BMI (kg/m²)	26.3	26.1	−0.23	NS	26.0	25.7	−0.39	0.004	−0.16	NS
						49.3	BW (kg)	67.5	66.9	−0.61	NS	67.2	66.2	−0.99	<0.01	−0.38	NS
Nagao (2009)	0	0	0	0	0	ND	BMI (kg/m²)	27.7	27.5	−0.1	NS	27.7	27.1	−0.6	<0.05	−0.5	<0.05
						297	BW (kg)	75.6	75.3	-0.3	NS	75.8	74.3	−1.5	<0.05	−1.2	<0.05
Ayton (2009)	−2	−2	−2	0	−2	200	BW (kg)	77.4	77.3	−0.12	ND	76.7	75.3	−1.35	ND	−1.23	<0.05
						81											

Note: High, −2; middle, −1; low, 0; BW, body weight; ND, not described; NS, not significant.

reported, but body weight and the body fat ratio were significantly improved compared with the placebo group. Ayton Global Research carried out a similar study in England [20], in which a coffee beverage containing 200 mg of Svetol was ingested by subjects with a BMI of 25–30 kg/m^2 for 4 weeks. As a result, body weight showed a significant decrease.

There have been two clinical studies of Asian subjects. Yeon et al. [21] used GCBE supplied by our company, which contains 45% chlorogenic acid derivatives, 24% chlorogenic acid, and approximately 10% caffeine. Subjects with a BMI >23 kg/m^2 or body fat ratio >27% took 100 mg of GCBE twice a day for 8 weeks. While body weight and BMI were not reduced compared with the placebo group, a significant decrease of abdominal fat at the L1 level was noticed in computerized tomography CT scans. Nagao et al. [22] conducted a large-scale clinical study on 106 Japanese subjects with a BMI range of 25 to 30 kg/m^2 who drank a coffee beverage containing 297 mg of chlorogenic acid derivatives for 12 weeks. As a result, BMI, body weight, and the body fat ratio all showed significant improvement. Considering the results of these clinical studies, more than 400 mg/day of GCBE is required to significantly improve BMI and body weight compared with placebo. The results of our meta-analysis of the effects of GCBE on BMI and body weight are summarized in Figure 7.5. Data from three and five studies were combined for analysis of the effect on BMI and body weight, respectively. While GCBE significantly ($p < .00001$) reduced both BMI and body weight, very high heterogeneity was detected by the χ^2 test and I^2 statistics (Figure 7.5).

7.4 VARIATION OF CHLOROGENIC ACID DERIVATIVES IN GCBE

Regarding GCBE used in clinical trials, Svetol (Naturex Inc., France) is caffeine-free whereas the other types of GCBE contain caffeine. Green coffee bean extract-P (Oryza Oil & Fat Chemical Co. Ltd., Japan) contains 5%–15% caffeine. However, the composition of chlorogenic acid derivatives has not been determined. Therefore, we compared HPLC chromatograms of the chlorogenic acid derivatives in Svetol, green coffee bean extract-P, and a coffee beverage (Kao Co. Ltd., Japan) [23]. As shown in Figure 7.6 and Table 7.6, the chlorogenic acid peaks in green coffee extract-P and Svetol were highest among the peaks of chlorogenic acid derivatives. The chromatograms of these two types of GCBE were quite similar, but the chromatogram of the coffee beverage from Kao was different. The highest peak in this coffee beverage was that of 3-caffeoyl quinic acid, while the peaks of 4-caffeoylquinic acid and 3-feruloylquinic acid were higher than in the other two types of GCBE and the peaks of dicaffeoylquinic acids were lower.

7.5 CONCLUSION

The active components and antiobesity mechanisms of GCBE have been clarified. However, a relatively high daily dose of GCBE, approximately 400 mg/day or more, is required for efficacy. Clinical trials of GCBE performed so far have not been satisfactory with regard to design and the number of subjects. Thus,

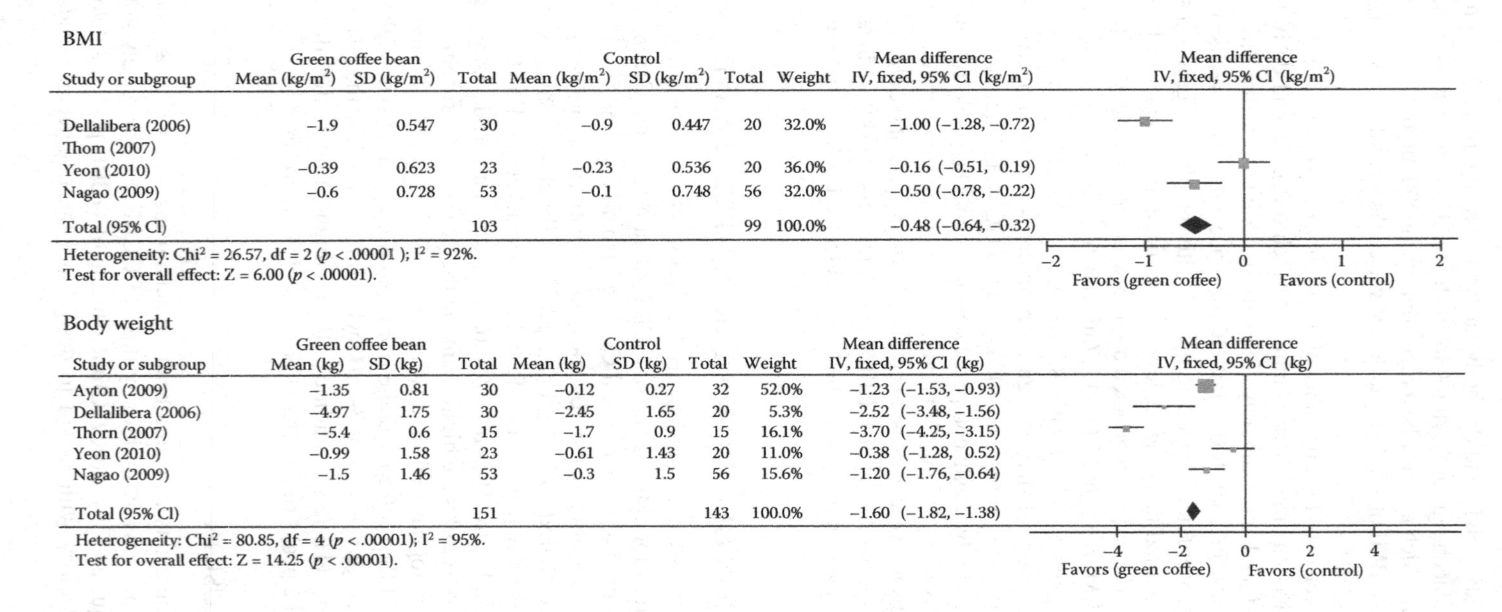

FIGURE 7.5 Forest plots for the influence of GCBE on changes in BMI and body weight.

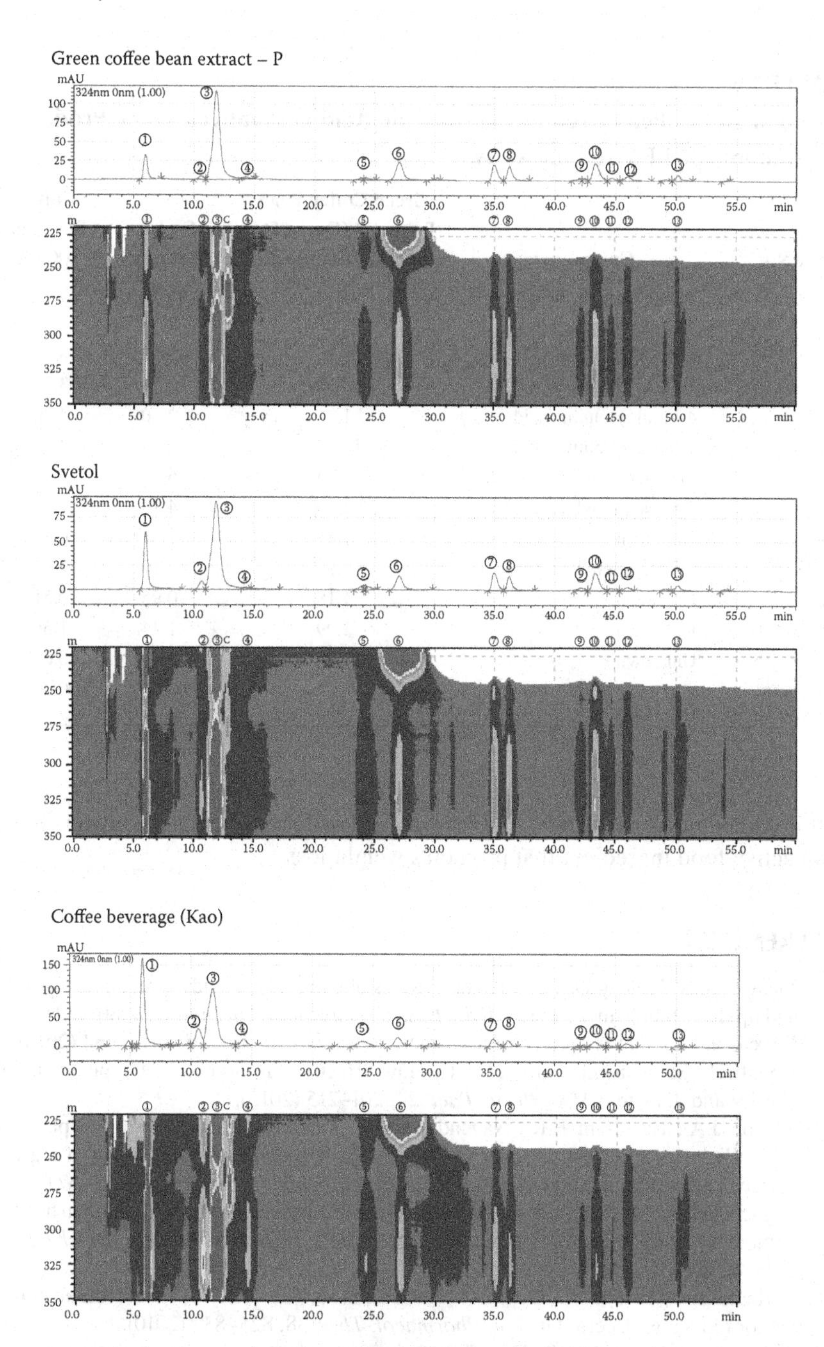

FIGURE 7.6 (See color insert.) Comparison of HPLC chromatograms of GCBE products used for the clinical trials. Peak 1: 3-caffeoylquinic acid; 2: 4-caffeoylquinic acid; 3: chlorogenic acid; 4: 3-feruloylquinic acid; 5: 4-feruloylquinic acid; 6: 5-feruloylquinic acid; 7: 3,4-dicaffeoylquinic acid; 8: 3,5-dicaffeoylquinic acid; 10: 4,5-dicaffeoylquinic acid; C: caffeine; Peaks 9, 11–13: unknown peaks.

TABLE 7.6
Comparison of Peak Area of Chlorogenic Acid Derivatives in the Products Containing GCBE Used for RCTs

Peak No.	Compound	Green Coffee Bean Extract-P (Oryza Oil & Fat Chemical)	Svetol (Naturex)	Coffee Beverage (Kao)
1	3-Caffeoyl quinic acid	7.45	15.59	29.72
2	4-Caffeoyl quinic acid	1.28	2.58	7.93
3	Chlorogenic acid	51.10	48.59	38.79
4	3-Feruloyl quinic acid	0.53	0.23	3.29
5	4-Feruloyl quinic acid	1.70	2.60	4.20
6	5-Feruloyl quinic acid	10.20	6.03	4.35
7	3,4-Dicaffeoyl quinic acid	6.35	6.14	3.09
8	3,5-Dicaffeoyl quinic acid	5.70	4.70	2.12
9	Unknown	1.43	1.31	0.88
10	4,5-Dicaffeoyl quinic acid	8.73	7.70	2.83
11	Unknown	1.18	0.95	0.51
12	Unknown	2.09	1.44	1.66
13	Unknown	2.26	2.11	0.63
Total (%)		100.00	100.00	100.00

well-designed trials performed on a larger scale will be required to confirm GCBE as an active food ingredient that promotes weight loss.

REFERENCES

1. Meng S., Cao J., Feng Q., Peng J., Hu Y. Roles of chlorogenic acid on regulating glucose and lipids metabolism: A review. *Evid. Based Complement Alternat. Med.* 801459 (2013).
2. Marcason W. What is green coffee extract? *J. Acad. Nutr. Dietetics* 113, 364 (2013).
3. Abdali D., Samson S.E., Grover A.K. How effective are antioxidant supplements in obesity and diabetes? *Med. Princ. Pact.* 24, 201–215 (2015).
4. Vinson J.A., Burnham B.R., Nagendran M.V. Randomized, double-blind, placebo-controlled, linear dose, crossover study to evaluate the efficacy and safety of a green coffee bean extract in overweight subjects. *Diabetes Metab. Syndr. Obes.* 7, 467 (2014).
5. Soga S., Ota N., Shimotoyodome A. Stimulation of postprandial fat utilization in healthy humans by daily consumption of chlorogenic acids. *Biosci. Biotechnol. Biochem.* 77, 1633–1636 (2013).
6. Chikama A., Watanabe T., Ochiai R., Katashima M. The safety of excess intake of coffee for reducing visceral fat. *Jpn. Pharmacol. Ther.* 38, 825–832 (2010).
7. Song S.J., Choi S., Park T. Decaffeinated green coffee bean extract attenuates diet-induced obesity and insulin resistance in mice. *Evid. Based Complement Alternat. Med.* 718379 (2014).
8. Ghadieh H.E., Smiley Z.N., Kopfman M.W., Najjar M.G., Hake M.J., Najjar S.M. Chlorogenic acid/chromium supplement rescues diet-induced insulin resistance and obesity in mice. *Nutr. Metabol.* 12, 19 (2015).

9. Jia H., Aw W., Egashira K., Takahashi S., Aoyama S., Saito K., Kishimoto Y., Kato H. Coffee intake mitigated inflammation and obesity-induced insulin resistance in skeletal muscle of high-fat diet-induced obese mice. *Genes Nutr.* 9, 389 (2014).
10. Li K.C.J.D., Croft K.D., Henry P.D., Matthews V., Hodgson J.M., Ward N.C. Green coffee polyphenols do not attenuate features of the metabolic syndrome and improve endothelial function in mice fed a high fat diet. *Arch. Biochem. Biophys.* 559, 46–52 (2014).
11. Mubarak A., Hodgson J.M., Considine M.J., Croft K.D., Matthews V.B. Supplementation of a high-fat diet with chlorogenic acid is associated with insulin resistance and hepatic lipid accumulation in mice. *J. Agric. Food Chem.* 61, 4371–4378 (2013).
12. Shimoda H., Ski E., Aitani M. Inhibitory effect of green coffee bean extract on fat accumulation and body weight gain in mice. *BMC Complement. Altern. Med.* 6, 9 (2006).
13. Tanaka K., Nishizono S., Tamaru S., Kondo M., Shimoda H. Tanaka J., Okada T. Antiobesity and hypotriglyceridemic properties of coffee bean extract in SD rats. *Food Sci. Technol. Res.* 15, 147–152 (2009).
14. Murase Y., Misawa K., Minegishi Y., Aoki M., Ominami H., Suzuki Y., Hase Y. Coffee polyphenols suppress diet-induced body fat accumulation by downregulating SREBP-1c and related molecules in C57BL/6J mice. *Am. J. Physiol. Endocrinol. Metab.* 300, E122–133 (2011).
15. Zheng G., Qiu Y., Zhang Q.F., Li D. Chlorogenic acid and caffeine in combination inhibit fat accumulation by regulating hepatic lipid metabolism-related enzymes in mice. *Br. J. Nutr.* 112, 1034–1040 (2014).
16. Onakpoya I., Terry R., Ernst E. The use of green coffee extract as a weight loss supplement: A systematic review and meta-analysis of randomised clinical trial. *Gastroenterol. Res. Practice.* ID382852, 6 (2011).
17. Hausenblas H., Hynh B. Effect of green coffee bean extract on weight loss. *Natural Med. J.* 6, 3 (2014).
18. Dellalibera O., Lemaire B., Lafai S. Svetol, green coffee extract induces weight loss and increases the lean to fat mass ratio in volunteers with overweight problem. [French] *Phytotherapie* 4, 1–4 (2006).
19. Thom E. The effect of chlorogenic acid enriched coffee on glucose absorption in healthy volunteers and its effect on body mass when used long-term in overweight and obese people. *J. Int. Med. Res.* 35, 900–908 (2007).
20. Ayton Global Research. The effect of chlorogenic acid enriched coffee (Coffee shape) on weight when used in overweight people. Independent market study on the effect of coffee shape on weight loss. June (2009).
21. Yeon P.J., Young K.J., Pyo L.S., Ho LJ. The effect of green coffee bean extract supplementation on body fat reduction in over weight/obese woman. *Korean J. Nutr.* 43, 374–381 (2010).
22. Nagao T., Ochiai R., Watanabe T., Kataoka K., Komikado M., Tokimitsu I, Tsuchida T. Visceral fat-reducing effect of continuous coffee beverage consumption in obese subjects. *Jpn. Pharm. Ther.* [Japanese] 37, 333–344 (2009).
23. Stalmach A., Mullen W., Nagai C., Croizer A. On-line HPLC analysis of the antioxidant activity of phenolic compounds in brewed, paper-filtered coffee. *Braz. J. Plant Physiol.* 18, 253–262 (2006).

8 Antihypertension Effects of Green Coffee Bean Extract and Chlorogenic Acids

Ichiro Tokimitsu and Atsushi Suzuki

CONTENTS

8.1 INTRODUCTION

Coffee is one of the most widely consumed beverages in the world; therefore, even potentially small health benefits associated with coffee intake may have important implications for public health.

In a recent National Institutes of Health-AARP Diet and Health Study, 229,119 men and 173,141 women were monitored from 1995 to 2008 to examine the association of coffee drinking with subsequent total and cause-specific mortality [1]. Participants were 50–71 years of age at baseline. During 5,148,760 person-year of follow-up from 1995 to 2008, a total of 33,731 men and 18,784 women died. In age-adjusted models, the risk of death was increased among coffee drinkers. However, coffee drinkers were also more likely to smoke, and after adjustment for smoking status and other potential confounders, there was a significant inverse association between coffee consumption and mortality. Inverse associations were observed for deaths due to heart disease, respiratory disease, stroke, injuries and accidents, diabetes, and infections, but not for cancer-related deaths.

From a cardiovascular standpoint, several reviews have summarized the effects of coffee consumption on coronary heart disease [2,3], and many epidemiological studies have generally shown neutral effects. However, a meta-analysis of 21 independent prospective cohort studies from January 1966 to January 2008 suggested that moderate coffee consumption may decrease the long-term risk of coronary heart disease [4].

Among cardiovascular risk factors, hypertension is a strong independent risk factor. In the past, coffee was often viewed as a risk factor of hypertension. However, evidence analyzed from several epidemiological studies showed no clinically important effects of long-term coffee consumption on hypertension [5,6].

Most of the data on coffee's health effects are based on observational data, with very few randomized, controlled studies; association does not prove causation. Moreover, as coffee is a complex beverage containing hundreds of biologically active components, it remains unknown what components impact on cardiovascular risk factors. In this chapter, we introduce the antihypertension effects of green coffee bean extract (GCBE) and chlorogenic acids (CGA), major polyphenol components of GCBE, and discuss the different roles of coffee components in hypertension.

8.2 ANTIHYPERTENSION EFFECTS OF GREEN COFFEE BEAN EXTRACT

The antihypertension effect of GCBE was first reported by Suzuki et al. in 2002 [7]. In spontaneously hypertensive rats (SHR), a single oral administration of GCBE (180, 360, and 720 mg/kg) reduced blood pressure in a dose-dependent manner. Systolic blood pressure was reduced by 10–15 mmHg from baseline 10 h after the ingestion of GCBE at 720 mg/kg. However, GCBE had no significant effect on the normotensive counterparts (control rat Wistar-Kyoto [WKY]). Furthermore, chronic administration of GCBE mixed in rodent feed to young SHR for 6 weeks reduced the magnitude of high blood pressure development in a dose-dependent manner. Systolic blood pressure was 211 ± 2 in rats fed a control diet versus 199 ± 2, 186 ± 3, and 179 ± 4 mmHg in rats fed diets containing 0.25%, 0.5%, and 1% GCBE, respectively (Figure 8.1). Similar to the results of single oral administration, GCBE had no effect in the WKY control rats.

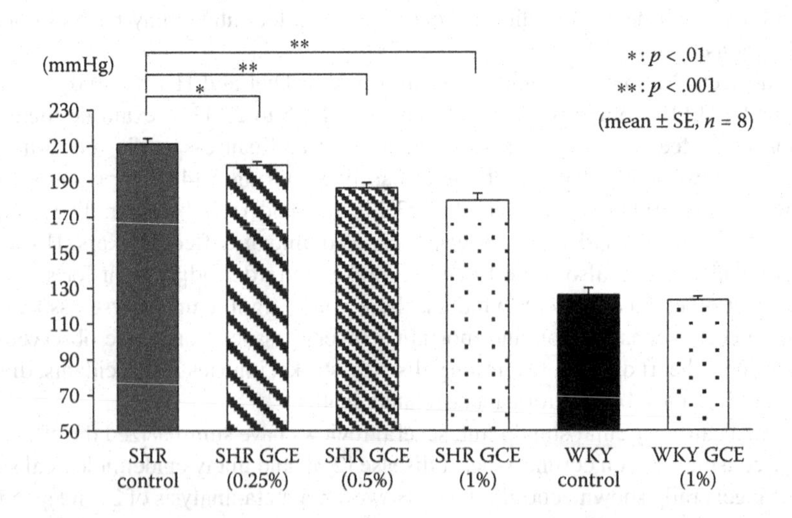

FIGURE 8.1 Systolic blood pressure after the 6-week experimental period in SHR or WKY rats. (Modified from Suzuki A, et al. *Hypertens Res.*, 2002; 25: 99–107.)

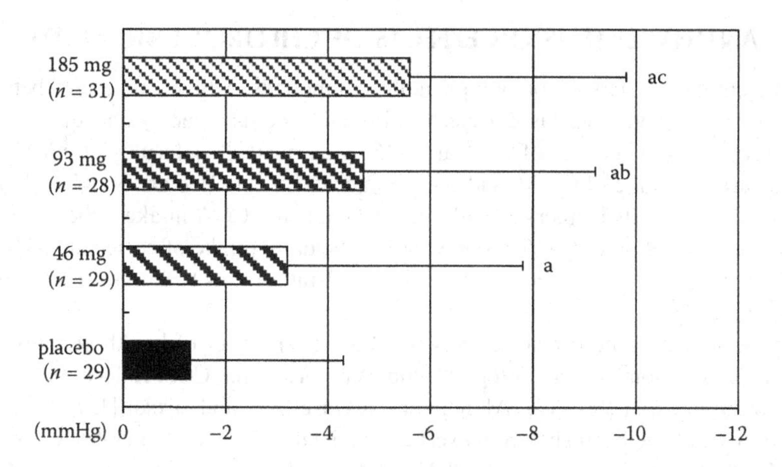

FIGURE 8.2 Mean (±SD) change in systolic blood pressure from baseline at 28 days after ingestion. [a] $p > .01$ compared with the baseline (one-way ANOVA); [b] $p < .05$, [c] $p < .01$ compared with the placebo (two-way ANOVA). (Modified from Kozuma K, et al. *Hypertens. Res.*, 2005; 28: 711–718.)

These findings in animals were later confirmed by studies in human patients with mild hypertension. Kozuma et al. reported the dose-dependent relationship of GCBE in 117 male volunteers with mild hypertension [8]. Subjects were randomized into four groups: a control group, and three drug groups that received 46, 93, or 185 mg of GCBE once a day. After 28 days, systolic blood pressure in the control, 46 mg, 93 mg, and 185 mg groups was reduced by −1.3 ± 3.0, −3.2 ± 4.6, −4.7 ± 4.5, and −5.6 ± 4.2 mmHg from the baseline, respectively. The decreases in systolic blood pressure in the 93 mg group and 185 mg group were statistically significant compared with the placebo group (Figure 8.2). Diastolic blood pressure in the control, 46 mg, 93 mg, and 185 mg groups was reduced by −0.8 ± 3.1, −2.9 ± 2.9, −3.2 ± 3.2, and −3.9 ± 2.8 mmHg from the baseline, respectively, and significant effects were observed in the 93 mg and 185 mg groups compared with the placebo group.

In another randomized clinical trial, Watanabe et al. reported similar effects of GCBE on systolic and diastolic blood pressure, which decreased significantly during the ingestion period in subjects (N = 28) with mild hypertension randomized to receive treatment with 480 mg GCBE per day for 12 weeks [9]. Moreover, Ochiai et al. [10] investigated the effects of GCBE on blood vessels in healthy males. The subjects were 20 healthy males with reduced vasodilation responses to ischemic reactive hyperemia, measured by strain gauge plethysmogram. Of the 20 subjects, 10 subjects ingested a test drink containing 500 mg GCBE every day for 4 months, and the other 10 subjects ingested a control drink. During the ingestion period, strain gauge plethysmogram, acceleration plethysmogram, pulse wave velocity, and serum biochemical parameters were measured. The reactive hyperemia ratio in the test drink group began to increase 1 month after ingestion, and was significantly higher than that of the control group after 3 and 4 months of ingestion. These results suggested that GCBE improved vasoreactivity.

8.3 ANTIHYPERTENSION EFFECTS OF CHLOROGENIC ACIDS

GCBE contains a family of polyphenolic compounds, which are esters between transcinnamic acid (such as caffeic, ferulic, and coumaric acid) and quinic acid. The three major subclasses of CGA are caffeoylquinic (CQA), feruloylquinic (FQA), and dicaffeoylquinic (diCQA) acids. The major CGA in coffee are 5-caffeoylquinic acid (5-CQA) and its isomers 3- and 4-CQA [11]. Daily CGA intake in heavy coffee drinkers is approximately 0.5–1.0 g, whereas the daily intake of coffee abstainers is <100 mg [12]. Thus, the majority of dietary CGA intake may be influenced by coffee consumption [11].

In recent years, the potential roles of CGA in a number of health benefits have been explored. Some epidemiological studies reported that CGA reduce the relative risks of type 2 diabetes [13], Alzheimer's disease [14], and stroke [15]. In animal studies, CGA have been shown to exert a beneficial influence on metabolic diseases [16]. Special attention was paid to CGA's effect on insulin resistance and the underlying molecular mechanisms [17].

During the last decade, investigations have demonstrated that CGA have an antihypertension effect in both SHR and humans. Recently, Onakpoya et al. reported the effect of CGA on blood pressure, by meta-analysis of randomized clinical trials (7 eligible studies, 364 participants) [18]. They suggested that CGA intake causes statistically significant reductions in systolic and diastolic blood pressure, although the size of the effects was moderate.

In SHR, Suzuki et al. reported that a single oral ingestion (50–200 mg/kg) of 5-CQA dose-dependently decreased blood pressure [7], and they suggested that 5-CQA was the underlying reason for this antihypertensive effect. Furthermore, Suzuki et al. examined the effects of 5-CQA on blood pressure and vascular function in age-matched normotensive WKY rats and SHR in detail [19], reporting that a single ingestion of 5-CQA (30–600 mg/kg) reduced blood pressure in SHR, and its effect was blocked by the administration of a nitric oxide (NO) synthase inhibitor, N(G)-nitro-L-arginine methyl ester. When SHR were fed diets containing 0.5% 5-CQA for 8 weeks (approximately 300 mg/kg per day), the development of hypertension was inhibited compared with the control diet group. 5-CQA increased urinary excretion of NO metabolites and decreased urinary excretion of hydrogen peroxide; decreased nicotinamide adenine dinucleotide phosphate (NADPH)-dependent superoxide anion production in the aorta, suggesting that dietary 5-CQA inhibited vascular NADPH oxidase activity; significantly improved acetylcholine-induced endothelium-dependent vasodilation in the aorta; and markedly reduced the degree of immunohistochemical staining for nitrotyrosine and media hypertrophy in aorta sections. A positive relationship between oxidative stress and blood pressure was demonstrated in some models of experimental hypertension [20], and NADPH oxidase-derived superoxide was shown to have a pivotal role in the regulation of vascular tone [21]. Suzuki et al. suggested that dietary 5-CQA may reduce oxidative stress and improve NO bioavailability by inhibiting excessive production of reactive species in the vasculature, leading to the attenuation of endothelial dysfunction, vascular hypertrophy, and hypertension in SHR [19].

It was also reported that because significant increases in caffeic acid or ferulic acid were detected in plasma after oral ingestion of 5-CQA in SHR, these acids (2.5, 5, 10 μmol/kg) were intravenously injected into SHR under anesthesia and the carotid arterial pressure was measured, which demonstrated that ferulic acid had a stronger depressor effect than caffeic acid [7]. Suzuki et al. reported the effect of ferulic acid on blood pressure in SHR, and demonstrated that after oral administration of ferulic acid (1–100 mg/kg) to SHR, systolic blood pressure significantly decreased in a dose-dependent manner [22]. When oral ferulic acid (50 mg/kg) was administrated to SHR, blood pressure was lowest after 1 h, and returned to basal levels after 6 h. There was a significant correlation between ferulic acid content in SHR plasma and changes in the systolic blood pressure of the tail artery. When 7-week-old SHR were given 10 and 50 mg/kg per day of ferulic acid for 6 weeks, increases in blood pressure were significantly attenuated compared with SHR on the control diet. Furthermore, the depressor effect of intravenous ferulic acid (1 mg/kg) was significantly attenuated by pretreatment of SHR with the NO synthase inhibitor N(G)-nitro-L-arginine methyl ester. This suggested that the hypotensive effect of ferulic acid in SHR is associated with NO-mediated vasodilation. Suzuki et al. also suggested that ferulic acid restores endothelial function through the enhancement of the bioavailability of basal and stimulated NO in SHR aortas [23].

Other mechanisms by which 5-CQA or its metabolites exert their antihypertension effects were also presented. Ferulic acid may interact with the renin-angiotensin-aldosterone system by inhibiting angiotensin-converting enzyme activity, demonstrated both *in vitro* and *in vivo* [24]. In the stroke-prone SHR, systolic blood pressure was decreased 30 mmHg lower than baseline in response to a single oral administration of ferulic acid at a dose of 9.5 mg/kg, corresponding with a simultaneous reduction of plasma angiotensin-converting enzyme activity from 20.6 to 16.9 mU/mL 2 h after administration. Taken together, these results warrant more detailed experimentation to determine the mechanism of action of 5-CQA and its metabolites.

Several pharmacokinetics studies reported that the small intestine was the site where quinic acid is cleaved from CQA and FQA, as well as the site of caffeic and ferulic acid release, whereas the colon was important for the conversion of both ferulic and caffeic acid to dihydroferulic acid and its absorption [11,25,26]. Because it has been shown that beverage components appear to influence the bioaccessibility and intestinal absorption of CGA [27], future research efforts should consider the extent to which beverage composition impacts absorption efficiency and processes as well as the metabolism of CGA.

8.4 ANTIHYPERTENSION EFFECTS DIFFER BETWEEN GCBE AND REGULAR ROASTED COFFEE

The consumption of regular roasted coffee does not reduce blood pressure, despite the 5-CQA content of roasted coffee falling within the range that demonstrated antihypertension effects in the previously mentioned studies [5,6]. As GCBE reduced

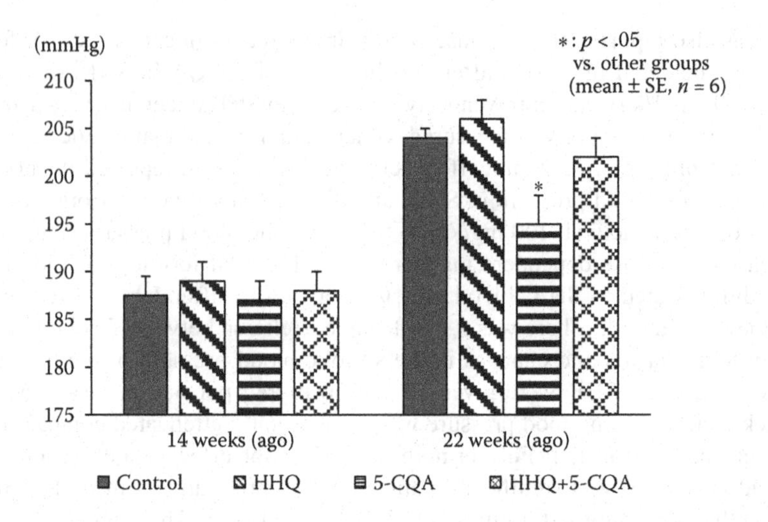

FIGURE 8.3 Systolic blood pressure during the 8-week experimental period in SHR rats. (Modified from Suzuki A, et al. *Am. J. Hypertens*, 2008; 21: 23–27.)

blood pressure in human hypertensive subjects despite a caffeine content equal to that in roasted coffee, caffeine content alone does not convincingly explain the discrepancy in the antihypertension effects of GCBE versus regular roasted coffee.

It has been hypothesized that the antihypertension effects of GCBE are not observed with roasted coffee consumption due to the production of pro-oxidant components such as hydroxyhydroquinone (HHQ), which can neutralize the effects of GCBE in the roasted coffee (Figure 8.3) [28]. Suzuki et al. reported that HHQ inhibited the CQA-induced improvement in hypertension, urinary NO metabolites or hydrogen peroxide excretion, endothelial dysfunction, and nitrotyrosine deposits in SHR aortas. However, it was also reported that the administration of HHQ alone had little effect on these processes.

Indeed, findings from an SHR study showed that the removal of low-molecular-weight components from roasted coffee, including HHQ, by treatment with activated charcoal may allow the CQA present to exert its antihypertension effect; and the attenuation of hypertension by HHQ-reduced coffee was associated with the suppression of NADPH oxidase mRNA expression including the improvement in endothelium-dependent vasodilation in SHR aortas [29]. Recently, several studies in humans have suggested that HHQ-reduced coffee with comparable levels of caffeine have an antihypertension effect, as shown in Table 8.1. Although the mechanism of HHQ is not fully understood and the data relating to its function are still preliminary, HHQ-reduced coffee may have potential for providing cardiovascular benefits.

8.5 CONCLUSIONS

Lifestyle improvements such as undertaking an exercise regimen and developing healthy eating habits are important for the prevention of hypertension, but the

TABLE 8.1
Effects of HHQ-Reduced Coffee on Blood Pressure in Human Studies

Authors, Year	Duration	Population	Treatment	Results
Chikama et al., 2006 [30]	12 w	41 high normal 59 mildly hypertensive	Randomized double-blind parallel trial • Active coffee CQA; 299 mg/184 mL, HHQ; 0.05 mg/184 mL • Control coffee CQA; 0 mg/184 mL, HHQ; 0.02 mg/184 mL	SBP was significantly decreased in the active group compared with the control group.
Nagao et al., 2007 [31]	12 w	120 high normal 95 mildly hypertensive	Randomized double-blind parallel trial • Active milk coffee CQA; 168 mg/100 g, HHQ; 0.019 mg/100 g • Control milk coffee CQA; 0 mg/100 g, HHQ; 0.004 mg/100 g	The decreases in SBP and DBP were significantly greater in the active group than in the control group.
Yamaguchi et al., 2007 [32]	12 w	88 high normal	Randomized double-blind parallel trial • Active coffee CQA; 300 mg/184 mL, HHQ; 0.03 mg/184 mL • Control coffee CQA; 0 mg/184 mL, HHQ; 0.03 mg/184 mL	The decreases in SBP and DBP were significantly greater in the active group than in the control group.
Chikama et al., 2008 [33]	12 w	38 high normal 60 mildly hypertensive	Randomized double-blind parallel trial • Active coffee CQA; 299 mg/184 mL, HHQ; 0.05 mg/184 mL • Control coffee CQA; 299 mg/184 mL, HHQ; 1.69 mg/184 mL	SBP was significantly lower in the active group than in the control group throughout the intake period.

(Continued)

TABLE 8.1 (CONTINUED)
Effects of HHQ-Reduced Coffee on Blood Pressure in Human Studies

Authors, Year	Duration	Population	Treatment	Results
Ochiai et al., 2008 [34]	4 w	31 patients with essential hypertension undergoing treatment with antihypertensive drugs	Randomized double-blind crossover trial • Active coffee CQA; 299 mg/184 mL, HHQ; 0.05 mg/184 mL • Control coffee CQA; 299 mg/184 mL, HHQ; 1.69 mg/184 mL	HHQ-reduced coffee did not significantly change SBP or DBP compared with the control coffee.
Yamaguchi et al., 2008 [35]	4 w	203 mildly hypertensive	Randomized double-blind parallel trial • Test coffee CQA; 0 mg/184 mL, HHQ; 0.02 mg/184 mL CQA; 82 mg/184 mL, HHQ; 0.03 mg/184 mL CQA; 172 mg/184 mL, HHQ; 0.04 mg/184 mL CQA; 299 mg/184 mL, HHQ; 0.05 mg/184 mL • Control coffee CQA; 299 mg/184 mL, HHQ; 1.7 mg/184 mL	CQA has an antihypertensive effect in a dose-dependent manner in HHQ-reduced coffee, and ordinary coffee showed almost no effect.
Ochiai et al., 2009 [36]	8 w	21 mildly hypertensive	Randomized double-blind parallel trial • Active coffee CQA; 300 mg/184 mL, HHQ; 0.03 mg/184 mL • Control coffee CQA; 0 mg/184 mL, HHQ; 0.03 mg/184 mL	In the active group, SBP was significantly decreased from the baseline, but not in the control group.

adoption of these practices is often difficult. GCBE or CGA, in particular their metabolite ferulic acid, have been shown to have antioxidative and antihypertension effects, which are more pronounced in the absence of HHQ. As a source of antioxidants and as a potential lifestyle modification, HHQ-reduced coffee may hold promise in the pursuit of a healthy blood pressure.

REFERENCES

1. Freedman ND, Park Y, Abnet CC, Hollenbeck AR, Sinha R. Association of coffee drinking with total and cause-specific mortality. *N. Engl. J. Med.*, 2012; 366: 1891–1904.
2. Rebello SA, van Dam RM. Coffee consumption and cardiovascular health: Getting to the heart of the matter. *Curr. Cardiol. Rep.*, 2013; 15: 403–415.
3. O'Keefe JH, Bhatti SK, Patil HR, DiNicolantonio JJ, Lucan SC, Lavie CJ. Effects of habitual coffee consumption on cardiometabolic disease, cardiovascular health, and all-cause mortality. *J. Am. Coll. Cardiol.*, 2013; 62: 1043–1051.
4. Wu JN, Ho SC, Zhou C, Ling W, Chen W, Wang C, Chen Y. Coffee consumption and risk of coronary heart diseases: A meta-analysis of 21 prospective cohort studies. *Int. J. Cardiol.*, 2009; 137: 216–225.
5. Guessous I, Eap CB, Bochud M. Blood pressure in relation to coffee and caffeine consumption. *Curr. Hypertens. Rep.*, 2014; 16: 468–477.
6. Zhang Z, Hu G., Caballero B, Appel L, Chen L. Habitual coffee consumption and risk of hypertension: A systematic review and mata-analysis of prospective observational studies. *Am. J. Clin. Nutr.*, 2011; 93: 1212–1219.
7. Suzuki A, Kagawa D, Ochiai R, Tokimitsu I, Saito I. Green coffee bean extract and its metabolites have a hypotensive effect in spontaneously hypertensive rats. *Hypertens Res.*, 2002; 25: 99–107.
8. Kozuma K, Tsuchiya S, Kohori J, Hase T, Tokimitsu I. Antihypertensive effect of green coffee bean extract on mildly hypertensive subjects. *Hypertens. Res.*, 2005; 28: 711–718.
9. Watanabe T, Arai Y, Mitsui Y, Kusaura T, Okawa W, Kajihara Y, Saito I. The blood pressure-lowering effect and safety of chlorogenic acid from green coffee bean extract in essential hypertension. *Clin. Exp. Hypertens.*, 2006; 28: 439–449.
10. Ochiai R, Jokura H, Suzuki A, Tokimitsu I, Ohishi M, Komai N, Rakugi H, Ogihara T. Green coffee bean extract improves human vasoreactivity. Green coffee bean extract improves human vasoreactivity. *Hypertens. Res.*, 2004; 27: 731–737.
11. Zhao Y, Wang J, Ballerre O, Luo H, Zhang W. Antihypertensive effects and mechanisms of chlorogenic acids. *Hypertens. Res.*, 2012; 35: 370–374.
12. Olthof MR, Hollman PC, Katan MB. Chlorogenic acid and caffeic acid are absorbed in humans. *J. Nutr.*, 2001; 131: 66–71.
13. van Dam RM, Hu FB. Coffee consumption and risk of type 2 diabetes: A systematic review. *JAMA*, 2005; 294: 97–104.
14. Lindsay J, Laurin D, Verreault R, Helliwell B, Hill GB, McDowell I. Risk factors for Altzheimer's disease: A prospective analysis from the Canadian Study of Health and Aging. Am. J. *Epdermiol.*, 2002; 156: 445–453.
15. Larsson SC, Virtamo J, Wolk A. Coffee consumption and risk of stroke in women. *Stroke*, 2011; 42: 908–912.
16. Cho SC, Jeon SM, Kim MJ, Yeo J, Seo KI, Choi MS, Lee MK. Chlorogenic acid exhibits anti-obesity property and improves lipid metabolism in high-fat diet-induced-obese mice. *Food Chem. Toxicol.*, 2011; 48: 937–943.

17. Ma Y, Gao M, Liu D. Chlorogenic acid improves high fat diet-induced hepatic steatosis and insulin resistance in mice. *Pharm. Res.*, 2015; 32: 1200–1209.
18. Onakpoya IJ, Spencer EA, Thompson MJ, Heneghan CJ. The effects of chlorogenic acid on blood pressure: A systematic review and meta-analysis of randomized clinical trials. *J. Hum. Hypertens.*, 2015; 29: 77–81.
19. Suzuki A, Yamamoto N, Jokura H, Yamamoto M, Fujii A, Tokimitsu I, Saito I. Chlorogenic acid sttenuates hypertension and improves endothelial function in spontaneously hypertensive rat. *J. Hypertens.*, 2006; 24: 1065–1073.
20. Banday AA, Muhammad AB, Fazili FR, Lokhandwala M. Mechanisms of oxidative stress-induced increase in salt sensitivity and development of hypertension in Sprague-Dawley rats. *Hypertension*, 2007; 49: 664–671.
21. Lambeth JD. NOX enzymes and the biology of reactive oxygen. *Nat. Rev. Immunol.*, 2004; 4: 181–189.
22. Suzuki A, Kagawa D, Fujii A, Ochiai R, Tokimitsu I, Saito I. Short- and long-term effects of ferulic acid on blood pressures in spontaneously hypertensive rats. *Am. J. Hypertens.*, 2002; 15: 351–357.
23. Suzuki A, Yamamoto M, Jokura H, Fujii A, Tokimitsu I, Hase T, Saito I. Ferulic acid restores endothelium-dependent vasodilation in aortas of spontaneously hypertensive rats. *Am. J. Hypertens.*, 2007; 20: 508–513.
24. Ardiansyah, Ohsaki Y, Shirakawa H, Koseki T, Komai M. Novel effects of a single administration of ferulic acid on the regulation of blood pressure and the hepatic lipid metabolic profile in stroke-prone spontaneously hypertensive rats. *J. Agric. Food Chem.*, 2008; 56: 2825–2830.
25. Renouf M, Guy PA, Marnet C, Fraering AL, Lonet K, Moulin J, Ensien M, Barron D, Dionisi F, Cavin C, Williamson G, Steiling H. Measurement of caffeic and ferulic acid equivalents in plasma after coffee consumption: Small intestine and colon are key sites for coffee metabolism. *Mol. Nutr. Food Res.*, 2010; 54: 760–766.
26. Stalmach A, Mullen W, Barron D, Uchida K, Yokota T, Cavin C, Steiling H, Williamson G, Crozier A. Metabolite profiling of hydroxycinnamate deriatives in plasma and urine after the ingestion of coffee by humans: Identification of biomarkers of coffee consumption. *Drug Metab. Dispos.*, 2009; 37: 1749–1758.
27. Renouf M, Marmet C, Guy P, Fraering AL, Longet K, Moulin J, Enslen M, Barron D, Cavin C, Dionisi F, Rezzi S, Kochhar S, Steiling H, Williamson G. Nondairy creamer, but not milk, delays the appearance of coffee phenolic acid equivalents in human plasma. *J. Nutr.*, 2010; 140: 259–263.
28. Suzuki A, Fujii A, Jokura H, Tokimitsu I, Hase T, Saito I. Hydroxyhydroquinone interferes with the chlorogenic acid-induced restoration of endothelial function in spontaneously hypertensive rats. *Am, J. Hypertens.*, 2008; 21: 23–27.
29. Suzuki A, Fujii A, Yamamoto N, Yamamoto M, Ohminami H, Kameyama A, Shibuya Y, Nishizawa Y, Tokimitsu I, Saito I. Improvement of hypertension and vascular dysfunction by hydroxyhydroquinone-free coffee in a genetic model of hypertension. *FEBS Lett.*, 2006; 580: 2317–2322.
30. Chikama A, Yamaguchi T, Watanabe T, Mori K, Katsuragi Y, Tokimitsu I, Kajimoto O, Kitakaze M. Effects of chlorogenic acids in hydroxyhydroquinone-reduced coffee on blood pressure and vascular endothelial function in humans. *Prog. Med.*, 2006; 26: 1723–1736.
31. Nagao T, Ochiai R, Katsuragi Y, Hayakawa Y, Kataoka K, Komikado M, Tokimitsu I, Tsuchida T. Hydroxyhydroquinone-reduced milk coffee decreases blood pressure in individuals with mild hypertension and high-normal blood pressure. *Prog. Med.*, 2007; 11: 2649–2664.
32. Yamaguchi T, Chikama A, Inaba M, Ochiai R, Katsuragi Y, Tokimitsu I, Tsuchida T, Saito I. Antihypertensive effects of hydroxyhydroquinone-reduced coffee on high-normal blood pressure subjects. *Prog. Med.*, 2007; 27: 683–694.

33. Chikama A, Yamaguchi T, Ochiai R, Kataoka K, Tokimitsu I. Effects of hydroxyhydroquinone-reduced coffee on blood pressure in high-normotensives and mild hypertensives. *J. Health Sci.*, 2008; 54: 162–173.
34. Ochiai R, Nagao T, Katsuragi Y, Tokimitsu I, Funatsu K, Nakamura H. Effects of hydroxyhydroquinone-reduced coffee in patients with essential hypertension. *J. Health Sci.*, 2008; 54: 302–309.
35. Yamaguchi T, Chikama A, Mori K, Watanabe T, Shioya Y, Katsuragi Y, Tokimitsu I. Hydroxyhydroquinone-free coffee: A double-blind, randomized controlled dose-response study of blood pressure. *Nutr. Metab. Cardiovasc. Dis.*, 2008; 18: 408–414.
36. Ochiai R, Chikama A, Kataoka K, Tokimitsu I, Maekawa Y, Ohishi M, Rakugi H, Mikami H. Effects of hydroxyhydroqinone-reduced coffee on vasoreactivity and blood pressure. *Hypertens. Res.*, 2009; 32: 969–974.

9 Therapeutic Potential of Green Coffee Bean in Nonalcoholic Fatty Liver Disease

Rama P. Nair, Debasis Bagchi, Anand Swaroop, and Sreejayan Nair

CONTENTS

ABSTRACT

Nonalcoholic fatty liver disease (NAFLD) is emerging as a leading cause of liver disease globally. The increase in the incidence of NAFLD is closely associated to the epidemic of obesity and its associated metabolic consequences. Recent studies have shown that consumption of coffee can lower the risks associated with a host of chronic conditions including NAFLD. This chapter will focus on the published studies that demonstrate a link between green coffee bean consumption and reduced risks associated with the development of NAFLD.

Keywords: green coffee bean, liver, fat

9.1 INTRODUCTION

Nonalcoholic fatty liver disease (NAFLD) is a major cause of morbidity and mortality and afflicts about 30% of the U.S. population. According to data from the National Health and Nutrition Examination Survey cases of NAFLD showed a steady increase, accounting for 75.1% of all cases of chronic liver disease between 2005 and 2008, although the prevalence of major causes of chronic liver diseases remained stable during this period [1]. The increase in NAFLD during recent years is attributed to the emerging epidemic of obesity and its related metabolic anomalies [1]. A recent report indicates that 66% of subjects older than 50 years with diabetes or obesity are thought to have steatohepatitis (a subtype of NAFLD) [2]. Another report shows that 85% of subjects who develop NAFLD exhibit at least one characteristic of metabolic syndrome [3]. Both genetic and dietary factors have been implicated in the pathophysiology of NAFLD [4]. Consequently, diet and exercise have been shown to have beneficial effects in curtailing NAFLD, although compliance is a major problem. As there are currently no drugs that are approved by the Food and Drug Administration (FDA), it is important to identify and characterize natural products and supplements that have beneficial attributes in treating NAFLD.

9.2 PATHOPHYSIOLOGY

NAFLD is characterized by triglyceride accumulation in the hepatocytes (steatosis) and is often associated with obesity, metabolic disease, and diabetes. When steatosis is associated with inflammatory changes and fibrosis, the condition is referred to as nonalcoholic steatohepatitis (NASH) [5,6]. Subjects with NASH are predisposed to cirrhosis, hepatocellular carcinoma, and early atherosclerosis [7]. NAFLD is a multifactorial disease and the molecular mechanisms leading to it are still unclear, although a number of postulates have been proposed to explain the progression of the disease [7,8]. As NAFLD often coexists with obesity and metabolic syndrome, mechanisms including insulin resistance, glucose intolerance, glucotoxicity, and lipotoxicity have been implicated in the pathogenesis of NAFLD [9]. Hepatic insulin resistance, defined as the reduced sensitivity of the liver cells to insulin, results in impaired insulin signal transduction, which results in dysregulation of glucose evidenced as an increase in gluconeogenesis and hyperglycemia. Under normal circumstances, insulin binding to insulin receptor results in the phosphorylation of the insulin receptor, which acts as a tyrosine kinase that subsequently stimulates and activates a variety of downstream substrates including insulin receptor substrate (IRS-1), phosphatidylinositol-3-kinase (PI3K), and protein kinase B (Akt/PKB). Phosphorylated Akt mediates the translocation of GLUT-4 vesicles from the cytoplasm to the cell membrane, which facilitates glucose uptake. Akt also phosphorylates and deactivates glycogen synthase kinase 3 (GSK3), which restores glycogen synthase activity, resulting in hepatic glycogen synthesis. Activated Akt can also phosphorylate the transcription factor FOXO1 (forkhead box protein), which results in the translocation of FOXO from the nucleus to the cytoplasm, thereby restricting its involvement in the transcription of gluconeogenic genes such as phosphoenolpyruvate carboxykinase (PEPCK) and glucose-6-phosphatase (G6Pase). In addition to insulin resistance, persistent oxidative stress and resultant low-grade inflammation are hallmarks of NAFLD. Resistance to insulin signaling is thought to be mediated by the availability of excessive free fatty acids and inflammatory cytokines associated with obesity. Recent evidence suggests that hepatic endoplasmic reticulum (ER) stress, which is a consequence of protein mishandling (due to excessive cargo supplied to the ER in states of obesity), contributes to insulin resistance [10], which may also potentially represent a common pathway leading to NAFLD. Studies have shown that obesity-induced ER stress is mediated via the activation of the c-Jun N-terminal kinase (JNK) pathway, which leads to the phosphorylation of a serine residue on IRS-1, thus facilitating its ubiquitination [11]. The observations that subjects with fatty liver exhibited elevated levels of JNK phosphorylation together with increased ER stress, and weight reduction in obese subjects reduced JNK phosphorylation and reduced ER stress further substantiates the view that cross talk between the insulin signaling pathway and ER stress may have an important role in the pathogenesis of the disease [12,13].

In addition to causing insulin resistance, excessive lipid accumulation in liver and fat tissues can result in an "overspill" of fatty acids or its toxic metabolites, causing lipotoxicity [14]. Lipotoxicity can induce an increase in systemic proinflammatory cytokines, which can continue a vicious cycle leading to further hepatic damage. Hyperglycemia, elevated free fatty acids, and proinflammatory cytokines can also induce the generation of noxious reactive oxygen free radicals (ROS), which can further lead to tissue damage and fibrosis [15]. The major source of ROS is the mitochondria, wherein hepatic β-oxidation is elevated under increased availability of free fatty acids resulting in an increase of electron flux in the electron transport chain [16]. Overcompensation by the mitochondria will eventually result in decompensation, leading to mitochondrial dysfunction [16].

9.3 PHARMACOTHERAPY

As there are no FD approved drugs to treat NAFLD, lifestyle modification through diet and exercise is the mainstay of the treatment for this disease. Studies by Dixon and coworkers have reported that weight loss improves abnormal liver histological features in obese subjects with metabolic syndrome [17]. Although insulin sensitizers such as thiazolidinediones have been shown to improve hepatic steatosis [18,19], cardiovascular adverse effects associated with these classes of drugs are a major deterrent to their use. In another recent trial, where low-dose metformin plus dietary treatment was compared with dietary treatment alone over a period of 6 months, metformin was found to be more effective than dietary treatment alone in normalizing several metabolic parameters in NAFLD patients [20]. Although several other treatment options such as ursodeoxycholic acid, statins, and poly- and monounsaturated fatty acids have been proposed, none have been demonstrated to be of consistent benefit in treating NAFLD. Natural products and phytochemicals, owing to their pluripotent properties including protection against oxidative stress, attenuation of insulin resistance, improving glucose disposal, and reducing lipotoxicity may find application in the management of NAFDL.

9.4 COFFEE AND NAFLD

Several recent studies have suggested the beneficial effects of coffee on NAFLD. In a recently published excellent systematic review, Saab and coworkers conclude (based on epidemiologic studies) that consumption of approximately three or more cups of coffee daily reduces hepatotoxicity due to a variety of underlying pathologic processes [21]. Catalano and coworkers studied the effect of coffee consumption on bright liver in subjects with NAFLD and compared it to body mass index and insulin resistance, and found that coffee drinking was inversely associated with bright liver, insulin resistance (assessed as homeostatic model assesment [HOMA] IR), and obesity [22]. In another study, Birerdinc and coworkers, using data from four continuous cycles of the National Health and Nutrition Examination Surveys (NHANES 2001–2008), found that caffeine intake is independently associated with a lower risk of NAFLD [23]. Yamashita and coworkers have demonstrated that coffee consumption is associated with elevated adiponectin levels, which they speculate as the potential explanation for the benefits of coffee in hepatobiliary disease [24]. Gutiérrez-Grobe and coworkers demonstrated that a high intake of coffee has a protective effect against NAFLD, although they did not observe any alteration in antioxidant status in the subjects who consumed coffee [25]. More recently, Xiao and coworkers performed a cross-sectional study to demonstrate an association between coffee consumption and hepatic enzymes with a special emphasis on decaffeinated coffee [26]. This study involved 27,793 subjects obtained through the 1999–2010 NHANES database. Interestingly, this study found an inverse relationship between liver enzyme levels and decaf intake, suggesting that coffee components other than caffeine may also have an important role in the beneficial effects on the liver.

9.5 GREEN COFFEE BEAN EXTRACT

Recent evidence suggests that coffee roasting can alter the polyphenolic components in the coffee and thereby its biological activity [27]. Emerging evidence suggests that green coffee bean extract, rich in chlorogenic acid, may have potential in reducing weight gain [28]. Using freshly isolated human-derived adipocytes, Flanagan and coworkers showed that a commercial green coffee bean extract causes the release of free fatty acids, crediting lipolytic properties to green coffee bean extract [29]. Shimoda and coworkers found that treating ddY mice with green coffee bean extract for 14 days in response to olive oil loading resulted in a suppression of body weight and visceral fat accumulation. Furthermore, green coffee bean lowered the levels of triglycerides accumulated in the liver and enhanced the activity of carnitine palmitoyltransferase (CPT), suggesting that the extract enhances fat metabolism by the liver [30]. Song and coworkers investigated the effect of decaffeinated green coffee bean on obesity and insulin resistance in mice subjected to a high-fat diet and demonstrated that green coffee bean extract reduced weight gain, downregulated genes involved in adipogenesis, attenuated proinflammatory pathway, and augmented the translocation of GLUT4 from the cytoplasm to the plasma membrane in white adipose tissues [31].

In contrast however, Li Kwok Cheong and colleagues failed to see any alterations in high-fat-diet-induced obesity, glucose intolerance, insulin resistance, or systemic oxidative stress in C57BL6 mice subjected to a high-fat diet [32]. In studies conducted in our laboratory using a similar model of a high-fat diet, we found a marginal improvement in insulin tolerance associated with green coffee bean extract but failed to see any changes in the rate of glucose disposal [33]. However, mice treated with green coffee bean exhibited significant reduction in hepatic steatosis. Interestingly, chlorogenic acid partially rescued insulin signaling, as evidenced by the levels of Akt phosphorylation in the liver of mice, which was blunted following high-fat diet feeding. This effect of chlorogenic acid on insulin signaling was surprising in that it did not translate into improving whole-body glucose tolerance. Furthermore, we failed to observe any alterations in the phosphorylation of IRβ, suggesting that the changes in Akt phosphorylation may be downstream of the insulin receptor.

There is a paucity of human studies that focus on the effects of green coffee bean in subjects with obesity and NAFLD. Bakuradze and coworkers conducted a 12-week interventional study aimed at characterizing the DNA-protective and antioxidant potential of coffee, rich in both roast products and green coffee bean constituents, and concluded that coffee consumption reduces oxidative damage, body fat mass, and energy/nutrient uptake [34]. A study by Thom in 12 healthy volunteers demonstrated that ingestion of coffee enriched with chlorogenic acid (but not normal or decaffeinated coffee) resulted in lower glucose absorption and a significant reduction in body mass [35].

CONCLUSION

Studies in experimental animals and in cultured cells suggest that green coffee bean extract and/or its components may attenuate weight gain, alleviate hepatic fat accumulation, increase lipolysis, and improve oxidative stress. However, there also are published studies that did not find any benefits, necessitating further studies with standardized extract and established animal models to determine the effect of green coffee bean on obesity and fatty liver disease. Long-term clinical studies in a larger population are warranted to attribute causality to the large amounts of epidemiological data that demonstrate an association between liver health and coffee consumption.

REFERENCES

1. Younossi, Z. M., Stepanova, M., Afendy, M., Fang, Y., Younossi, Y., Mir, H., Srishord, M. (2011) Changes in the prevalence of the most common causes of chronic liver diseases in the United States from 1988 to 2008. *Clin Gastroenterol Hepatol*, 9, 524–530.
2. Rinella, M. E. (2015) Nonalcoholic fatty liver disease: A systematic review. *JAMA*, 313, 2263–2273.
3. Gariani, K., Philippe, J., Jornayvaz, F. R. (2013) Non-alcoholic fatty liver disease and insulin resistance: From bench to bedside. *Diabetes Metab*, 39, 16–26.
4. Pearlman, M., Loomba, R. (2014) State of the art: Treatment of nonalcoholic steatohepatitis. *Curr Opin Gastroenterol*, 30, 223–237.
5. Gastaldelli, A., Kozakova, M., Hojlund, K., Flyvbjerg, A., Favuzzi, A., Mitrakou, A., Balkau, B., Investigators, R. (2009) Fatty liver is associated with insulin resistance, risk of coronary heart disease, and early atherosclerosis in a large European population. *Hepatology*, 49, 1537–1544.
6. Paredes, A. H., Torres, D. M., Harrison, S. A. (2012) Nonalcoholic fatty liver disease. *Clin Liver Dis*, 16, 397–419.
7. Higuera-de la Tijera, F., Servin-Caamano, A. I. (2015) Pathophysiological mechanisms involved in non-alcoholic steatohepatitis and novel potential therapeutic targets. *World J Hepatol*, 7, 1297–1301.
8. Hassan, K., Bhalla, V., El Regal, M. E., A-Kader, H. H. (2014) Nonalcoholic fatty liver disease: A comprehensive review of a growing epidemic. *World J Gastroenterol*, 20, 12082–12101.

9. Asrih, M., Jornayvaz, F. R. (2015) Metabolic syndrome and nonalcoholic fatty liver disease: Is insulin resistance the link? *Mol Cell Endocrinol*, 418, 55–65.
10. Cnop, M., Foufelle, F., Velloso, L. A. (2012) Endoplasmic reticulum stress, obesity and diabetes. *Trends Mol Med*, 18, 59–68.
11. Hotamisligil, G. S. (2007) Endoplasmic reticulum stress and inflammation in obesity and type 2 diabetes. In *Fatty Acids and Lipotoxicity in Obesity and Diabetes*, Novartis Foundation Symposium, 286, 86–94; discussion 94–88, 162–163, 196–203.
12. Gregor, M. F., Yang, L., Fabbrini, E., Mohammed, B. S., Eagon, J. C., Hotamisligil, G. S., Klein, S. (2009) Endoplasmic reticulum stress is reduced in tissues of obese subjects after weight loss. *Diabetes*, 58, 693–700.
13. Puri, P., Mirshahi, F., Cheung, O., Natarajan, R., Maher, J. W., Kellum, J. M., Sanyal, A. J. (2008) Activation and dysregulation of the unfolded protein response in nonalcoholic fatty liver disease. *Gastroenterology*, 134, 568–576.
14. Cusi, K. (2012) Role of obesity and lipotoxicity in the development of nonalcoholic steatohepatitis: Pathophysiology and clinical implications. *Gastroenterology*, 142, 711–725 e716.
15. Robertson, G., Leclercq, I., Farrell, G. C. (2001) Nonalcoholic steatosis and steatohepatitis. II. Cytochrome P-450 enzymes and oxidative stress. *Am J Physiol Gastrointest Liver Physiol*, 281, G1135–1139.
16. Rolo, A. P., Teodoro, J. S., Palmeira, C. M. (2012) Role of oxidative stress in the pathogenesis of nonalcoholic steatohepatitis. *Free Radic Biol Med*, 52, 59–69.
17. Dixon, J. B., Bhathal, P. S., Hughes, N. R., O'Brien, P. E. (2004) Nonalcoholic fatty liver disease: Improvement in liver histological analysis with weight loss. *Hepatology*, 39, 1647–1654.
18. Neuschwander-Tetri, B. A., Brunt, E. M., Wehmeier, K. R., Oliver, D., Bacon, B. R. (2003) Improved nonalcoholic steatohepatitis after 48 weeks of treatment with the PPAR-gamma ligand rosiglitazone. *Hepatology*, 38, 1008–1017.
19. Aithal, G. P., Thomas, J. A., Kaye, P. V., Lawson, A., Ryder, S. D., Spendlove, I., Austin, A. S., Freeman, J. G., Morgan, L., Webber, J. (2008) Randomized, placebo-controlled trial of pioglitazone in nondiabetic subjects with nonalcoholic steatohepatitis. *Gastroenterology*, 135, 1176–1184.
20. Garinis, G. A., Fruci, B., Mazza, A., De Siena, M., Abenavoli, S., Gulletta, E., Ventura, V., Greco, M., Abenavoli, L., Belfiore, A. (2010) Metformin versus dietary treatment in nonalcoholic hepatic steatosis: A randomized study. *Int J Obes (Lond)*, 34, 1255–1264.
21. Saab, S., Mallam, D., Cox, G. A., 2nd, Tong, M. J. (2014) Impact of coffee on liver diseases: A systematic review. *Liver Int*, 34, 495–504.
22. Catalano, D., Martines, G. F., Tonzuso, A., Pirri, C., Trovato, F. M., Trovato, G. M. (2010) Protective role of coffee in non-alcoholic fatty liver disease (NAFLD). *Dig Dis Sci*, 55, 3200–3206.
23. Birerdinc, A., Stepanova, M., Pawloski, L., Younossi, Z. M. (2012) Caffeine is protective in patients with non-alcoholic fatty liver disease. *Aliment Pharmacol Ther*, 35, 76–82.
24. Yamashita, K., Yatsuya, H., Muramatsu, T., Toyoshima, H., Murohara, T., Tamakoshi, K. (2012) Association of coffee consumption with serum adiponectin, leptin, inflammation and metabolic markers in Japanese workers: A cross-sectional study. *Nutr Diabetes*, 2, e33.
25. Gutiérrez-Grobe, Y., Chávez-Tapia, N., Sánchez-Valle, V., Gavilanes-Espinar, J. G., Ponciano-Rodríguez, G., Uribe, M., Méndez-Sánchez, N. (2012) High coffee intake is associated with lower grade nonalcoholic fatty liver disease: The role of peripheral antioxidant activity. *Ann Hepatol*, 11, 350–355.
26. Xiao, Q., Sinha, R., Graubard, B. I., Freedman, N. D. (2014) Inverse associations of total and decaffeinated coffee with liver enzyme levels in National Health and Nutrition Examination Survey 1999–2010. *Hepatology*, 60, 2091–2098.

27. Priftis, A., Stagos, D., Konstantinopoulos, K., Tsitsimpikou, C., Spandidos, D. A., Tsatsakis, A. M., Tzatzarakis, M. N., Kouretas, D. (2015) Comparison of antioxidant activity between green and roasted coffee beans using molecular methods. *Mol Med Rep* 12, 7293–7302.
28. Mullin, G. E. (2015) Supplements for weight loss: Hype or help for obesity? Part II. The inside scoop on green coffee bean extract. *Nutr Clin Pract*, 30, 311–312.
29. Flanagan, J., Bily, A., Rolland, Y., Roller, M. (2014) Lipolytic activity of Svetol(R), a decaffeinated green coffee bean extract. *Phytother Res*, 28, 946–948.
30. Shimoda, H., Seki, E., Aitani, M. (2006) Inhibitory effect of green coffee bean extract on fat accumulation and body weight gain in mice. *BMC Complement Altern Med*, 6, 9.
31. Song, S. J., Choi, S., Park, T. (2014) Decaffeinated green coffee bean extract attenuates diet-induced obesity and insulin resistance in mice. *Evid Based Complement Alternat Med*, 2014, 718379.
32. Li Kwok Cheong, J. D., Croft, K. D., Henry, P. D., Matthews, V., Hodgson, J. M., Ward, N. C. (2014) Green coffee polyphenols do not attenuate features of the metabolic syndrome and improve endothelial function in mice fed a high fat diet. *Arch Biochem Biophys*, 559, 46–52.
33. Hua, Y., Ren, S. Y., Guo, R., Rogers, O., Nair, R. P., Bagchi, D., Swaroop, A., Nair, S. (2015) Furostanolic saponins from Trigonella foenum-graecum alleviate diet-induced glucose intolerance and hepatic fat accumulation. *Mol Nutr Food Res*, 59, 2094–2100.
34. Bakuradze, T., Boehm, N., Janzowski, C., Lang, R., et al. (2011) Antioxidant-rich coffee reduces DNA damage, elevates glutathione status and contributes to weight control: Results from an intervention study. *Mol Nutr Food Res*, 55, 793–797.
35. Thom, E. (2007) The effect of chlorogenic acid enriched coffee on glucose absorption in healthy volunteers and its effect on body mass when used long-term in overweight and obese people. *J Int Med Res*, 35, 900–908.

10 Caffeic Acid and Its Biological Effects on Brain Function

Myra O. Villareal, Yuki Sato, and Hiroko Isoda

CONTENTS

ABSTRACT

The health benefits of consumption of green coffee has been the subject of several studies. Coffee is a rich source of polyphenol caffeic acid. Here we present our findings on the benefits on brain health of consumption of green coffee and foods rich in caffeic acid and its derivatives. For example, caffeic acid and its derivatives, caffeoylquinic acid and its isomers, alleviate symptoms of Alzheimer's disease by increasing the energy available to the brain and improving learning and memory *in vivo*. Moreover, the caffeic acid derivative rosmarinic acid has the antidepressant effect of modulating signaling in the brain, specifically hypothalamic–pituitary–adrenal axis activity. How pigment cells can be used to screen compounds for their neuroprotective effect is also discussed.

10.1 INTRODUCTION

The strong influence of diet on health and alleviation of the symptoms of neurodegenerative diseases has long been recognized, and the effect of various food and beverage components—vitamins, minerals, and phenolic compounds—on health has been widely investigated (Spencer et al. 2008). *In vivo* and clinical studies have

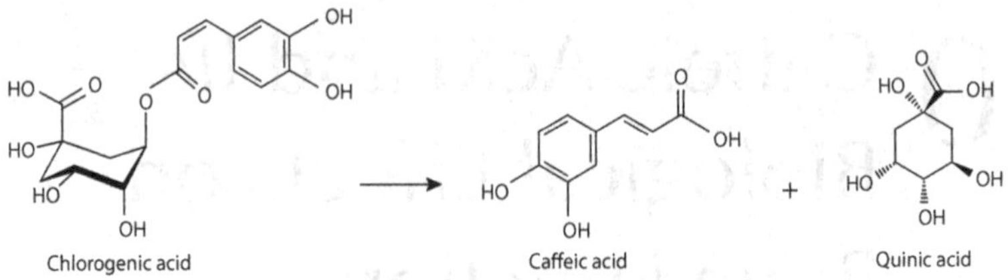

FIGURE 10.1 CGA hydrolysis yields caffeic acid and quinic acid.

reported that consumption of certain foods has therapeutic or preventive effects on the development of certain diseases. In our previous reports, for example, the therapeutic effects of olives (*Olea europea*), argan (*Argania spinosa*), sweet potato (*Ipomoea batatas*), and rosemary (*Rosmarinus officinalis*), as oils, leaves, or fruits are largely attributed to the high polyphenolic content of these foods (Samet et al. 2015; Villareal et al. 2013; Sasaki et al. 2013; Kondo et al. 2015). Alone or in synergy with the other components, these foods have provided antiallergy, anticancer, melanogenesis regulation, and antiobesity effects, as well as significant beneficial effects for brain health.

Green coffee is a functional food rich in chlorogenic acid (CGA), an ester formed between caffeic acid and quinic acid. Following hydrolysis, CGA readily yields caffeic acid and quinic acid (Figure 10.1). Reports have classified caffeic acid (3,4-dihydroxy-cinnamic acid) as a superior antioxidant in inhibiting low-density lipoprotein (LDL) oxidation and quenching radicals and singlet oxygen, making it a very potent antioxidant (Meyer et al. 1998; Kikuzaki et al. 2002; Foley et al. 1999). Foods that contain caffeic acid hold enormous potential in improving brain function and overall brain health.

Brain aging and most neurodegenerative diseases of the elderly are usually caused by oxidative damage, making the use of food rich in antioxidants such as polyphenols very attractive. Recent reports have shown that food polyphenols have great potential regarding antiaging and neuroprotective bioactivities (Rossi et al. 2008). Here, we review the effect of caffeic acid on brain health, exploring different caffeic acid derivatives and similar compounds. We also present the results of our screening for its effect on cell proliferation using B16 cells as the model cell line.

10.2 GREEN COFFEE PHENOLIC COMPOUNDS

Plants adapt to environmental stressors by producing secondary metabolites, mostly phenolic compounds. Coffee, one of the most popular beverages in the world, is classified as a functional beverage owing to its beneficial effect on health, due to the composition of the green beans (Esquivel and Jimenez 2012). Around 14% of coffee is made up of phenolic fraction with CGAs and related compounds caffeoylquinic (CQA), feruloylquinic (FQA), and dicaffeoylquinic (diCQA) as the main components (Farah et al. 2008). Its minor components include other phenolic compounds, such as tannins, lignans, and anthocyanins present in the coffee seeds. CGA has a very strong antioxidant activity, which provides beneficial health effects (Moreira et al. 2005) including beneficial effects on brain function (Farah and Donangelo 2006).

Oral administration of dietary polyphenols in animals and humans can affect various physiologic and physiopathologic processes, but to understand how these compounds can modulate signaling pathways associated with diseases and physiological processes, it is essential to determine if the polyphenols and their metabolites can effectively reach the target tissues and, more importantly, if they are degraded in the gut or hydrolyzed following absorption or exposure to the intestinal microflora (Gonthier et al. 2003).

The major CGA compounds present in coffee are differentially absorbed and/or metabolized in humans, as demonstrated by clinical trials with participants drinking brewed coffee, which identified three CQA isomers and three diCQA isomers in the plasma of all subjects, whereas two FQA were identified in only one subject. Moreover, dihydrocaffeic, gallic, isoferulic, ferulic, vanillic, caffeic, 5-CQA, sinapic, *p*-hydroxybenzoic, and *p*-coumaric acids were identified in the subjects' urine, with gallic and dihydrocaffeic acids showing highest levels (Monteiro et al. 2007).

Related studies on the absorption of phenolic acids from coffee done by Nardini et al. (2002), which analyzed coffee brew for free and total phenolic acids, also found that CGA was present in coffee at high levels, while free phenolic acids were undetectable. However, releasing bound phenolic acids by alkaline hydrolysis enabled the detection of ferulic acid and *p*-coumaric acid and high levels of caffeic acid, showing that intake of CGA-rich coffee results in increased caffeic acid concentration in the plasma, with an absorption peak at 1 h. Caffeic acid, mainly in the glucuronate/sulfate forms, is therefore the only phenolic acid found in plasma samples following coffee consumption, while CGA cannot be detected. However, there are also reports that all major CGA compounds in coffee are bioavailable in humans (Monteiro et al. 2007). Eight hours after consumption of decaffeinated green coffee extract containing 170 mg CGA, Farah et al. (2008) reported shows three CQA, three diCQA, and caffeic, ferulic, isoferulic, and p-coumaric acids in the plasma.

10.3 EFFECT OF CAFFEIC ACID AND CAFFEIC ACID DERIVATIVES ON BRAIN HEALTH

The caffeic acid (3,4-dihydroxycinnamic acid) chemical structure contains a double C=C bond that participates in stabilizing the radical by resonance (Cuvelier et al. 1992). Phenolic compounds are naturally occurring molecules known for their antioxidative properties. Their antioxidative potency is attributed to their structure, in particular to electron delocalization of the aromatic nucleus, with polyphenols such as caffeic acid being more effective than monophenols owing to the introduction of a second hydroxyl group in the *ortho* or *para* position, which is known to increase antioxidative activity (Shahidi and Wanasundara, 1992; Chen and Ho 1997).

We have evaluated caffeic acid and its derivatives for their effect on brain health and from what we have observed and as reported elsewhere, caffeic acid is a very strong antioxidant, the use of which can help prevent the development of Alzheimer's disease (AD) by promoting learning and memory, increasing adenosine triphosphate (ATP) production, and alleviating depression.

10.3.1 Prevention of Alzheimer's Disease (AD)

Advancement in medical science has improved the longevity of humans, but it cannot directly affect or improve the quality of life if it cannot prevent or delay the onset of age-related diseases. Most people aged 60 years and older suffer more from dementia than from stroke, cardiovascular diseases, and cancer according to the World Health report in 2003 (WHO report 2003; Ferri et al. 2006). AD is a progressive neurodegenerative disease characterized by the deposition of amyloid β-peptide into plaques and the accumulation of neurofibrillary tangles in neurons, neuronal loss, and synaptic pathology that can affect several parts of the brain. Evidence has shown that the density of plaques and the levels of amyloid β-peptide correlate with the severity of dementia (Religa et al. 2003).

AD is the most common dementia disorder in elderly people and it is projected that in 50 years, approximately 1 in 45 Americans will be afflicted with AD. Therefore, any therapeutic strategies or means of intervention that could delay the onset of AD would have a major public health impact (Religa et al. 2003; Brookmeyer et al. 1998). The Aβ plaque has been reported to cause oxidative damage, inflammation, and neurotoxicity. Another pathological hallmark of AD includes intracellular aggregates of hyperphosphorylated tau or neurofibrillary tangles (Sul et al. 2009). The protective effect of caffeic acid against the cytotoxicity of beta-amyloid, the plaques of which are recognized as one of the major causes of AD, has been reported (Sul et al. 2009).

10.3.1.1 Promotion of ATP (Energy) Production

The brain relies on glucose metabolism for its main source of energy, and the brain function is specifically dependent on ATP. It is a known fact that the human brain's neurons have the highest energy demand, requiring continuous delivery of glucose from blood. Moreover, the level of the energy available to the brain dictates its ability to process information, processing power, and generation of functional imaging signals (Howarth et al. 2012). We evaluated synthetic CQAs and CQA-rich food known for their various bioactivities such as antioxidant, anticancer, antiallergy, and other biological effects. Treatment with 3,5-di-*O*-caffeoylquinic acid increased the mRNA expression level of glycolytic enzymes and the intracellular ATP level, providing neuroprotection against amyloid β_{1-42}-induced cellular toxicity on human neuroblastoma SH-SY5Y cells (Han et al. 2010). At the same time, synthetic 1,4,5-tri-*O*-caffeoylquinic acid, 4,5-di-*O*-caffeoylquinic acid, 3,4,5-tri-*O*-caffeoylquinic acid, and other derivatives were evaluated for their differences in their effect on ATP production *in vitro*. Results showed that among the CQA compounds, 3,4,5-tri-*O*-caffeoylquinic acid was the most effective in promoting ATP production, suggesting that caffeoyl groups bound to quinic acid are the most bioactive form of CQA and that a compound containing more caffeoyl groups bound to quinic acid are more bioactive (Miyamae et al. 2011). AD is a disease with an increasing number of patients having age-related neurodegenerative disorders, and is a degenerative disorder of the CNS, which causes mental deterioration and progressive dementia. In our study on CQA-rich purple sweet potato (PSP), treatment with PSP increased the intracellular ATP production *in vitro* and significantly increased the ATP production by 73% following 4 h of treatment. The increase in ATP was accompanied by an increase in the levels of glycolysis metabolites acetyl-CoA divalent (AcCoA), citric acid, cis-aconitic acid, and succinic acid in response to PSP treatment. Like green coffee, PSP is rich in phenolic compounds such as anthocyanins and caffeoylquinic acids (CQA), also referred to as chlorogenic acid (3-*O*-caffeoylquinic acid or 3-CQA), 4-*O*-caffeoylquinic acid or crypto-chlorogenic acid (4-CGA), 5-*O*-caffeoylquinic acid (neochlorogenic acid or 4-CGA), 1,5-diCQA, 3,4-diCQA, 3,5-diCQA, and 5,5-diCQA (Sasaki et al. 2013; Farah et al. 2008).

10.3.1.2 Improvement of Learning and Memory

One of the hallmarks of AD is mental deterioration and progressive dementia caused by the presence of senile plaques of amyloid-β_{1-42}. Following reports on the ability of natural and synthetic CQAs to increase ATP production, we evaluated the protective effect of 3,5-di-O-CQA against amyloid-β^{1-42} cytotoxicity and whether this had beneficial effects or improved spatial learning and memory of mice subjected to the Morris Water Maze (MWM) test, the standard method for the evaluation of the spatial learning and memory (Han et al. 2010). In the MWM test, senescence-accelerated mice SAMP8 were placed inside a tank with water with an escape platform in the middle and spatial clues placed on the wall of the tank. SAMP8 mice are one of the animal models for studying aging. The mice were trained to find the platform for a week, after which they were evaluated for their ability to find the escape platform, and the time it takes for the mice to get to the platform was measured (escape latency time). Results showed that oral administration of 3,5-di-O-CQA (6.7 mg/kg/day) significantly decreased the escape latency time of SAMP8 mice compared to the control.

Moreover, CQA-rich purple sweet potato (PSP) extract orally administered to SAMP8 mice at 20 mg/kg/day, for example, can also significantly improve the spatial learning and memory of SAMP8 (Sasaki et al. 2013). This effect was attributed to the overexpression of antioxidant-, energy metabolism-, and neuronal plasticity-related proteins in the brain of SAMP8 following consumption of PSP extract, providing evidence that PSP has a neuroprotective effect on mouse brain and can improve the brain health of SAMP8, attributed to the polyphenols contained in PSP.

10.3.2 Antidepressant Effect

Depression is a common mental disorder, with more than 350 million people of all ages suffering from this disease globally (WHO 2012). Depression is a serious public health problem; it is very disabling and has a disease burden comparable to chronic diseases such as arthritis, asthma, and diabetes. At the same time, individuals suffering from these chronic diseases have increased risk of depression, with the combination of diabetes and depression being the most disabling (Moussavi et al. 2007). Although considered nonfatal, depressive episodes result in loss of productivity and poor health-related quality of life (Strine et al. 2004). Without treatment, it has the tendency to assume a chronic course, be recurrent, and over time be associated with increasing disability (Solomon et al. 2000; Andrews 2001).

Disturbances in oxidative metabolism are reported to be involved in anxiety disorders, high anxiety levels, and depression. That is why the effect of polyphenols with antioxidant properties on anxiety disorders, anxiety, and depression has been the subject of reports proposing the use of these natural compounds against diseases of the brain and the central nervous system (Bouayed 2010). We have recently reported that polyphenols have great potential as neuroprotective agents, helping to reduce stress and manage depression. Rosemary (*R. officinalis*), an edible aromatic plant, has been demonstrated to exert an antidepressant effect. Rosemary has antioxidant activity attributed mainly to its carnosic acid, carnosol, and rosmarinic acid (RA) components (Thorsen and Hildebrandt 2003).

In our previous study, we demonstrated *in vivo* that RA, an ester of caffeic acid and one of the bioactive compounds of rosemary, has an antidepression effect (Kondo et al. 2015). ICR mice were orally administered RA and subjected to a depression-inducing tail suspension test (TST). Changes in the levels of corticosterone and levels of catecholamines in the cerebrum were determined, and the effect on the hypothalamic–pituitary–adrenal (HPA) axis was evaluated by determining the expressions of the brain-derived neurotrophic factors (*Bdnf*), mitogen-activated protein kinase phosphate-1 (*Mkp-1*), tyrosine hydroxylase (*Th*), and pyruvate carboxylase (*Pc*) genes in the cerebrum. Results showed that RA significantly decreased the serum corticosterone level while increasing the dopamine level in the mice brain. Furthermore, it modulates depression at the molecular level by downregulating *Mkp-1* and upregulating *Bdnf* gene expression. Major depressive disorders are believed to be a result of repeated stress episodes and hyperactivity of the HPA axis. The corticotropin-releasing hormone (CRH) and locus ceruleus–norepinephrine (LC/NE)-autonomic systems, their peripheral effectors, the pituitary–adrenal axis, and the limbs of the autonomic system are part of the stress system that coordinates organisms' adaptive responses to stressors of any kind. Behavioral and peripheral changes, such as alleviation of depression, occur in response to the activation of the stress system, increasing the organism's chances for survival (Tsigos and Chrousos 2002). That RA can regulate the HPA suggests that RA may be used to treat or alleviate the symptoms of depression, postpartum depression, fibromyalgia, andchronic fatigue syndrome, which are all characterized by a low HPA axis and LC/NE activity.

10.4 FUTURE PERSPECTIVE: USE OF PIGMENT CELLS FOR EVALUATING COMPOUNDS FOR THEIR EFFECT ON NEURONAL FUNCTION

Melanocytes and neurons are neural crest-derived cells and cell lines used to study the bioactivities of functional compounds use melanoma cells for pigmentation-related studies, while neurotypic cells (e.g., SH-SY5Y cells) are used for assays related to neuronal activities such as the production and secretion of L-DOPA, a hormone-like bioregulator and a protential neurotransmitter. However, it has been demonstrated that pigment cells also have the ability to transform L-tryptophan to serotonin (Slominski 2009; Slominski et al. 2002) and can express elements of the hypothalamic-pituitary-thyroid axis and cholinergic system (Grando et al. 2006). B16 cells are relatively easier to culture compared to SH-SY5Y cells as they do not require special tissue culture plate (with coating), which is costly.

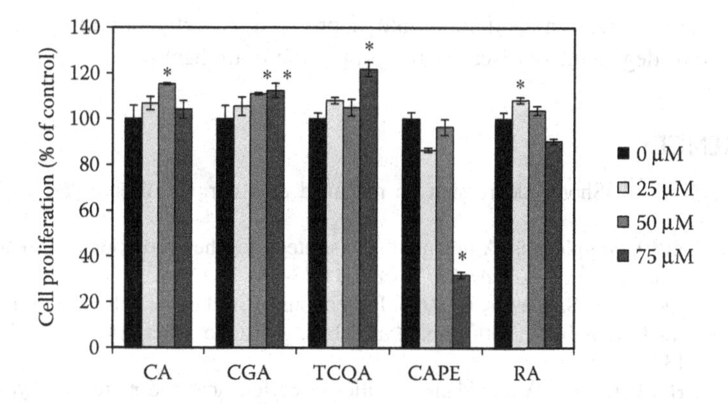

FIGURE 10.2 Effect of caffeic acid (CA) and its derivatives—CGA, caffeic acid phenetyl ester (CAPE), RA, and tricaffeoylquinic acid (TCQA)—on the proliferation of B16 murine melanoma cells determined using the MTT assay.

Here we determined the effect of caffeic acid (CA) and its derivatives CGA, tricaffeoylquinic acid (TCQA), caffeic acid phenetyl ester (CAPE), and RA on the proliferation of B16 murine melanoma cells, the model cell line for pigment cell research. Cells were seeded at 5×10^5 cells/100 mm petri dish and treated with CA, CGA, TCQA, CAPE, or RA (all obtained from Sigma) and the cells incubated for 24 h prior to the determination of the effect on cell proliferation using the 3-(4,5-dimethylthiazol-2-yl)-2,5-diphenyltetrazolium bromide tetrazolium reduction (MTT) assay. As shown in Figure 10.2, the phenolic compounds increased the cell proliferation, in a dose-dependent manner, with significant increase at up to 50 μM treatment. Treatment with 75 μM CAPE was cytotoxic to the cells. A general tendency to increase the cell proliferation was observed which is similar to what we have reported previously. Phenolic compounds have cytoprotective effect and promotes cell proliferation (Han et al. 2010; Sasaki et al. 2013).

Although there are reports that the efficiency of RA, an ester of caffeic acid and dihydrocaffeic acid, is greater than that of caffeic acid, here, the proliferation of the cells treated with CA was actually higher than RA-treated cells. Among the tested compounds, RA, TCQA, CGA, and CA have been reported to have significant beneficial effects on brain health. Further studies will be done to compare the effect of the RA and the other derivatives of caffeic acids on neuronal function and at the same time, evaluate the suitability of B16 cells for evaluating phenolic compounds for their effect on brain health. The use of pigment cells, either melanocytes or B16 cells, will enable us to screen more compounds in shorter time period.

10.5 CONCLUSION

Green coffee is a functional food that is a rich source of caffeic acid (CA) following hydrolysis of CGA and other caffeoylquinic acid derivatives. CA has a very strong antioxidant effect and consumption of caffeic acid, and caffeic acid derivates-rich foods such as green coffee increases the amount of energy available in the brain, provide neuroprotection, and modulate depression, thereby providing protection against neurodegenerative diseases and promoting brain health.

REFERENCES

Andrews, G. 2001. Should depression be managed as a chronic disease? *Br Med J* 322: 419–421.

Bouayed, J. 2010. Polyphenols: A potential new strategy for the prevention and treatment of anxiety and depression. *Curr Nut Food Sci* 6:13–18.

Brookmeyer, R., Gray, S., Kawas, C. 1998. Projections of Alzheimer's disease in the United States and the public health impact of delaying disease onset. *Am J Pub Health* 88: 1337–1342.

Chen, J.H., Ho, C.T. 1997. Antioxidant activities of caffeic acid and its related hydroxycinnamic acid compounds. *J Agric Food Chem* 45: 2374–2378.

Cuvelier, M.E., Richard, H., Berset, C. 1992. Comparison of the antioxidative activity of some acid-phenols: Structure-activity relationship. *Biosci Biotechnol Biochem* 56: 324–325.

Esquivel, P., Jiménez, V. M. 2012. Functional properties of coffee and coffee by-products. *Food Res Int* 46: 488–495.

Farah, A., Donangelo, C. M. 2006. Phenolic compounds in coffee. *Braz J Plant Physiol* 18: 23–36.

Farah, A., Monteiro, M., Donangelo C.M., Lafay, S. 2008. Chlorogenic acids from green coffee extract. *J Nutr* 138: 2309–2315.

Ferri, C., Prince, M., Brayne, C., et al. 2006. Global prevalence of dementia: A Delphi consensus study. *The Lancet* 366: 2112–2117.

Foley, S., Navaratnam, S., McGarvey, D.J., Land, E.J. Truscott, T.G., Rice-Evans, C.A. 1999. Singlet oxygen quenching and the redox properties of hydroxycinnamic acids, *Free Rad Biol Med* 26: 1202–1208.

Gonthier, M.P., Verny, M.A., Besson, C., Remesy, C. Scalbert, A., 2003. Chlorogenic acid bioavailability largely depends on its metabolism by the gut microflora in rats. *J Nutr* 133: 1853–1859.

Grando, S., Pittelkow, M.R. Schallreuter, K.U. 2006. Adrenergic and cholinergic control in the biology of epidermis: Physiological and clinical significance. *J Invest Dermatol* 126: 1948–1965.

Han, J., Miyamae, Y., Shigemori, H., Isoda, H. 2010. Neuroprotective effect of 3,5-di-*O*-caffeoylquinic acid on SH-SY5Y cells and senescence-accelerated-prone mice 8 through the up-regulation of phosphoglycerate kinase-1. *Neuroscience* 169: 1039–1045.

Howarth, C., Gleeson, P., Attwell, D. 2012. Updated energy budgets for neural computation in the neocortex and cerebellum *J Cereb Blood Flow Metab* 32: 1222–1232.

Kikuzaki, H., Hisamoto, M., Hirose, K., Akiyama, K., Taniguchi, H. 2002. Antioxidant properties of ferulic acid and its related compounds. *J Agric Food Chem* 50: 2161–2168.

Kondo, S., El Omri, A., Han, J., Isoda, H. 2015. Antidepressant-like effects of rosmarinic acid through mitogen-activated protein kinase phosphatase-1 and brain-derived neurotrophic factor modulation. *J Functional Foods* 14: 758–766.

Meyer, A.S., Heinonen, M., Frankel, E.N. 1998. Antioxidant interactions of catechin, cyanidin, caffeic acid, quercetin, and ellagic acid on human LDL oxidation. *Food Chem* 61: 71–75.

Miyamae, Y., Kurisu, M., Han, J., Isoda, H. 2011. Structure–activity relationship of caffeoylquinic acids on the accelerating activity on ATP production. *Chem Pharm Bul* 59: 502–507.

Monteiro, M., Farah, A., Perrone, D., Trugo, L. C., Donangelo, C. 2007. Chlorogenic acid compounds from coffee are differentially absorbed and metabolized in humans. *J Nutr* 137: 2196–2201.

Moreira, D.P., Monteiro, M.C., Ribeiro-ALves, M., Donangelo, C.M., Trugo, L.C. 2005. Contribution of chlorogenic acids to the iron-reducing activity of coffee beverages. *J Agric Food* 53: 1399–1402.

Moussavi, S., Chatterji, S., Verdes, E., Tandon, A., Patel, V., Ustun, B. 2007. Depression, chronic diseases, and decrements in health: Results from the World Health Surveys. *Lancet* 370: 851–58.

Nardini, M., Cirillo, E., Natella, F., Scaccini, C. 2002. Absorption of phenolic acids in humans after coffee consumption. *J Agric Food Chem* 50: 5735–5741.

Religa, D., Laudon, H., Styczynska, M., Winblad, B., Näslund, J., Vahram Haroutunian, V. 2003. Amyloid-β pathology in Alzheimer's disease and schizophrenia. *Am J Psychiatry* 160: 867–872.

Rossi, L., Mazzitelli, S., Arciello, M., Capo, C.R., Rotilio, G. 2008. Benefits from dietary polyphenols for brain aging and Alzheimer's disease. *Neurochem Res* 33: 2390–2400.

Samet, I., Villareal, M.O., Motojima, H., Han, J., Sayadi, S., Isoda, H. 2015. Olive leaf components apigenin 7-glucoside and luteolin 7-glucoside direct human hematopoietic stem cell differentiation towards erythroid lineage. *Differentiation* 89: 146–155.

Sasaki, K., Han, J., Shimozono, H., Villareal, M.O., Isoda, H. 2013. Caffeoylquinic acid-rich purple sweet potato extract, with or without anthocyanin, imparts neuroprotection and contributes to the improvement of spatial learning and memory of SAMP8 mouse. *J Agric Food Chem* 61: 5037–5045.

Shahidi, F., Wanasundara, P.K.J.P.D. 1992. Phenolic antioxidants. *Crit Rev Food Sci Nut* 32: 67–103.

Slominski, A. 2009. Neuroendocrine activity of the melanocyte. *Exp Dermatol* 18: 760–763.

Slominski, A., Semak, I., Pisarchik, A., Sweatman, T., Szczesniewski, A., Worstman, J. 2002. Conversion of L-tryptophan to serotonin and melatonin in melanoma cells. *FEBS Lett* 511: 102–106.

Solomon, D.A., Keller, M.B., Leon, A.C. et al. 2000. Multiple recurrences of major depressive disorder. *Am J Psychiatry* 157: 229–233.

Spencer, J.P.E., Abd El Mohsen, M.M., Minihane, A.M., Mathers, J.C. 2008. Biomarkers of the intake of dietary polyphenols: Strengths, limitations and application in nutrition research. *Br J Nut* 99: 12–22.

Strine, T.W., Chapman, D.P., Kobau, R., Balluz, L., Mokdad, A.H. 2004. Depression, anxiety, and physical impairments and quality of life in the US non-institutionalized population. *Psychiatr Serv* 55: 1408–1413.

Sul, D., Kim, H., Lee, D., Joo, S.J., Hwang, K.W., Park, S.-Y. 2009. Protective effect of caffeic acid against beta-amyloid-induced neurotoxicity by the inhibition of calcium influx and tau. *Life Sci* 84: 9–10.

Thorsen, M.A., Hildebrandt, K.S. 2003. Quantitative determination of phenolic diterpenes in rosemary extracts. Aspects of accurate quantification. *J Chromatog A* 995: 119–125.

Tsigos, C., Chrousos, G.P. 2002. Hypothalamic–pituitary–adrenal axis, neuroendocrine factors and stress. *J Psychosomatic Res* 53: 865–871.

Villareal, M., Kume, S., Bourhim, T., Bakhtaoui, F.Z., Kashiwagi, K., Han, J., Gadhi, C., Isoda, H. 2013. Activation of MITF by argan oil leads to the inhibition of the tyrosinase and dopachrome tautomerase expressions in B16 murine melanoma cells. *Evid Based Complementary Alternative Med* 2013: 9.

World Health Organization. 2003. Depression. Fact sheet No. 369, October 2012.

11 Coffee and Cognition
Extending Our Understanding beyond Caffeine

Karen Nolidin, Christina Kure, Andrew Scholey, and Con Stough

CONTENTS

ABSTRACT

Coffee is one of the most popular drinks in the world with more than two-billion cups consumed each day. Within each coffee bean there are many interesting compounds but the most researched compound is caffeine. There has been significant research examining the effect of caffeine on cognition with most research showing an enhancement of a limited number of cognition domains, particularly arousal and attention, even after the ingestion of small amounts of caffeine, although some researchers have argued that this is primarily a reversal of a caffeine-related withdrawal effect on cognition. Nevertheless, there is a growing view that other compounds in coffee may also improve cognition and perhaps could be used to ameliorate cognitive decline. This has given rise to research into other active components of coffee. These components, collectively termed polyphenols, have among other biochemical properties strong antioxidant and anti-inflammatory properties. Although the availability of some of these noncaffeine compounds such a chlorogenic acid are reduced in coffee drinks due to the roasting process, many researchers are now examining these compounds for their cardiovascular and cognitive effects. This has also led many food manufacturers to systematically examine a range of compounds found in green coffee beans for their beneficial effects on neurocognition.

11.1 INTRODUCTION

11.1.1 Coffee and Health?

Coffee is one of the most popular drinks in the world, being the third most consumed beverage behind water and tea (Wang et al. 2009). Coffee is a brewed drink made by infusing roasted coffee beans in hot water. There is significant variation in how coffee is prepared depending upon how the beans are processed, but irrespective of the brewing method, coffee brew and roasted coffee share most compounds (Belitz et al. 2009). The roasting of the coffee beans also changes the chemical composition and the availability of a range of compounds, for example, chlorogenic acid, which may be of interest for health promotion and in particular neurocognition although this area is particularly understudied. The international popularity of coffee and coffee extracts, along with its long history of consumption worldwide, has made coffee a common target for health-related research with many studies outlining both the beneficial and potentially harmful effects of coffee consumption. However, most studies have examined the role of caffeine on health and have generally neglected the many other compounds found in coffee beans.

Coffee as a whole substance has been investigated for its potential ability to affect numerous health factors and medical conditions. For instance, coffee consumption has been linked to positive outcomes for diabetes (Ding et al. 2014; Kempf et al. 2010; Palatini 2015; van Dam et al. 2005), and gout (Choi et al. 2007, 2010). Findings from epidemiological studies also suggest that coffee may confer a protective effect against age-related cognitive decline and Alzheimer's disease (AD) (Carman et al. 2014).

11.1.2 What Is in Coffee?

11.1.2.1 Active Ingredients of Coffee

Other than caffeine, roasted coffee also contains lipids, protein, carbohydrates, trigonelline, niacin, aliphatic acids, chlorogenic acids, minerals, melanoidins, and up to 950 different compounds (Belitz et al. 2009). Polyphenols represent a significant component of active compounds in coffee. The major polyphenols in coffee are flavonoids, particularly flavanols (catechins and proanthocyanidins), and phenolic acids (caffeic and ferulic) (Wang et al. 2009). The most abundant phenolic compounds in coffee are the chlorogenic acids (Ludwig et al. 2012). Chlorogenic acids are a family of compounds, and in coffee its main classes are caffeoylquinic acids, feruloylquinic acids, p-coumaroylquinic acids, dicaffeoylquinic acids, and caffeoylferuloylquinic acids (Stalmach et al. 2014).

The aforementioned active components of coffee have been shown to have antioxidant properties and epidemiological studies have linked them to a reduced incidence of a range of diseases. However most of these compounds have not been subjected to clinical trials in humans, particularly for cognitive and brain outcomes.

Many techniques involve boiling ground-roasted coffee beans in water or, alternatively, pouring, dripping, or spraying hot water through ground-roasted coffee, and then finally filtering it (Esquivel et al. 2012). Mills et al. (2013) found that a single cup of coffee (200 mL) prepared from commercially available coffees could contain roughly 30–120 mg of CGA. They found that decaffeination did not seem to affect the CGA levels, nor was there a difference between instant and plunger (French Press) coffee. However, coffees with lower levels of roasting or blends containing unroasted coffee had higher CGA levels.

11.1.3 Coffee and Cognition Studies

Epidemiological studies have shown that caffeine consumption reduces the risk of cognitive decline including AD (Arab et al. 2011; Eskelinen et al. 2009; Maia et al. 2002). Moderate coffee consumption of three to five cups per day at midlife was associated with the lowest risk of developing dementia and AD in later life (Eskelinen et al. 2009). Furthermore, there is evidence among tea and coffee drinkers that these reduced rates of cognitive decline is gender specific with longitudinal studies demonstrating protection in women but not men (Arab et al. 2011; Ritchie et al. 2007). In women, greater rates of caffeine consumption in the form of tea or coffee (>3 cups per day) demonstrated reduced cognitive decline with less decline seen in verbal retrieval and visuospatial memory (Ritchie et al. 2007). However another study, which assessed elderly men only, showed that greater coffee consumption reduced age-associated cognitive decline in these subjects (van Gelder et al. 2006). These studies suggest that while coffee and/or caffeine may protect older individuals from cognitive decline, these effects may be gender specific and further studies are needed to better understand these gender differences.

11.1.4 Caffeine and Cognition

Coffee has long been considered a cognitive enhancer. As the major active component of coffee, caffeine has been targeted as the driving force behind coffee's numerous effects and has been extensively researched.

Studies in animal models have shown positive effects of coffee on cognitive functioning (Arendash et al. 2006, 2010; Shukitt-Hale et al. 2013). In rat models, daily caffeine intake equivalent to five cups of coffee per day (500 mg/day) has shown cognitive benefits (Arendash et al. 2006, 2010). Rodents administered caffeine performed significantly better than controls on spatial learning, reference memory, working memory, and recognition/identification (Arendash et al. 2006). Additionally, in these studies, consuming the equivalent of five cups of coffee per day from young adulthood to older age protected against cognitive impairment and amyloid beta (Aβ) neuropathology (Arendash et al. 2010), reversed working memory impairment following a long-term treatment, and affected plasma levels of Aβ in AD mice and humans (Arendash et al. 2010). Furthermore, aged rats supplemented with a coffee diet that was equivalent to drinking up to 10 cups of coffee per day, performed better in psychomotor function and in cognitive function compared with the control rats. In their study, Shukitt-Hale et al. (2013) found that drinking an equivalent of 3 cups of coffee per day improved long-term memory, whereas drinking an equivalent of 7–10 cups improved working memory suggesting a dose-dependent effect on cognitive functioning. Furthermore, in a longitudinal study assessing coffee habits of elderly individuals, Araújo et al. (2015) showed that drinking 2–3 cups of coffee per day was associated with a better performance on verbal memory and an efficiency of recall in long-term memory. Collectively these findings suggest that daily caffeine consumption may reduce the motor coordination and the cognitive deficits associated with aging, and the risk of developing diseases associated with cognitive decline such as AD (Arendash et al. 2006; Shukitt-Hale et al. 2013).

However, studies investigating dietary caffeine intake do not necessarily take into consideration caffeine from sources other than coffee such as tea or chocolate. Caffeine only partially explains the effect of coffee on cognition. Additionally, the negative physical and psychological effects of caffeine (jitteriness, anxiety) are somewhat diminished when consumed in coffee (Camfield et al. 2013). This suggests that there are other components in coffee which offset these symptoms. This appears to be the case in studies that have investigated the combined effects of caffeine and tea components such as L-theanine (Dodd et al. 2015). These other active components are now attracting research and commercial attention. This chapter will focus on these components.

11.1.5 Chlorogenic Acid and Cognition

Chlorogenic acid (CGA) has been earmarked by some researchers as the main candidate for cognitive effects, outside of caffeine. Two recent randomized controlled trials (RCTs) have investigated the effects of CGA on cognition in humans. Both are acute studies, yet their results suggest that CGA is able to elicit mood and cognitive effects soon after consumption. A chronic RCT with CGA examining changes in cognition is now underway with this group.

Cropley et al. (2011), from Swinburne University, conducted research in older adults aged 53–79 years to determine if CGA-enriched coffee modulated brain function. The sample consisted of light coffee drinkers: a minimum of 1 cup to maximum of 8 cups consumed per week. Recruited participants were relatively healthy—exclusion criteria included previous diagnosis with any significant medical conditions, regular use of psychotropic medications, and untreated clinically high blood pressure. All participants were tested under the following four treatment conditions: decaffeinated coffee with normal CGA levels; decaffeinated coffee with high CGA levels; caffeinated coffee with normal CGA levels; and a placebo. The 6 g soluble coffee servings given to participants were equivalent to three standard servings. Participants were tested before and after drinking the coffee. The results of the study revealed that compared to decaffeinated coffee with normal CGA levels, decaffeinated coffee with high CGA levels had some positive effects on mood-related processes including an increase in alertness and a decrease in mental fatigue and headaches.

The second study from the same group at Swinburne University (Camfield et al. 2013) extended previous studies by investigating whether CGA affected cognition and mood differently when isolated from decaffeinated coffee. The three administered treatments were a decaffeinated green blend coffee, a treatment with CGA levels matched to the decaffeinated coffee, and a placebo. They found significant acute effects of the decaffeinated green blend coffee when compared with the placebo on select mood and cognitive processes such as reaction time and accuracy. However, the CGA treatment did not elicit these effects. Some of the results showed significance and the authors suggested a larger sample size is required in future RCTs in this area.

11.1.6 Other Coffee Compounds and Cognition

Trigonelline is another active constituent found in coffee beans which may contribute to the cognitive enhancing effects of coffee. In rodent models, Trigonelline has shown to regenerate dendritic and axonal cortical neurons in axonal cortical neurons and improve memory retention (Tohda et al. 2005). This is an important action of treatment for cognitive impairment as brain disorders are associated with neurodegeneration that is characterized by neuronal loss in brain tissues (Butt et al. 2011).

11.1.7 Possible Modes of Action

Coffee's mechanisms of action on cognitive functioning can be determined by examining its individual constituents. There may be additional biochemical processes involved in modulating cognition in coffee compounds other than the antioxidant, anti-inflammatory, and neuroprotective processes. Caffeine for instance increases acetylcholine and dopamine transmission in the brain by inhibiting the adenosine (A1 and A2a) receptors, which are the neurotransmitters involved in attention, arousal, and higher cognitive functions (Camfield et al. 2014 for review). Furthermore, in animal models caffeine decreases the hippocampal beta-amyloid levels and reduces alpha beta production, which may explain the mechanism by which caffeine protects cognition (Arendash et al. 2006).

Furthermore, prolonged oxidative stress associated with aging and reduced antioxidant capacity have been associated with conditions linked with cognitive impairments. An increase in free radial formation and lipid peroxidation as a result of oxidative stress are mechanisms contributing to AD pathology (Ansari et al. 2010). Parras and colleagues (2007) found that regardless of cost, origin of coffee bean, or brew method, commercially available coffees had good antioxidant capacity, and were very effective as scavengers of lipoperoxyl and OH– radicals. Chronic brewed-coffee consumption has shown to modulate the antioxidant system in rodent brains (Abreu et al. 2011). In particular, coffee consumption decreased the lipid peroxidation, increased the antioxidant concentration (glutathione), and increased the antioxidant enzyme activity (glutahione reductase and superoxide dismutase) (Abreu et al. 2011). Hoelzl et al. (2010) found that, compared with drinking water, participants during a 5-day intervention consuming CGA-enriched instant coffee had improved protection of certain macromolecules against oxidative damage. Corrêa et al. (2012) found that healthy adults drinking either medium-light roast or medium roast filter coffee over a 4-week period had a significantly improved antioxidant capacity (increased plasma total antioxidant status, catalase, superoxide dismutase, glutathione peroxidase) compared to baseline, however they did not observe improvements in the lipid peroxidation biomarkers.

11.2 METHODOLOGICAL ISSUES: COFFEE WITHDRAWAL AND COGNITION

The withdrawal effects of coffee have been attributed mainly to its caffeine content, and usually occurs 12–24 h following abstinence and peaks between 20 and 51 h (Juliano et al. 2004). Withdrawal symptoms mainly include headaches, fatigue, reduced alertness, clear headedness, jitteriness, and some cognitive impairment (Juliano et al. 2004; Lane 1997; Rogers et al. 1998, 2005; Stafford et al. 2005). These withdrawal symptoms tend to be worse following acute deprivation (Rogers et al. 2005). In a crossover study Lane (1997) showed that the effects of caffeine deprivation impacted the performance of serial memory tasks with a decrease in the number of correct responses in those who were caffeine deprived. Yet these effects were only seen in participants who were deprived of caffeine in the first testing session, suggesting an interaction effect. Moreover, acute deprivation (overnight) has shown to be associated with greater cognitive impairments including attention, reasoning, and response time than long-term deprivation at 3 weeks (Rogers et al. 2005). Furthermore, while caffeine abstinence also affects choice reaction time (Addicott et al. 2009), memory and selective attention do not seem to be affected (Addicott et al. 2009; Rogers et al. 2005). These studies have generally recruited individuals who consume caffeinated beverages (tea, coffee) and have examined the effects following withdrawal from caffeinated beverages. However, coffee is composed of various other constituents such as polyphenols and chlorogenic acid and their contribution, if any, of these individual molecules on withdrawal symptoms is currently unknown.

11.3 PROBLEMS IN MEASURING COGNITION ACROSS DIFFERENT COFFEE STUDIES

One of the current problems facing research on cognition and nutrition is the use of a wide range of different cognitive measures. This has recently been discussed by Stough and Pase (2015) and Pase and Stough (2014), who have argued that synthesizing RCTs involving nutritional supplements is difficult because of the different measures used in different studies, and the current lack of a systematic process to classify and aggregate the cognitive outcome data. They argued that research examining the effect of supplements, diet, and nutrition on cognition requires a new evidence-based method for grouping cognitive test data into broader cognitive abilities. The Cattell–Horn–Carroll (CHC) model of intelligence provides empirically based taxonomies of human cognition (Carroll 1993). This model provides a cognitive map that can be used to guide the handling and analysis of cognitive outcomes in clinical trial research. The cognitive processes described within the CHC model allows researchers, industry, and consumers to better understand which cognitive domains have been used in each research study. Different research studies utilize different tests of cognition and only a small part of the total number of cognitive domains that could be measured. Therefore, it is difficult to compare the results of different studies utilizing different cognitive measures without a comprehensive model of cognition. The CHC model provides this comprehensive model outlining different cognitive domains (Figure 11.1). Using this framework we might infer that the effects of coffee are consistently seen in processing speeds and this is probably due to the effects of caffeine. However more research on noncaffeine compounds and cognition are currently underway.

11.4 IDEAS FOR THE FUTURE, PROBLEMS IN THE PAST

Many epidemiological studies have found benefits from both short- and long-term regular consumption of coffee. However, epidemiological studies rely on accurate self-reports from participants, and the ability of questionnaires to capture relevant data rather than to measure actual cognitive processes. In addition, epidemiological studies do not properly control for the amount of coffee ingested over a period of time. While all coffee has overlapping chemical components, their amounts can vary depending on how the bean was processed, and how the coffee was brewed. If participants report drinking several cups of coffee per day, researchers may use a standard to calculate estimates of nutritional intake that may not truly reflect participants' actual intake. Differences in the quantities of components have also been found between coffees with different countries of origin and type of bean used (*Coffea arabica* and *Coffea robusta*) (Ludwig et al. 2012), and this sort of information may be difficult to obtain.

Additionally, many studies have been limited by how much information was captured. There are many factors that affect how coffee is absorbed into the human body. Epidemiological studies gather data relating to daily coffee consumption through food frequency questionnaires. However, as mentioned earlier, there are differences in the composition of differently prepared coffee. So even quantitative questionnaires are not able to effectively capture the differences of coffee. There are also other food sources that provide overlapping compounds found in coffee. A few RCTs measuring the effect of noncaffeine compounds found in coffee on cognition have been conducted, and to our knowledge none have been long-term studies. There have been RCTs that control the polyphenol intake in a washout period before coffee intervention. Research studies also cannot fully control for extraneous sources of polyphenols in the diet of participants. Instigating a washout period before coffee intervention by placing participants on a low-polyphenol diet would be ideal, however there would be a variation in how long participants would need to be on this diet in order to excrete residual polyphenols and their by-products. The addition of sweeteners and dairy to coffee can also affect the bioavailability of coffee polyphenols and their metabolites in humans as measured in plasma (Renouf et al. 2010) and in urine (Duarte et al. 2011). Polyphenols are more complex in their actions. While caffeine is largely understood and primarily metabolized by cytochrome P450 1A2–CYP1A2 in the liver, more research is needed on the bioavailability of coffee polyphenols after digestion. A mixture of human enzymes and gut microbiota may be involved in the digestion of coffee polyphenols (Calani et al. 2012), so individual differences between people may be influenced by gut health as well.

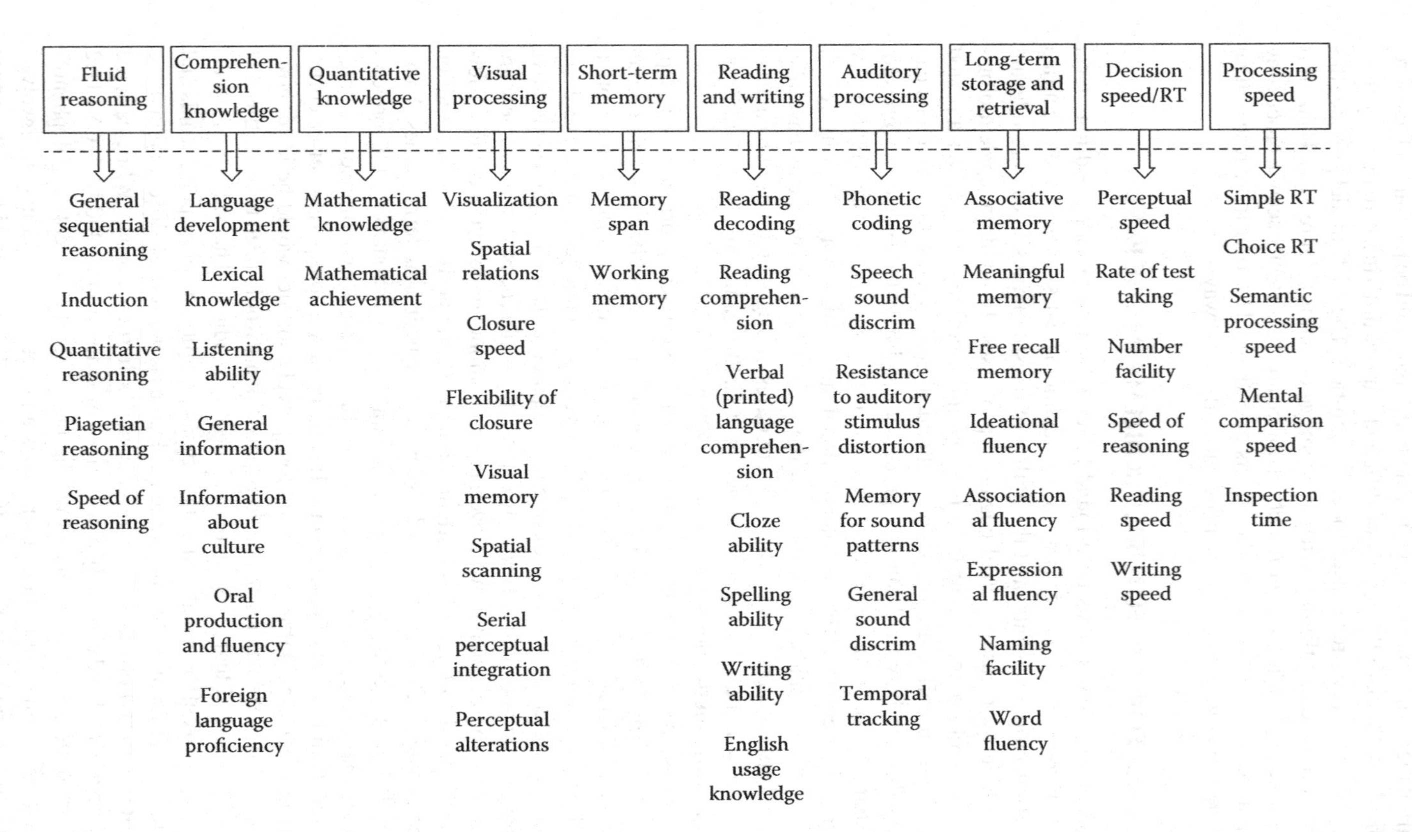

FIGURE 11.1 The broad and narrow abilities of the Cattell–Horn–Carroll model based on the writing of McGrew (2009). Some additional narrow abilities are omitted owing to space. Reproduced from Pase, M. P., Stough, C. (2014) An evidence-based method for examining and reporting cognitive processes in nutrition research. *Nutr Res Rev*, 27, 232–241.

Future studies are urgently required to assess the role of different compounds found in coffee on cognitive processes using cognitive measures that can be understood using a standardized model of cognition such as the CHC. There are significant opportunities for researchers and the industry in examining the role of noncaffeine compounds in coffee on cognition and related neurocognitive outcomes across the lifespan.

REFERENCES

Abreu, R. V., Silva-Oliveira, E. M., Moraes, M. F. D., Pereira, G. S., and Moraes-Santos, T. (2011). Chronic coffee and caffeine ingestion effects on the cognitive function and antioxidant system of rat brains. *Pharmacology Biochemistry and Behavior 99*(4), 659–664.

Addicott, M. A., and Laurienti, P. J. (2009). A comparison of the effects of caffeine following abstinence and normal caffeine use. *Psychopharmacology 207*(3), 423–431.

Ansari, M. A., and Sheff, S. W. (2010). Oxidative stress in the progression of Alzheimer disease in the frontal cortex. *Journal of Neuropathology and Experimental Neurology* 69(2), 155-167.

Arab, L., Biggs, M. L., O'Meara, E. S., Longstreth, W. T., Crane, P. K., and Fitzpatrick, A. L. (2011). Gender differences in tea, coffee, and cognitive decline in the elderly: The cardiovascular health study. *Journal of Alzheimer's Disease 27*(3), 553–566.

Araújo, L. F., Giatti, L., Padilha Dos Reis, R. C., Goulart, A. C., Schmidt, M. I., Duncan, B. B., and Ikram, M. A. (2015). Inconsistency of association between coffee consumption and cognitive function in adults and elderly in a cross-sectional study (ELSA-Brasil). *Nutrients 7*(11), 9590–9601.

Arendash, G. W., and Chuanhai, C. (2010). Caffeine and coffee as therapeutics against Alzheimer's disease. *Journal of Alzheimer's Disease 20*(Suppl. 1), S117–S126.

Arendash, G. W., Schleif, W., Rezai-Zadeh, K., Jackson, E. K., Zacharia, L. C., Cracchiolo, J. R., Shippy, D., and Tan, J. (2006). Caffeine protects Alzheimer's mice against cognitive impairment and reduces brain beta-amyloid production. *Neuroscience 142*(4), 941–952.

Belitz, H.-D., Grosch, W., and Schieberle, P. (2009). Coffee, tea, cocoa in *Food Chemistry* (4th ed., pp. 938–970), Berlin: Springer.

Butt, M. S., and Sultan, M. T. (2011). Coffee and its consumption: Benefits and risks. *Critical Reviews in Food Science and Nutrition 51*(4), 363–373.

Calani, L., Dall'Asta, M., Derlindati, E., Scazzina, F., Bruni, R., and Del Rio, D. (2012). Colonic metabolism of polyphenols from coffee, green tea, and hazelnut skins. *Journal of Clinical Gastroenterology 46*, S95–S99.

Camfield, D. A., Silber, B. Y., Scholey, A. B., Nolidin, K., Goh, A., and Stough, C. (2013). A randomised placebo-controlled trial to differentiate the acute cognitive and mood effects of chlorogenic acid from decaffeinated coffee. *PLoS ONE 8*(12), e82897.

Camfield, D. A., Stough, C., Farrimond, J., and Scholey, A. B. (2014). Acute effects of tea constituents L-theanine, caffeine, and epigallocatechin gallate on cognitive function and mood: A systematic review and meta-analysis. *Nutrition Reviews 72*(8), 507–522.

Carman, A. J., Dacks, P. A., Lane, R. F., Shineman, D. W., and Fillit, H. M. (2014). Current evidence for the use of coffee and caffeine to prevent age-related cognitive decline and Alzheimer's disease. *The Journal of Nutrition, Health & Aging 18*(4), 383–392.

Carroll, J. B. (1993). *Human Cognitive Abilities: A Survey of Factor Analytic Studies.* New York: Cambridge University Press.

Choi, H. K., and Curhan, G. (2007). Coffee, tea, and caffeine consumption and serum uric acid level: The third national health and nutrition examination survey. *Arthritis Care & Research 57*(5), 816–821.

Choi, H. K., and Curhan, G. (2010). Coffee consumption and risk of incident gout in women: The Nurses' Health Study. *American Journal of Clinical Nutrition 92*(4), 922–927.

Corrêa, T. A. F., Monteiro, M. P., Mendes, T. M. N., de Oliveira, D. M., Rogero, M. M., Benites, C. I.,Vinagre, C. G., et al. (2012). Medium light and medium roast paper-filtered coffee increased antioxidant capacity in healthy volunteers: Results of a randomized trial. *Plant Foods for Human Nutrition 67*(3), 277–282.

Cropley, V., Croft, R., Silber, B., Neale, C., Scholey, A., Stough, C., and Schmitt, J. (2011). Does coffee enriched with chlorogenic acids improve mood and cognition after acute administration in healthy elderly? A pilot study. *Psychopharmacology 219*(3), 737–749.

Ding, M., Bhupathiraju, S. N., Chen, M., van Dam, R. M., and Hu, F. B. (2014). Caffeinated and decaffeinated coffee consumption and risk of type 2 diabetes: A systematic review and a dose-response meta-analysis. *Diabetes Care 37*(2), 569–586.

Dodd, F., Kennedy, D., Riby, L., and Haskell-Ramsay, C. (2015). A double-blind, placebo-controlled study evaluating the effects of caffeine and L-theanine both alone and in combination on cerebral blood flow, cognition and mood. *Psychopharmacology (Berlin) 232*(14), 2563–2576.

Duarte, G. S., and Farah, A. (2011). Effect of simultaneous consumption of milk and coffee on chlorogenic acids' bioavailability in humans. *Journal of Agricultural and Food Chemistry 59*(14), 7925–7931.

Eskelinen, M. H., Ngandu, T., Tuomilehto, J., Soininen, H., and Kivipelto, M. (2009). Midlife coffee and tea drinking and the risk of late-life dementia: A population-based CAIDE study. *Journal of Alzheimer's Disease 16*(1), 85–91.

Esquivel, P., and Jiménez, V. M. (2012). Functional properties of coffee and coffee by-products. *Food Research International 46*(2), 488–495.

Hoelzl, C., Knasmüller, S., Wagner, K. H., Elbling, L., Huber, W., Kager, N., Ferk, F., et al. (2010). Instant coffee with high chlorogenic acid levels protects humans against oxidative damage of macromolecules. *Molecular Nutrition & Food Research 54*(12), 1722–1733.

Juliano, L. M., and Griffiths, R. R. (2004). A critical review of caffeine withdrawal: Empirical validation of symptoms and signs, incidence, severity, and associated features. *Psychopharmacology (Berl) 176*(1), 1–29.

Kempf, K., Herder, C., Erlund, I., Kolb, H., Martin, S., Carstensen, M., Koenig, W., et al. (2010). Effects of coffee consumption on subclinical inflammation and other risk factors for type 2 diabetes: A clinical trial. *The American Journal of Clinical Nutrition 91*(4) 950–957.

Lane, J. D. (1997). Effects of brief caffeinated-beverage deprivation on mood, symptoms, and psychomotor performance. *Pharmacology Biochemistry and Behavior 58*(1), 203–208.

Ludwig, I. A., Sanchez, L., Caemmerer, B., Kroh, L. W., De Peña, M. P., and Cid, C. (2012). Extraction of coffee antioxidants: Impact of brewing time and method. *Food Research International 48*(1), 57–64.

Maia, L., and de Mendonca, A. (2002). Does caffeine intake protect from Alzheimer's disease? *European Journal of Neurology 9*(4), 377–382.

Mills, C. E., Oruna-Concha, M. J., Mottram, D. S., Gibson, G. R., and Spencer, J. P. E. (2013). The effect of processing on chlorogenic acid content of commercially available coffee. *Food Chemistry 141*(4), 3335–3340.

Palatini, P. (2015). Coffee consumption and risk of type 2 diabetes. *Diabetologia 58*(1), 199–200.

Parras, P., Martínez-Tomé, M., Jiménez, A. M., and Murcia, M. A. (2007). Antioxidant capacity of coffees of several origins brewed following three different procedures. *Food Chemistry 102*(3), 582–592.

Pase, M. P., and Stough, C. (2014). An evidence-based method for examining and reporting cognitive processes in nutrition research. *Nutrition Research Reviews* 27, 232–241.

Renouf, M., Marmet, C., Guy, P., Fraering, A. L., Longet, K., Moulin, J., Enslen, M., et al. (2010). Nondairy creamer, but not milk, delays the appearance of coffee phenolic acid equivalents in human plasma. *Journal of Nutrition 140*(2), 259–263.

Ritchie, K., Carriere, I., de Mendonca, A., Portet, F., Dartigues, J. F., Rouaud, O., Barberger-Gateau, P., Ancelin, M. L. (2007). The neuroprotective effects of caffeine: A prospective population study (the Three City Study). *Neurology 69*(6), 536–545.

Rogers, P. J., and Dernoncourt, C. (1998). Regular caffeine consumption: A balance of adverse and beneficial effects for mood and psychomotor performance. *Pharmacology Biochemistry and Behavior 59*(4), 1039–1045.

Rogers, P. J., Heatherley, S. V., Hayward, R. C., Seers, H. E., Hill, J., and Kane, M. (2005). Effects of caffeine and caffeine withdrawal on mood and cognitive performance degraded by sleep restriction. *Psychopharmacology 179*(4), 742–752.

Shukitt-Hale, B., Miller, M. G., Chu, Y.-F., Lyle, B. J., and Joseph, J. A. (2013). Coffee, but not caffeine, has positive effects on cognition and psychomotor behavior in aging. *Age 35*(6) 2183–2192.

Stafford, L. D., and Yeomans, M. R. (2005). Caffeine deprivation state modulates coffee consumption but not attentional bias for caffeine-related stimuli. *Behavioural Pharmacology 16*(7), 559–571.

Stalmach, A., Williamson, G., and Crozier, A. (2014). Impact of dose on the bioavailability of coffee chlorogenic acids in humans. *Food and Function 5*(8), 1727–1737.

Stough, C., and Pase, M. P. (2015). Improving cognition in the elderly with nutritional supplements. *Current Directions in Psychological Science* 24, 177-183.

Tohda, C., Kuboyama, T., and Komatsu, K. (2005). Search for natural products related to regeneration of the neuronal network. *NeuroSignals 14*(1–2), 34–45.

van Dam, R. M., and Hu, F. B. (2005). Coffee consumption and risk of type 2 diabetes: A systematic review. *JAMA 294*(1), 97–104.

van Gelder, B. M., Buijsse, B., Tijhuis, M., Kalmijn, S., Giampaoli, S., Nissinen, A., and Kromhout, D. (2006). Coffee consumption is inversely associated with cognitive decline in elderly European men: The FINE Study. *European Journal of Clinical Nutrition 61*(2), 226–232

Wang, Y., and Ho, C.-T. (2009). Polyphenolic chemistry of tea and coffee: A century of progress. *Journal of Agricultural and Food Chemistry 57*(18), 8109–8114.

12 Nontargeted Metabolomics Reveal Changes in Chlorogenic Acids in Ripening *Coffea arabica* Green Beans

Koichi Nakahara, Keiko Iwasa, and Chifumi Nagai

CONTENTS

ABSTRACT

Green coffee beans contain various bioactive compounds and potently functional compounds that contribute to the overall beverage bioactivity and flavor quality. However, little is known about the relationship between the metabolomic compounds in green beans and the functional characteristics of coffee.

Previous metabolomic studies in our laboratory were performed on green beans using liquid chromatography–mass spectrometry (LC–MS)-based nontargeted analysis. The association between the metabolites and beverage flavor quality was investigated. Since the chemical composition of green beans is known to be closely linked to the ripeness of the coffee cherries, the metabolites at four stages of ripeness in three cultivars of *Coffea arabica* green beans were investigated. The immature marker tryptophan was identified as a causative agent in the development of the off-flavor in coffee beverages.

The present study was carried out in three sections. The first set of trials on metabolic profiling revealed that chlorogenic acids (CGAs), which are antioxidants, are also key markers of ripening and that the CGA profile changed depending on the stage of ripeness.

The second investigation, an analysis of dynamic changes during the ripening process, revealed that CGAs with di- or tri-methylated hydroxycinnamoyl moieties are found in higher amounts in the riper beans of all three cultivars. Therefore, CGA profiling might be indicative of the metabolic processes taking place during the ripening stages. In the third trial, CGA profiling and metabolomic analysis of 36 *C. arabica* green bean samples from Guatemala were correlated with different cupping scores after roasting. This revealed that the contents of CGA with di-methylated hydroxycinnamoyl moieties were greater in green beans with higher cupping scores.

Metabolomics can characterize green coffee beans and will enable us to maximize the functional properties of coffee beans. Metabolomics might also allow us to identify new chemical indices of the functional properties in coffee.

12.1 INTRODUCTION

Over 800 flavor components have been identified in coffee, and people enjoy the varied flavor notes, such as chocolate, fruits, caramel, and honey. In addition, coffees have various bioactive characteristics [1] that are generated by chemical compounds in the beans. Recently, green beans as well as roasted bean extracts have been focused on as a source of these bioactive compounds. However, there have been very few studies on the relationship between the compounds in green beans (metabolites) and the resulting bioactivities and functional characteristics of green beans or coffee beverages.

Metabolomics, the study of metabolites, have been used in the medical, microbiology, and plant physiology fields [2], and have enabled us to reveal changes in chemical compounds during green bean ripening. Liquid chromatography–mass spectrometry (LC–MS), coupled with a statistical multivariate analysis of metabolome (LC–MS-based metabolic profiling), is a sensitive and comprehensive technique [3,4] that can be used to study the relationship between the compounds and their activities and functional characteristics. This technique can also clarify the novel markers of the bioactivities of coffee.

In coffee production, the ripeness of the coffee cherries has a strong impact on cupping quality. Fully mature beans provide good cupping quality, while, alternatively, a mixture of immature beans in a cup can produce a strong off-flavor. Contamination with immature beans is a serious problem in Brazilian coffee markets [5–7]. Since the chemical composition varies depending on the level of ripeness [8], green beans at four stages of ripening were studied. The marker in immature beans that lowered cup quality was previously identified [9].

Metabolic profiling techniques were employed to identify the metabolites correlated with beverage quality. The relationship between ripening and CGAs was studied. These acids have various bioactivities such as antioxidant, hepatoprotective, hypoglycemic, anti-inflammatory, and antiviral activities [10–18]. First, nontargeted metabolic profiling analysis was used to investigate CGA in ripening coffee beans (Section 12.2). Next, changes in diverse CGAs during ripening were studied in detail using LC–high-resolution (HR)-MS measurements (Section 12.3). Metabolomics of 36 green beans were scored to quality grade and the CGA was profiled. The association between the characterization of CGA and cupping scores was discussed in Section 12.4.

12.2 METABOLIC PROFILING IN RIPENING *Coffea arabica* GREEN BEANS

The aim of this study was to conduct a profiling of metabolites in ripening *C. arabica* beans, in particular focusing on CGA with various bioactivities. The design strategy of this work is shown in Figure 12.1.

12.2.1 MATERIALS AND METHODS

12.2.1.1 Green Bean Samples

To obtain reproducible quantitative analysis data, the cultivars and cherry ripeness was characterized.

All coffee cherry samples came from coffee trees in the same fields at the Hawaii Agriculture Research Center (HARC), Hawaii. Three cultivars, Typica, SL28, and Catuai [20–21], were used. The coffee cherries were hand-picked within two days on October 12 and 13, 2010, and were divided into four groups according to color (green, pink, red, and dark red) (Figure 12.2a). The hardnesses of 15 cherries from each group were measured with a duo meter model E (Asker, Japan), and the hardness values ($n = 15$) were averaged (Figure 12.2b). Then, wet processing and drying were

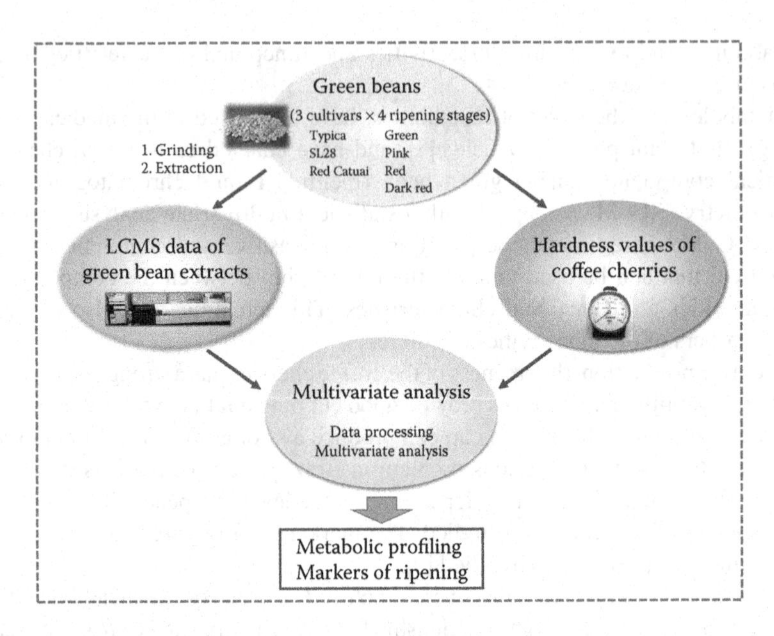

FIGURE 12.1 Our strategy of metabolic profiling.

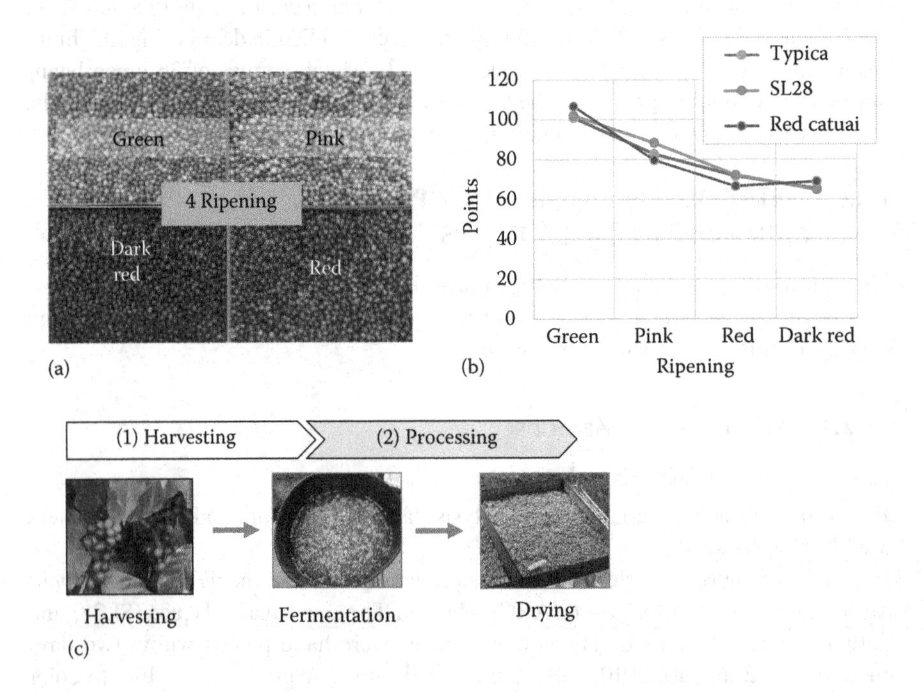

FIGURE 12.2 (See color insert.) Green *C. arabica* beans at four stages of ripening. (a) Coffee cherries of four ripening stages. (b) Hardness values of the coffee cherries. (c) The process from harvesting of coffee cherries to green beans.

carried out under uniform conditions for all samples (Figure 12.2c), as described in the previous report [9]. A total of 12 green coffee samples were collected at four ripening stages from three cultivars.

12.2.1.2 Metabolite Extraction and LC–MS Measurements for Metabolic Profiling

Metabolites were extracted from green beans and analyzed by LC–MS (LCMS-IT TOF, Shimadzu, Japan) on a Luna-C18 column (250 × 1.0 mm, 5 μm particle size; Phenomenex, CA) [9,22].

12.2.1.3 Data Processing and Multivariate Statistical Analysis

Data processing (peak picking and alignment), normalization, and filtering of the ion signals in negative mode were performed as described in [9–22]. They produced 581 valid ion signals. Subsequently, a multivariate statistical analysis was performed using the SIMCA P$^+$ ver. 13.0.3 software program (Umetrics, Sweden). An orthogonal projection to latent structure (OPLS) regression model analysis [23] was performed to identify the markers correlated with ripening (Figure 12.3b and c).

12.2.1.4 Sample Preparation of Green Coffee Beans and Setting the Index of Ripening for Metabolic Profiling

Three cultivars were used to identify the common markers in different cultivars growing in the same environmental condition. Cherries were grouped into four ripening stages (green, pink, red, and dark red) and then measured for hardness. Since hardness values (average value of $n = 15$) decrease during ripening regardless of cultivars (Figure 12.1c), they were used as an index of ripening for metabolic profiling analysis. Twelve green bean samples were used at four ripening stages from three cultivars.

12.2.1.5 LC–MS Analysis and Data Processing

Metabolite extracts were analyzed by the LCMS-IT TOF instrument in triplicate measurements ($n = 3$) (Figure 12.3a). The LC–MS spectra in negative ion modes were processed (peak picking, alignments, and filtering) to obtain 581 valid ion signals.

12.2.1.6 Metabolic Profiling

To study the relationship between the LC–MS data of green bean extracts at four ripening stages and hardness (an index of ripening stages), a multivariate statistical technique was used. OPLS regression analysis was applied to create the ripening predicting model (Figure 12.3b).

12.2.2 Results and Discussion

The multivariate statistical technique model showed that hardness values (ripening stages) were highly predicted by metabolites in green beans (Figure 12.3b). The quality of this model was good according to the value of the coefficient (R^2 of 0.99), the cross-validated correlation coefficient (Q^2 of 0.90), and the root mean squared

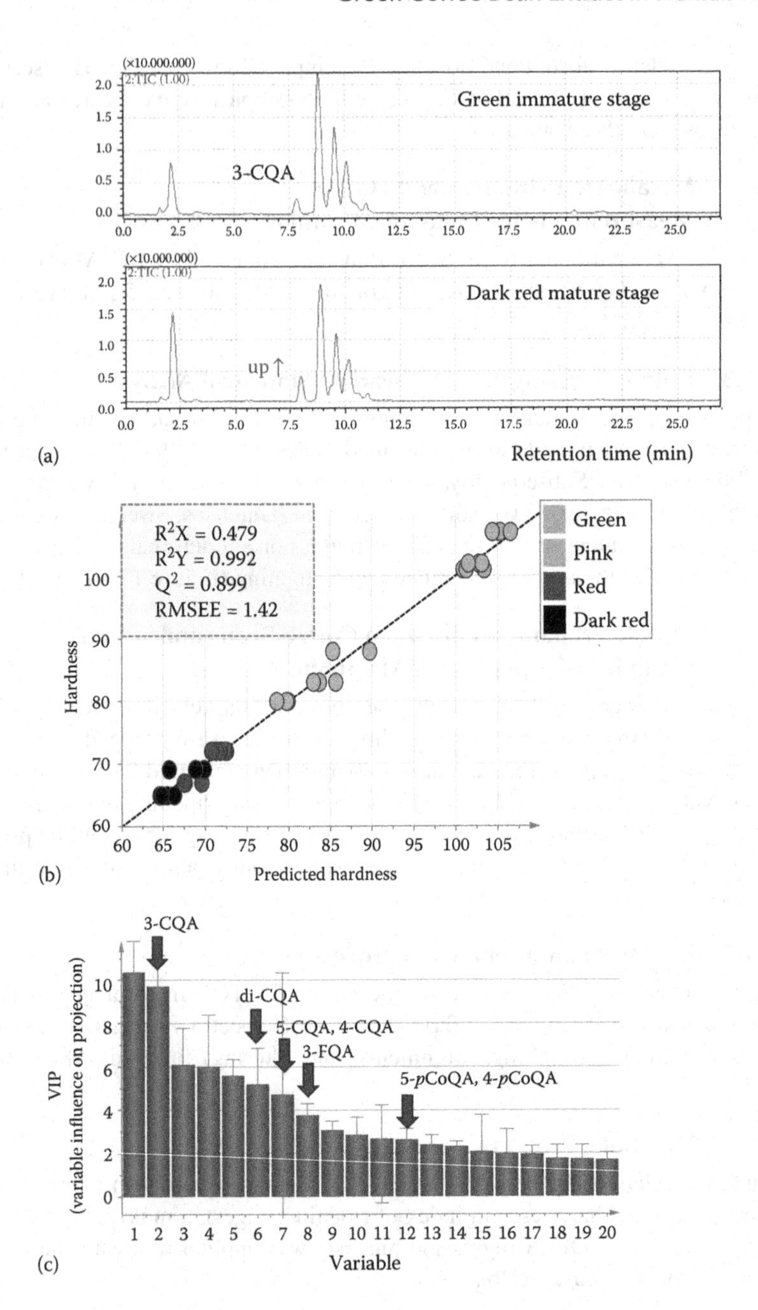

FIGURE 12.3 (See color insert.) Multivariate analyses. (a) Total ion chromatogram of bean extracts of Typica at green immature stage (upper) and dark red mature stage (lower) in negative ion mode by LC–MS measurements. The peak (3-CQA), which is more abundant in the bean extract (at dark red stage), is shown. (b) OPLS regression model. Hardness values (the ripening stages) were predicted by the metabolite information in the green beans. (c) The variable influence on projection (VIP) plots. The top 20 variables are shown. The arrowheads indicate CGA in the lists.

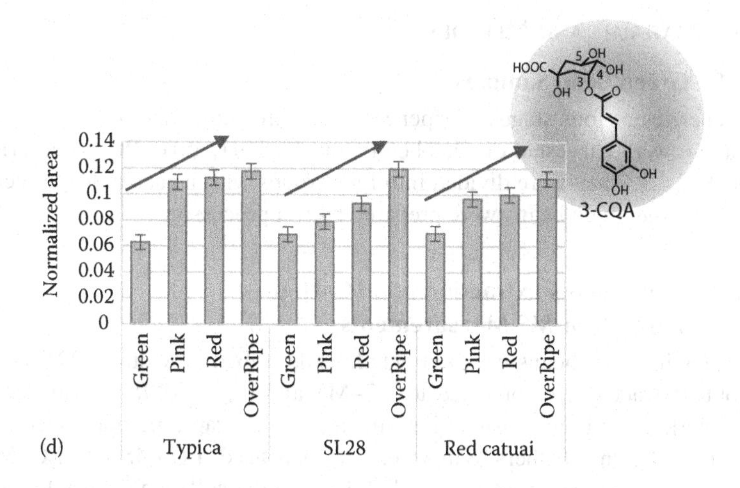

FIGURE 12.3 (Continued) Multivariate analyses. (d) 3-CQA exists in greater amounts in riper beans.

error of estimation (RMSEE of 1.42) [24]. The list of variables (metabolites ion signals) was plotted to strongly contribute to the regression, according to the variable influence on prediction (VIP) (Figure 12.3c). The higher ranked metabolites were assumed to be strongly associated with ripening.

The metabolites ion signals were characterized based on the *m/z* value. Interestingly, several CGA were present in the top 20 VIP lists (Figure 12.3c). The structural characterization of isomers of CGA was assumed by the LC elution-time data, compared with that of the literature [25,26]. In the VIP list, the second ranked metabolite was 3-caffeoylquinic acid (3-CQA), the sixth ranking metabolite was di-caffeoylquinic acid (diCQA, the 3,5-, 4,5-, and 3,4-isomers of which co-elute), the seventh was ion signals of co-eluted 5-CQA and 4-CQA, the eighth was 3-feruoylquinic acid (3-FQA), and the twelfth was ion signals co-eluted of 5-*p*-coumaroylquinic acid (5-*p*CoQA) and 4-*p*-coumaroylquinic acid (4-*p*CoQA). The International Union of Pure and Applied Chemistry (IUPAC) numbering system was used (data not shown). 3-CQA contents were plotted with increasing ripeness in the beans of three cultivars (Figure 12.3d). Thus, CQA are shown to be key markers of green coffee bean ripeness. This finding indicates that significant changes of CGA take place during the four ripening stages.

12.3 ANALYSES OF CHANGES OF DIVERSE CGA DURING RIPENING *COFFEA ARABICA* GREEN BEANS

In this chapter, changes of diverse CGA derivatives during ripening were studied. A comprehensive analysis was carried out on beans at four stages of ripeness using LC–HR-MS, and extracted ions corresponding to CGA.

12.3.1 Materials and Methods

12.3.1.1 Green Bean Samples

Coffee cherries at four stages of ripeness from three cultivars, Typica, SL28, and Red Catuai, were harvested on October 18 and 19, 2011, at HARC, as described in Section 12.2.1.1. They were divided into four groups within each cultivar according to color, and the green beans were prepared by wet processing.

12.3.1.2 Metabolites Extraction and LC–High-Resolution-MS Measurements

Metabolites in green beans were extracted, as described previously [22]. Then, the metabolite extracts were subjected to LC–MS and LC–MS/MS measurements. A high-resolution and high-sensitive instrument, an Orbitrap-type mass spectrometer (Q-Exactive; Thermo Fishers, San Jose, CA), was used. LC–MS and LC–MS/MS measurement conditions were recorded [22], while the collision energy for MS/MS analysis of 20%–35% (normalized) was used.

12.3.1.3 Analyses of Changes of Diverse CGA in Ripening *Coffea arabica* Beans

More than 60 CGA derivatives, a family of esters with (–)-quinic acid and certain transcinnamic acids, have been characterized in *C. canephora* green coffee beans [26–29]. However, studies on the changes of CGA in ripening are limited to the major constituents of CGA [30–33], and there is little information on the variation of these diverse CGA during ripening. In order to study the relationship between diverse CGA and ripening, four ripening coffee beans of three cultivars were analyzed by LC–HR-MS and LC–HR-MS/MS. Forty-one isomers were characterized (data not shown) on the basis of their theoretical masses, the fragment ions on MS/MS spectra, and LC retention time data (hydrophilicity), and compared with data from other studies [25–29]. A heat map was generated using a Multi-Experiment Viewer (MeV v4.9) (http://www.tm4.org/mev.html), by the Z-score values of 41 metabolite signals. A heat map illustrating the changes in CGA in Red Catuai during ripening is presented in Figure 12.4.

12.3.2 Results and Discussion

The results indicated that most of the diverse CGA derivatives varied during ripening (Figure 12.4). The common changes in CGA for all the three cultivars are summarized in Figure 12.5; the abbreviations are as follows: *p*-coumaroyl (*p*-Co), caffeoyl (C), feruloyl (F), dimethoxycinnamoyl (D), trimethoxycinnamoyl (T), and sinapoyl (Si). Numbers were assigned to regioisomers according to the LC elution order in the case of isomers, whose substitution sites of the cinnamoyl moiety on quinic acid were uncharacterized, for example, *p*CoCQA-1 and *p*CoCQA-2. We observed three findings. First, 5-*p*CoQA, 5-CQA, and F-CQA were higher in green immature beans, but their regioisomers 3-*p*CoQA, 3-CQA, 3-FQA were higher in dark red mature beans. Two isomers of 5-*p*CoQA and 4-*p*CoQA, two isomers of

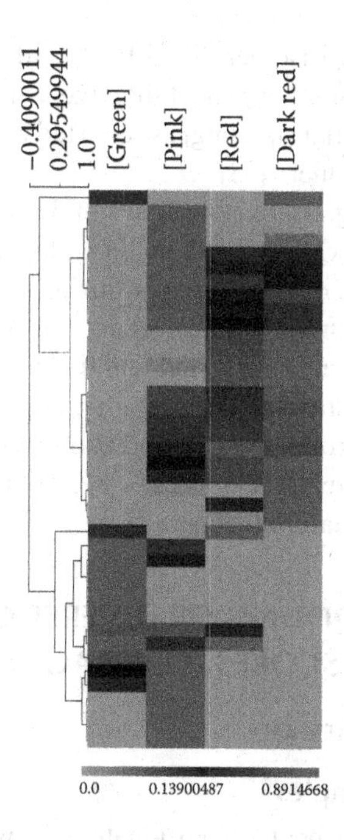

FIGURE 12.4 (See color insert.) Heat map of diverse CGA contents in ripening green coffee beans of Red Catuai.

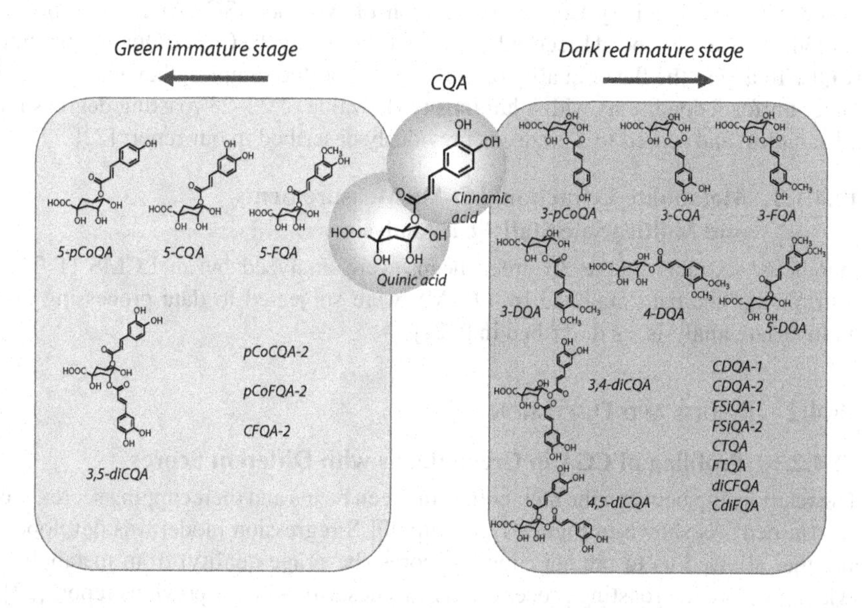

FIGURE 12.5 Changes of diverse CGA contents in ripening green coffee beans.

5-CQA and 4-CQA, and two isomers of 5-FQA and 4-FQA were co-eluted. The 5- isomers are known to be more prevalent than the 4- isomers, and an isomerization process might take place during ripening, as reported on the isomerization of 5-CQA and 5-FQA into its minor isomers [33].

Secondly, during ripening, decreasing levels of 3,5-diCQA was concomitant with increasing levels of 3,4-diCQA and 4,5-diCQA, suggesting that the transesterification of 3,5- into 3,4- and 4,5- progresses during ripening [33]. Finally, di- and tri-methylated hydroxycinnamoyl isomers of mono- and di-substituted CGA were higher in dark red mature beans. A second and third methylation of the hydroxyl in the cinnamoyl moiety might take place in later stages of ripening.

These results suggest a proposed CGA metabolic pathway based on the metabolites referred to in previous references [27,31]. Metabolites downstream in the pathway are higher in dark red mature beans.

12.4 METABOLIC PROFILING OF DIVERSE CGA CORRELATED WITH CUPPING SCORES (BEVERAGE FLAVOR QUALITY)

12.4.1 Materials and Methods

12.4.1.1 Green Bean Samples

Thirty-six samples of green beans from Guatemala were obtained commercially. These samples differed by variety of cultivar, production method, ripening, and processing method (wet processing or dry processing).

12.4.1.2 Sensory Evaluation of Beverage Flavor Quality

Sensory evaluation of coffee beverage from the 36 samples was performed in accordance with the Specialty Coffee Association of America (SCAA) cupping protocol [34] by an experienced Licensed Q grader, certified by the Coffee Quality Institute (CQI). To assess the flavor quality of the 36 green coffee samples, they were roasted under uniform conditions with a luminosity (L) value of 22–23 roasting degrees for all samples, and scored to a grade, as previously described in our report [22].

12.4.1.3 Metabolite Extraction, LC–MS Measurements, and Multivariate Statistical Analysis

Metabolite extracts of the 36 green beans were analyzed by an LCMS-IT TOF instrument. The data obtained by LC–MS were subjected to data processing and multivariate analysis, as described in [9,22].

12.4.2 Results and Discussion

12.4.2.1 Profiling of CGA in Green Beans with Different Scores

The relationship between the metabolites in green beans and their cupping scores was determined. As shown in Figure 12.7b, an OPLS regression model was developed, and that allowed us to predict cupping scores (beverage quality) from metabolites existing before the roasting process. This was described in our previous report [27].

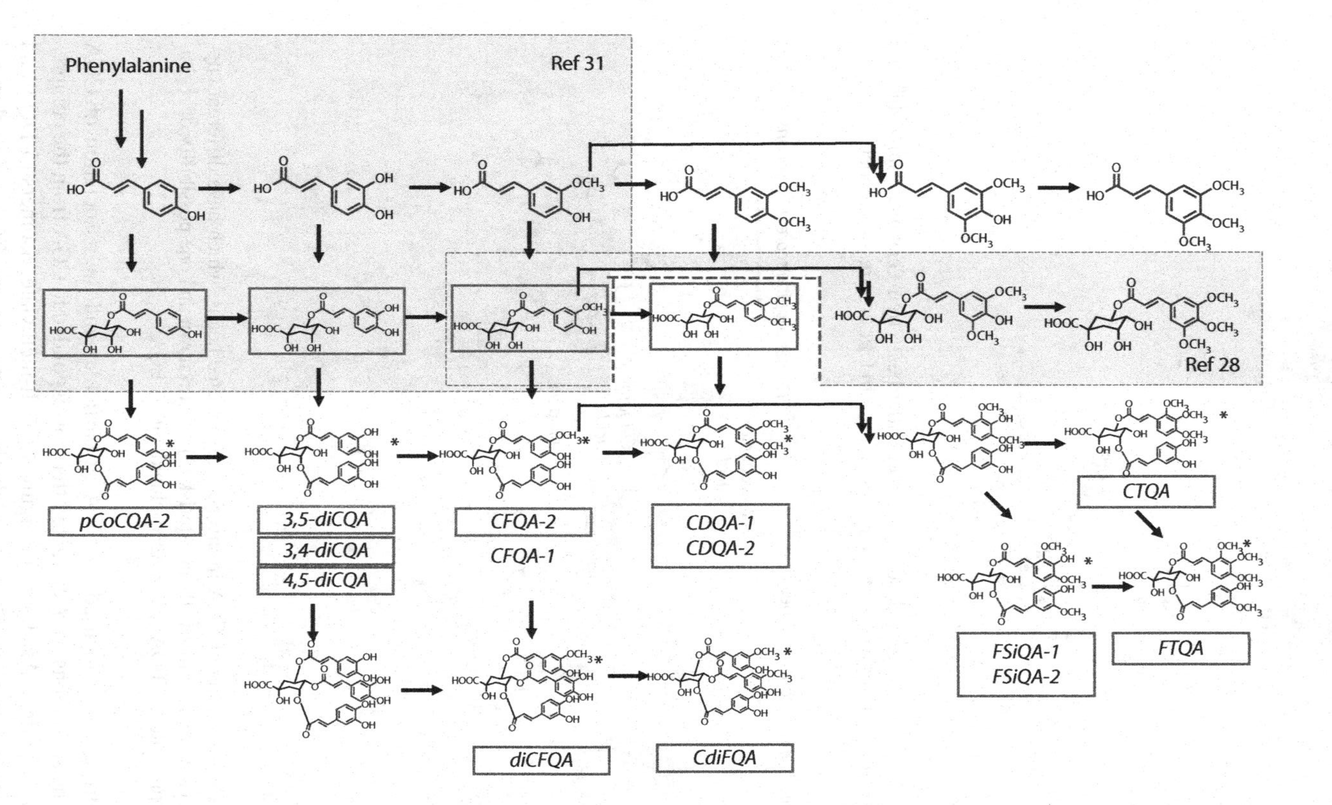

FIGURE 12.6 (See color insert.) Proposed CGA metabolic pathway and changes of diverse CGA contents in ripening. CGA isomers circled with a green line are present in higher amounts in the immature beans, and those circled with a red line are present in higher amounts in the mature beans. Isomer structures with an asterisk (*) are unknown and one possibility of regioisomers are presented. The pathways with gray circles were described in a previous report. (From Jaiswal et al., *J. Agric. Food Chem.* 2010, 58, 8722–8737; Koshiro et al., *Z Naturforsch C.*, 2007, 62, 731–742.)

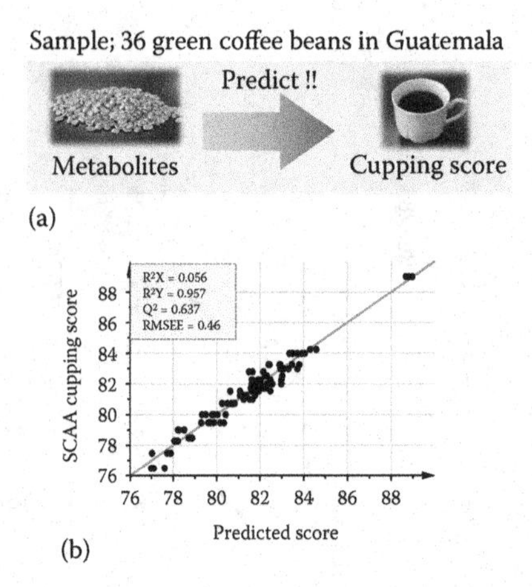

FIGURE 12.7 Multivariate analyses on 36 green coffee beans from Guatemala. (a) Metabolite data of green coffee beans can predict cupping scores. (b) OPLS regression model.

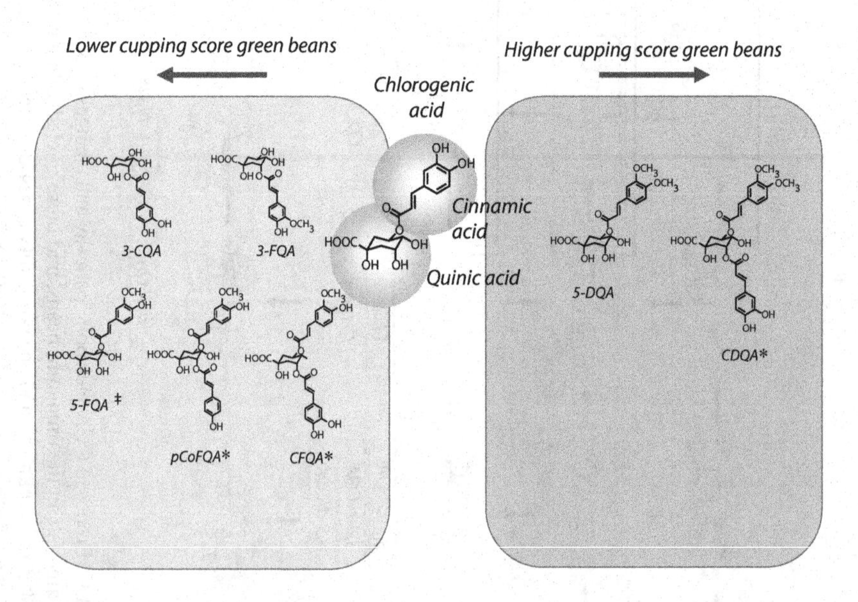

FIGURE 12.8 Profiling of CGA in diverse green coffee beans, which have different cupping score. Isomer structures with an asterisk (*) are unknown and one possibility of regioisomers are presented. 5-FQA (≠) were co-eluted with 4-FQA.

This current study focused on CGA in particular and the association of CGA with cupping score. Ions were extracted that corresponded to CGA from the comprehensive LC–MS data. As shown in Figure 12.8, di-methylated isomers (5-DQA and CDQA) were higher in green beans with higher cupping scores. CGA and its thermal products produced during roasting, such as lactones, vinylcatechol oligomers, and other phenol derivatives, influenced the coffee flavors and thereby the quality of beverage [19,35]. However, the contribution of the isomers that characterized high cupping score beans remains unclear.

12.5 CONCLUSION

CGA have various beneficial health properties. Their bioactive intensities depend on the CGA isomers. An LC–MS-based metabolomics technique was adopted to investigate changes of diverse CGA, including minor constituents of isomers, during bean ripening. Metabolic profiling revealed that most CGA varied during ripening, and were correlated with the ripening process. 3-CQA in particular is a good marker of ripening across all three cultivar beans. Studies of the variation of each of the isomers during ripening showed that biosynthesis of the second methylation and the third methylation on the hydroxyl group of cinnamoyl moiety, the isomerization of 5-*p*CoQA, 5-CQA, and 5-FQA into 3-*p*CoQA, 3-CQA, and 3-FQA, and the isomerization of 3,5-diCQA into 3,4-diCQA and 4,5-diCQA all took place in later ripening stages. These findings were observed in all three cultivars. Furthermore, dimethylated isomers are more prelavent in higher cupping score beans. A novel CGA derivative was found that correlated with a high cupping score.

Metabolomics is a powerful tool used to characterize the chemical compounds in green coffee beans. It could allow us to select beans with certain benefits, and to identify as yet unknown markers.

REFERENCES

1. Specialty Coffee Association of Japan; *Coffee Meister Training Course Text Book*; Tokyo, Japan, **2011**; pp. 116–117 (in Japanese).
2. Patti, G.J.; Yanes, O.; Siuzdak, G. Innovation: Metabolomics: The apogee of the omics trilogy. *Nat. Rev. Mol. Cell Biol.* **2012**, *13*, 263–269.
3. Fiehn, O. Metabolomics: The link between genotypes and phenotypes. *Plant. Mol. Biol.* **2002**, *48*, 155–171.
4. Dettmer, K.; Aronov, P.A.; Hammock, B.D. Mass spectrometry based metabolomics. *Mass Spectrom Rev.* **2007**, *26*, 51–78.
5. Agresti, P.D.C.M.; Franca, A.S.; Oliveria, L.S.; Augusti, R. Discrimination between defective and non-defective Brazilian coffee beans by their volatile profile. *Food Chem.* **2008**, *106*, 787–796.
6. Leroy, T.; Ribeyre, F.; Bertrand, B.; Charmetant, P; Dufour, M. et al. Genetics of coffee quality. *Braz. J. Plant Physiol.* **2006**, *18*, 229–242.
7. Santos, J.R.; Sarraguc, M.C.; Rangel, A.O.; Lopes, J.A. Evaluation of green coffee beans quality using near infrared spectroscopy: A quantitative approach. *Food Chem.* **2012**, *135*, 1828–1835.
8. De Vos, D.H.R.; Borem, F.M.; Bouwmeester, H.J.; Bino, R.J. Untargeted metabolomics as a novel tool in coffee research. *Proceedings, 21th Coll ASIC*, **2006**, Montpellier, France.
9. Setoyama, D.; Iwasa, K.; Seta, H.; Shimidzu, H.; Fujimura, Y.; Miura, D.; Wariishi, H.; Nagai, C.; Nakahara, K. High-throughput metabolic profiling of diverse green *Coffea arabica* beans identified tryptophan as a universal discrimination factor for immature beans. *PLoS One* **2013**, *8*, e70098.
10. Natella, F.; Nardimi, M.; Gianetti, I.; Dattilo, C.; Scaccini, C. Coffee drinking influences plasma antioxidant capacity in humans. *J. Agric. Food Chem.* **2002**, *50*, 6211–6216.

11. Pereira, A.S.; Pereira, A.F.M.; Trugo, L.C.; Neto, F.R.A. Distribution of quinic acid derivatives and other phenolic compounds in Brazilian propolis. *Z. Naturforsch.* **2003,** *58c*, 590–593.
12. Fujioka, K.; Shibamoto, T. Quantitation of volatiles and nonvolatile acids in an extract from coffee beverages: Correlation with antioxidant activity. *J. Agric. Food Chem.* **2006**, *54*, 6054–6058.
13. Grace, S.C.; Logan, B.A.; Adams, W.W. Seasonal differences in foliar content of chlorogenic acid, a phenylpropanoid antioxidant, in *Mahonia repens. Plant Cell Environ.* **1998**, *21*, 513–521.
14. Basnet, P.; Matsushige, K.; Hase. K.; Kadota, S.; Namba, T. Four di-o-caffeoyl quinic acid derivatives from propolis. Potent hepatoprotective activity in experimental liver injury models. *Biol. Pharm. Bull.* **1996**, *19*, 1479–1484.
15. Tatefuji, T.; Izumi, N.; Ohta, T.; Arai, S.; Ikeda, M.; Kurimoto, M. Isolation and identification of compounds from Brazilian propolis which enhance macrophage spreading and mobility. *Biol. Pharm. Bull.* **1996**, *19*, 966–970.
16. Hemmerle, H.; Burger, H-J.; Bellow, P.; Schubert, G.; Rippel, R.; Schindler, P.W.; Paulus, E.; Herling, A.W. Chlorogenic acid and synthetic chlorogenic acid derivatives: Novel inhibitors of hepatic glucose-6-phosphate translocase. *J. Med. Chem.* **1997**, *40*, 137–145.
17. Robinson, W.E. Jr.; Cordeiro, M.; Abdel-Malek, S.; Jia, Q.; Chow, S.A.; Reinecke, M.G.; Mitchell, W.M. Dicaffeoylquinic acid inhibitors of human immunodeficiency virus integrase: Inhibition of the core catalytic domain of human immunodeficiency virus integrase. *Mol. Pharmacol.* **1996**, *50*, 846–855.
18. Farah, A.; Monteiro, M.: Donangelo, C.M.; Lafay, S. Chlorogenic acids from green coffee extract are highly bioavailable in human. *J. Nutr.* **2007**, *137*, 2196–3301.
19. Farah, A.; Donangelo, C.M. Phenolic compounds in coffee. *Braz. J. Plant Physiol.* **2006**, *18*, 23–36.
20. Steiger, L.; Nagai, C.; Moore, H.; Morden, W.; Osgood, V. et al. AFLP analysis of genetic diversity within and among *Coffea arabica* cultivars. *Theor. Appl. Genet.* **2002,** *108*, 209–215.
21. Nagai, C.; Osgood, R.V.; Cavaletto, C.G.; Bittenbender, H.C.; Wiever, K., et al. Coffee breeding and selection in Hawaii. *Proceedings, the 19th ASIC, International Conference on Coffee Science.* **2001**, Trieste, Italy.
22. Iwasa, K.; Setoyama, D.; Seta, H.; Shimidzu, H.; Fujimura, Y.; Miura, D.; Wariishi, H.; Nagai, C.; Nakahara, K. Identification of 3-methylbutanoyl glycosides in green *Coffea arabica* beans as causative determinants for the quality of coffee. *J. Agric. Food Chem.* **2015**, *63*, 3742–3751.
23. Wiklund, S.; Johansson, E.; Sjostrom, L.; Mellerowicz, E.; Edlund, U.; Shockcor, J. P.; Gottfries, J.; Moritz, T.; Trygg, J. Visualization of GC/TOF-MS-based metabolomics data for identification of biochemically interesting compounds using OPLS class models. *Anal. Chem.* **2008**, *80*, 115–122.
24. Eriksson, L.; Johansson, E.; Kettaneh-Wold, N.; Trygg, J.; Wikstrom, C. et al. *Part I Multi- and Megavariate Data Analysis Basic Principles and Applications.* UMETRICS. Sweden. **2006**.
25. Perrone, D.; Farah, A.; Donangelo, C.M.; Paulis, T. de P.; Martin, Pe. R. Comprehensive analysis of major and minor chlorogenic acids and lactones in economically relevant Brazilian coffee cultivars. *Food Chem.* **2008**, *106*, 859–867.
26. Clifford, M.N.; Johnston, K.L.; Kuhnert, N. Hierarchical scheme for LC-MSn identification of chlorogenic acids. *J. Agric. Food Chem.* **2003**, *51*, 2900–2911.
27. Jaiswal, R.; Patras, M.A.; Eravuchira, P.J.; Kuhnert, N. Profile and characterization of the chlorogenic acids in green robusta coffee beans by LC-MSn: Identification of seven new classes of compounds. *J. Agric. Food Chem.* **2010**, *58*, 8722–8737.

28. Clifford, M.N.; Marks, S..; Knight, S.; Kuhnert, N. Characterization by LC-MSn of four new classes of p-coumaric acid-containing diacyl chlorogenic acids in green coffee beans. *J. Agric. Food Chem.* **2006**, *54*, 4095–4101.
29. Clifford, M.N.; Knight, S.; Surucu, B.; Kuhnert, N. Characterization by LC-MSn of four new classes of chlorogenic acids in green coffee beans: dimethoxycinnamoylquinic acids, diferuloylquinic acids, caffeoyl-dimethoxycinnamoylquinic acids, and feruloyl-dimethoxycinnamoylquinic acids. *J. Agric. Food Chem.* **2006**, *54*, 1957–1969.
30. Clifford, M.N.; Kazi, T. The influence of coffee bean maturity on the content of chlorogenic acids, caffeine and trigonelline. *Food Chem.* **1987**, *26*, 59–69.
31. Koshiro, Y.; Jackson, M.C.; Katahira, R.; Wang, M.L.; Nagai, C.; Ashihara, H. Biosynthesis of chlorogenic acids in growing and ripening fruits of *Coffea arabica* and *Coffea canephora* plants. *Z. Naturforsch. C.* **2007**, *62*, 731–742.
32. De Menezes, H.C. The relationship between the state of maturity of raw coffee beans and the isomers of caffeoylquinic acid. *Food Chem.* **1994**, *50*, 293–296.
33. Jöet, T.; Salmona, J.; Laffargue, A.; Descroix, F.; Dussert, S. Use of the growing environment as a source of variation to identify the quantitative trait transcripts and modules of co-expressed genes that determine chlorogenic acid accumulation. *Plant Cell Environ.* **2010**, *33*, 1220–1233.
34. Specialty Coffee Association of America. Cupping protocols. URL (http://www.scaa.org/?page=resources&d=cupping-protocols) (July 25, 2015).
35. Oliver Frank, O.; Blumberg, S.; Kunert, C.; Zehentbauer, G.; Hofmann, T. Structure determination and sensory analysis of bitter-tasting 4-vinylcatechol oligomers and their identification in roasted coffee by means of LC-MS/MS. *J. Agric. Food Chem.* **2007**, *55*, 1945–1954.

13 Effect of Green Coffee Bean Extract on Nrf2/ARE Pathway

Mirza Sarwar Baig and Raj K. Keservani

CONTENTS

ABSTRACT

Coffee (*Coffea arabica* L. and *Coffea canephora* var. robusta) is one of the most popular nonalcoholic beverages in the world. The phenolic acids (caffeic acid, ferulic acid, and p-coumaric acid), the chlorogenic acids [5-caffeoylquinic acid (5-CQA), and 5-feruloylquinic acid (5-FQA)], and other bioactive compounds present in coffee are capable of modulating the transcription of antioxidant enzymes. Taking this into account, both the chlorogenic acids and the free phenolic acids act as bioactive substances in the green coffee bean extract. Caffeine is the most abundant purine alkaloid present in green and roasted coffee, which is capable of modulating the transcription of antioxidant enzymes. But over consumption of caffeine can cause adverse effects such as caffeine intoxication, anxiety, and sleep disorders. In this chapter, we will discuss the effects of green coffee bean extract on the Nrf2/ARE pathway.

Keywords: green coffee, Nrf2/ARE pathway, phenolic acids, chlorogenic acids, Phase II enzymes, and antioxidant enzymes

13.1 INTRODUCTION

Coffee is one of the most popular nonalcoholic beverages in the world and an important commercially traded product. Coffee production is the primary livelihood for millions of small land-holders and farm workers worldwide. *C. arabica* (Arabica coffee) and *C. canephora* (Robusta coffee) are the two most common commercially cultivated coffee species, and together account for about 70% of world production (Hicks 2002; Davis et al. 2006; Enyan et al. 2013). Other less popular coffee species grown are *C. liberica, stenophylla, mauritiana*, and *racemosa*. According to Assi (1977) there are at least 32 wild species of coffee grown in Africa, and among them the *C. congensis, eugenoides, zanguebarrie,* and *excelsa* are more prevalent (Assi 1977). The coffee fruit contains two seeds, called beans, which are separately enclosed in a thin membrane called spermoderm or testa. This spermoderm is known as silver skin when it becomes dry, or known as chaff when it is roasted. The spermoderm or testa is surrounded by a layer of mucilage immediately inside the fleshy part of the cherry. After harvesting, the seeds are classified and then separated from the pulp either by wet or dry processing (Clarke 1976).

Hot or cold coffee beverages are prepared from roasted coffee beans, which are the seeds of berries obtained from the *Coffea* plants (Keservani et al. 2010; Keservani et al. 2015a; Keservani et al. 2015b). Coffee is slightly acidic (~pH 5.1) in nature and taking a sip stimulates the central nervous system (CNS) of humans (Keservani and Sharma 2014). Darker roasted coffees are less acidic—both in their flavor profile and in any actual acid content. *C. robusta* has been characterized as a neutral coffee, weak-flavored, and occasionally exhibits a strong or pronounced bitterness (Charrier and Berthaund 1985; Illy and Viani 1995). *C. arabica* coffee is higher-priced, milder, fruitier, and acidulous (Bertrand et al. 2003). *C. arabica* coffee is considered to be superior to *C. robusta* due to its organoleptic properties experienced via the senses including taste, sight, smell, and touch, and therefore it is more expensive (Enyan et al. 2013). The quality of coffee depends strongly on species and geographic origin, with consequent wide variations in its commercial value. Arabica coffees produced in Central America are traditionally the most highly appreciated, whereas Brazilian Arabica coffee is considered to be of lower quality, due to the methods of harvesting (strip-picking) and processing practices used in that country (Mancha-Agresti, 2008). The importance of the coffee market and its globalization has increased concern about species and origin, and producers have responded by labeling products with information relating to origin and species. Therefore, it is very important to guarantee the authenticity of species and geographic origins of the coffee beans.

13.2 GLOBAL CONSUMPTION OF GREEN COFFEE

Coffee is internationally traded in two forms, one is instant and the other is known as roasted. Trade between the producing and consuming countries consists mostly of green coffee beans (unroasted or raw product packed in 60 kg bags) and bulk instant coffee (McClumpha 1988). Once traded, the green coffee beans (unroasted) are roasted to varying degrees, depending on the desired flavor, before brewed to serve a cup of coffee. Bulk instant coffee imported from the producing countries is usually blended and repackaged in the consuming countries. The roasted coffee trade takes place almost exclusively between the consuming countries. Green coffee beans and instant coffees can be stored for a long periods of time, while roasted coffee loses its freshness much more quickly and has a shorter shelf life.

Historically, Brazil, and Colombia are the leading coffee producers in the world. In the 1990s, the situation changed with a rapid growth of coffee production in Vietnam. The International Coffee Organization (ICO) categorizes exports by type of coffee such as Mild Arabica coffees, Brazilian Naturals, and Robustas. Mild Arabica coffees are further divided into Colombian Milds and Other Milds. Colombian Milds are comprised of coffees produced in Colombia, Kenya, and Tanzania. The large producers in the Other Milds category are Guatemala, Mexico, and India. Brazilian Naturals basically consist of Hard Arabicas from Brazil and Ethiopia. The last category includes Robusta coffees from all origins whereby Vietnam is by far the main producer, but Côte d'Ivoire (Ivory Coast), Indonesia, and Uganda are also major producers. In normal supply conditions, the market prices are highest for the Colombian Milds category, followed by Other Milds, Brazilian Naturals, and finally the wide spectrum of Robustas. The Scandinavian countries and Germany, who prefer Mild Arabica coffees in their blends, are the biggest coffee consuming countries (level of consumption per capita in the world) in Europe. In Southern Europe, Robusta coffee is the key component in espresso blends and darker roasts. Coffee consumers in the United States and United Kingdom prefer lighter roasts in general, but require a wide spectrum of qualities.

The international trading, consumption, economical, and political rivalry among coffee producing countries is very interesting. Over 90% of coffee production takes place in developing countries, while consumption happens mainly in industrialized economies, with the exception of Brazil which is both the top producer and also the top consumer of coffee in the world. Since World War II unroasted green coffee beans have become the second most valuable traded commodity exported by developing countries after crude oil. From 1970 to circa 2000 commodities traded in an order of value was crude oil in first place, coffee in second, followed by sugar, cotton, and others (Talbot 2004; Pendergrast 2009). Attempts to control the international coffee trade have been taking place since 1902, making coffee one of the first regulated commodities (Friis-Hansen 2000; Akiyama 2001; Ponte 2002a). A number of developing countries, even those with a low share of the global export market, rely on coffee for a high proportion of their export earnings. The governments of these producing countries have treated coffee as a strategic commodity; they have either directly controlled domestic marketing and quality control operations, or have strictly regulated them—at least until market liberalization took place during the 1980s and 1990s (Raikes et al. 2000).

13.3 GREEN COFFEE BEAN EXTRACT AND ITS COMPOSITION

The chemical composition of coffee is very complex which includes more than 2000 substances of different chemical and physical properties. All the components of coffee are not yet known. Some of those chemical constituents that have been identified possess physiological effects, in which caffeine is the most well-known alkaloid that produces significant beneficial effects. In this chapter, we have attempted to compile most or all of the composing chemicals and elements of both green and roasted coffee beans (*C. arabica* and *C. robusta*) (Tables 13.1 through 13.11). In Table 13.1, all the major components such as minerals, caffeine, trigonelline, lipids, total chorogenic acids (CGA), aliphatic acids, carbohydrates (oligosaccharides and total polysaccharides), amino acids, proteins, and humic acids are expressed in a percentage of the dry basis (Clifford 1975). The mono- and polysaccharides carbohydrate content of *C. arabica* and *C. robusta* coffee is shown in Table 13.2. We have comparatively

TABLE 13.1
Chemical Compositions of Green, Roasted (Arabica and Robusta), and Instant Coffee Beans

	Arabica (% dmb)		Robusta (% dmb)		
Components	**Green**	**Roasted**	**Green**	**Roasted**	**Instant**
Minerals	3.0–4.2	3.5–4.5	4.0–4.5	4.6–5.0	9.0–10.0
Caffeine	0.9–1.2	~1.0	1.6–2.4	~2.0	4.5–5.1
Trigonelline	1.0–1.2	0.5–1.0	0.6–0.75	0.3–0.6	—
Lipids	12.0–18.0	14.5–20.0	9.0–13.0	11.0–16.0	1.5–1.6
Total chlorogenic acids	5.5–8.0	1.2–2.3	9.0–10.0	3.9–4.6	5.2–7.4
Aliphatic acids	1.5–2.0	1.0–1.5	1.5–2.0	1.0–1.5	—
Oligosaccahrides	6.0–8.0	0–3.5	5.0–7.0	0–3.5	0.7–5.2
Total polysaccharides	50.0–55.0	24.0–39.0	37.0–47.0	—	~6.5
Amino acids	2.0	0	2.0	0	0
Proteins	11.0–13.0	13.0–15.0	11.0–13.0	13.0–15.0	16.0–21.0
Humic acids	—	16.0–17.0	—	16.0–17.0	15.0

Note: % dmb, percentage of dry matter basis.

TABLE 13.2
Carbohydrate Content in Green Coffee (% dmb)

Constituents	**Arabica**	**Robusta**
Monosaccharides	0.2–0.5	0.2–0.5
Sucrose	6.0–9.0	3.0–7.0
Polysaccharides	43.0–45.0	46.9–48.3
Arabinose	3.4–4.0	3.8–4.1
Mannose	21.3–22.5	21.7–22.4
Glucose	6.7–7.8	7.8–8.7
Galactose	10.4–11.9	12.4–14.0
Rhamnose	0.3	0.3
Xylose	0–0.2	0.2

TABLE 13.3
Fatty Acid Composition of Oil from Green Coffee Beans (Expressed as a % of Total Lipids)

Researchers	Calzorali et al., 1963	Kroplien et al., 1963	Hartmann et al., 1968	Chassevent et al., 1974
Myristic acid C14:0	Traces	Traces	0.06–0.14	0.2
Palmitic acid C16:0	35.20–38.60	30.7–35.3	35.44–41.35	35.2–36.7
Palmitoleic acid C16:1	Traces	Traces	—	—
Margaric acid C17:0	—	Traces	—	—
Stearic acid C18:0	6.60–8.35	6.6–9.0	7.53–10.60	7.2–9.7
Oleic acid C18:1	7.55–10.90	7.6–10.1	8.07–9.58	9.5–11.9
Linoleic acid C18:2	38.40–43.0	43.2–45.9	36.64–43.08	41.2–42.6
Linolenic acid C18:3	?	1.1–1.7	—	1.3–2.7
Arachidic C20:0	4.05–4.75	2.7–3.3	X	0.3–1.5
Gadoleic C20:1	—	?	X	—
Behemic a. C22:0	0.65–2.60	0.3–0.5	X	—

Note: X, C20:0 and higher = 4.28–6.43.

TABLE 13.4
Lipid Composition of Green Coffee

Lipidic Fractions	Percentage of Total Lipids	Components
Triglycerides	70–80	Esters of linoleic and palmitic acids
Free fatty acids (in % of oleic acid)	0.5–2.0	Esters of linoleic and palmitic acids Cafestol (furokaurane) and (in Arabica) kahweol
Esters of diterpenes	15–18.5	(furokaurene), atractyligenine
Triterpenes, sterols, ester of methylsterols	1.4–3.2	sitosterol, stigmasterol, campesterol
Free diterpenes	0.1–1.2	—
Free triterpenes and sterols	1.3–2.2	Squalene and nonacosane
Phospholipids	0.1	Amides of arachidic, behenic and lignoceric acids
Hydrocarbons	Traces	—
5-Hydroxytriptamides	0.3–1.0	Alpha, beta and gamma isomers
Tocopherols	0.3–0.7	—

analyzed the experimental data of four studies (Calzorali et al. 1963; Kroplien et al. 1963; Hartmann et al. 1968; and Chassevent et al. 1974) who have independently identified different types of fatty acids. The fatty acid composition (expressed in % of total lipids) shows that linoleic acid, palmitic acid, oleic acid, and stearic acid are the major components of lipids present in green coffee beans (Table 13.3). Triglycerides, esters of linoleic and palmitic acids, compose the major lipidic fraction at 70%–80%

TABLE 13.5
Free and Total Amino Acids in Green Coffee (% of Dry Basis)

Amino Acids	Free Amino Acids		Total Proteins
	Arabica	Robusta	
Alanine	0.05	0.09	0.5
Arginine	0.01	0.02	0.5
Aspartic acid	0.05	0.09	**1.0**
Asparagine	0.05	0.09	—
Cysteine	0.001	0.001	0.3
Glutamic acid	0.13	0.08	**1.9**
Glycine	0.01	0.02	0.6
Histidine	0.01	Traces	0.2
3-Methyl histidine	Traces	Traces	—
Isoleucine	0.01	0.02	0.4
Leucine	0.01	0.02	**1.0**
Gamma-aminobutyric acid	0.05	0.10	—
Lysine	0.01	Traces	0.6
Methionine	0.004	0.004	0.2
Phenylalanine	0.02	0.04	**0.7**
Proline	0.03	0.04	0.6
Serine	0.03	0.04	0.5
Threonine	Traces	0.01	0.3
Tyrosine	0.01	0.02	0.4
Valine	0.01	0.02	0.5
Tryptophan	0.01	0.05	0.1

of total lipids, while phospholipids and hydrocarbons are present in trace amounts in green coffee beans (Table 13.4). Aspartic acid, glutamic acid, leucine, and phenylalanine are abundantly present (% of dry basis) in total amino acids in green coffee (Table 13.5). It is found that the roasting of green coffee beans causes a percentage increase in most of the amino acids except arginine, cysteine, lysine, serine, and threonine. It is also found that medium roasting of *C. arabica* and *C. robusta* coffees causes a higher increase in the percentage amount of most amino acids than dark roasting (Table 13.6). Caffeine is the most abundant purine alkaloid present in green and roasted coffee, although it contains several other purine alkaloids such as theobromine, theophylline, paraxanthine, theacrine, liberine, and methylliberine. The caffeine content of *C. robusta* (15,000–26,000 mg/kg/db) is generally higher than *C. arabica* (9,000–14,000 mg/kg/db). Theacrine and methylliberine are present in trace amounts in *C. robusta* while almost absent in *C. arabica* (Table 13.7). Similarly, the caffeine content of different non alcoholic beverages varies from species to species. For instance, the caffeine content of coffee, tea, cola, and cocoa are 60–90, 30–40, 16, and 4 mg/150 mL, respectively (Table 13.8).

TABLE 13.6
Amino Acid Composition (as % Total Proteins) of Green and Roasted Coffees after Hydrolysis

	Arabica			Robusta		
Amino Acids	**Green Bean**	**High Roasting**	**Moderate Roasting**	**Green Bean**	**High Roasting**	**Moderate Roasting**
Alanine	4.91	5.97	5.48	4.87	6.84	7.85
Arginine	4.72	0.00	0.00	2.28	0.00	0.00
Aspartic acid	**10.50**	**9.07**	**9.02**	**9.44**	**8.94**	**8.19**
Cysteine	3.44	0.38	0.34	3.87	0.14	0.14
Glutamic acid	**18.86**	**20.86**	**23.29**	**17.88**	**24.01**	**29.34**
Glycine	5.99	6.86	7.08	6.26	7.68	8.87
Histidine	2.85	1.99	2.17	1.79	2.23	0.85
Isoleucine	4.42	4.75	4.91	4.11	5.03	5.46
Leucine	**8.74**	**9.95**	**11.19**	**9.04**	**9.65**	**14.12**
Lysine	6.19	2.54	2.74	5.36	2.23	2.56
Methionine	2.06	2.32	1.48	1.29	1.68	1.71
Phenylalanine	5.79	6.75	6.05	4.67	7.26	6.82
Proline	**6.58**	**6.52**	**6.96**	**6.46**	**9.35**	**10.22**
Serine	5.60	1.77	1.26	4.97	0.14	0.00
Threonine	3.73	2.43	1.83	3.48	2.37	1.02
Tyrosine	3.54	4.31	3.54	7.45	9.49	8.87
Valine	**5.50**	**6.86**	**3.31**	**6.95**	**10.47**	**9.49**

TABLE 13.7
Purine Alkaloids in Green Coffee

Components	**Arabica (mg/kg/db)**	**Robusta (mg/kg/db)**
Caffeine	9,000–14,000	15,000–26,000
Theobromine	36–40	26–82
Theophylline	7–23	86–344
Paraxanthine	3–4	8–9
Theacrine	0	11
Liberine	5	7–110
Methylliberine	0	3

Coffee is one of the richest sources of phenolics, in which the chlorogenic acids (CGAs) are the most abundant class of phenolic compounds constituting up to 12% of the dry matter of green coffee beans. The most abundant CGAs in coffee are 5-chlorogenic acid (5-CGA) and its isomers 3- and 4-CGA. Additionally, the isomers of dicaffeoylquinic acids (3,4-, 3,5-, and 4,5-diCQA), feruloylquinic acids (3-, 4-, and

TABLE 13.8
Caffeine Content of Several Nonalcoholic Beverages

Beverages	Caffeine (in mg/150 mL)	Parts Per Million (PPM)
Roasted ground coffee	90	600
Instant soluble coffee	63	420
Decaffeinated coffee	3	20
Tea (leaf or bags)	42	280
Instant soluble tea	32	213
Cola	16	107
Chocolate or cocoa	4	27
Milk chocolate	3	20

TABLE 13.9
Chlorogenic Acids of Arabica and Robusta Raw Coffees (% db)

Components	Arabica	Robust
5-Chlorogenic acid	3.0–5.6	4.4–6.5
4-Cchlorogenic acid	0.5–0.7	0.7–1.1
3-Chlorogenic acid	0.3–0.7	0.6–1.0
Total	3.8–7.0	5.7–8.6
3,4-Dicaffeoylquinic acid	0.1–0.2	0.5–0.7
3,5-Dicaffeoylquinic acid	0.2–0.6	0.4–0.8
4,5-Dicaffeoylquinic acid	0.2–0.4	0.6–1.0
Total	0.5–1.2	1.5–2.5
3-Feruloylquinic acid	Traces	0.1
4-Feruloylquinic acid	Traces	0.1
5-Feruloylquinic acid	0.3	1.0
5-Feruloyl, 4-caffeoylquinic acid	0	Traces
Total	0.3	1.2
3- p-Coumaroylquinic acids	Traces	0.1
4- p-Coumaroylquinic acids	Traces	0.1
5- p-Coumaroylquinic acids	0.2	0.8
Total	0.2	1.0

5-FQA), diferuloylquinic acids (dFQA), and p-coumaroylquinic acids (3-, 4-, and 5-p-CoQA) are found in green coffee beans (Table 13.9).

Green coffee beans are mainly composed of insoluble polysaccharides like cellulose and hemicelluloses. They also contain soluble carbohydrates, such as the monosaccharides fructose, glucose, galactose, and arabinose; the oligosaccharides such as sucrose, raffinose, and stachyose; and polymers of galactose, mannose, arabinose, and glucose. Soluble carbohydrates act by binding aroma, stabilizing foam, and sedimenting and increasing the viscosity of the extract. In addition, nonvolatile aliphatic

TABLE 13.10
Aliphatic Acids in Coffee (% db)

Components		Green Coffee	Roasted Coffee
Volatile	Formic acid	Traces	0.06–0.15
	Acetic acid	0.01	0.25–0.34
	Propanoic acid	Traces	Traces-0.03
	Butanoic acid	Traces	Traces-0.03
	Hexanoic acid	Traces	Traces-0.03
	Decanoic acid	Traces	Traces-0.03
	Lactic acid	Traces	0.02–0.03
	Fumaric acid	Traces	0.01–0.03
	Oxalic acid	0–0.2	–
	Isovaleric acid	Traces	Traces-0.02
Nonvolatile	Citric acid	0.7–1.4	0.3–1.1
	Malic acid	0.3–0.7	0.1–0.4
	Quinic and quinidinic acid	0.3–0.5	0.6–1.2

TABLE 13.11
Typical Mineral Content of Green Coffee Beans (Values Expressed per 100 g Air-Dried Beans)

Major Components	Milligrams (mg)	Minor Components	Microgram (μg)
Sodium (Na)	2.3–17	Chromium (Cr)	74–1327
Potassium (K)	1350–1712	Vanadium (V)	70–110
Calcium (Ca)	76–120	Barium (Ba)	100–615
Magnesium (Mg)	142–176	Nickel (Ni)	11–388
Iron (Fe)	2.1–10.5	Cobalt (Co)	10–93
Manganese (Mn)	1.1–9.8	Lead (Pb)	18–27
Rubidium (Rb)	0.6–4.2	Molybdenum (Mo)	11–27
Zinc (Zn)	0.5–3.2	Titanium (Ti)	4–20
Copper (Cu)	0.5–2.3	Cadmium (Cd)	3
Strontium (Sr)	0.4–1.3		

acids such as citric acid, malic acid, and quinic acids, and volatile acids such as formic, acetic, propanoic, butanoic, isovaleric, hexanoic, and decanoic acids are also present (Table 13.10).

But the roasting of coffee causes differences in some ingredients including carbohydrates, melanoidins, lipids, proteins, minerals, CGA, aliphatic acids, and caffeine. Oils and waxes are also important constituents, accounting for 8%–18% of the dry mass, together with proteins and free amino acids at 9%–12% w/w, and minerals at 3–5% w/w (Clifford 1975; Quijano-Rico and Spettel 1975; Clifford 1985a) (Table 13.11).

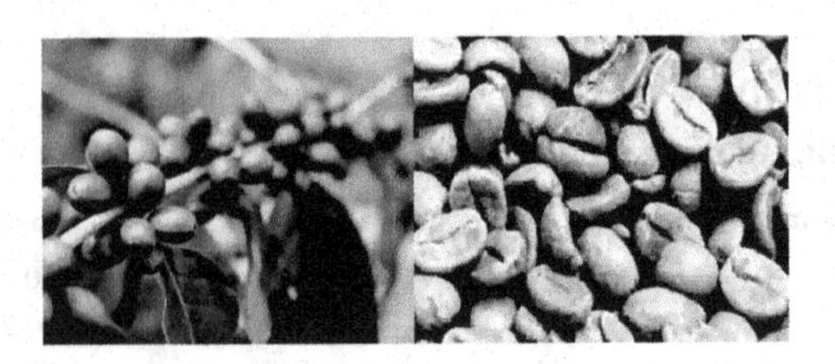

FIGURE 13.1 Green coffee bean.

Coffee is the major source of chlorogenic acids (CGA) in the human diet, with daily intake in coffee drinkers being 0.5–1 g, whereas coffee abstainers typically ingest <100 mg/day (Figure 13.1). Coffee is a good source of potassium, magnesium, and fluoride. A variety of analytical techniques with various degrees of sensitivity and specificity, such as (1) gas chromatography (GC), (2) high-performance liquid chromatography (HPLC), (3) isotope ratio mass spectrometry (IRMS), (4) visible micro-Raman spectroscopy, (5) ultraviolet–visible absorption spectroscopy (UV–VIS), (6) elemental analysis-like inductively coupled plasma–atomic emission spectrometry (ICP-AES), and (7) liquid chromatography–mass spectrometry (LC-MS) have been conducted during the past decade to find chemical components that can be used to differentiate coffee species and origins. However, all of these techniques are compound targeted; they can each assess differences in only one component or one class of components.

13.3.1 Carbohydrate Content of Green Coffee Beans

About 50%–60% of green coffee consists of carbohydrates, some of them are water-soluble and some are water-insoluble fractions (Goldoni 1979). These carbohydrates can be subdivided into low-molecular-mass carbohydrates, reserve polysaccharides, and structural polysaccharides, some of which are intimately associated with non-carbohydrate material such as lignin or proteins (Taylor 1975). The monosaccharide content of *C. arabica* and *C. robusta* is very low and almost equal at 0.2%–0.5% dmb, while the polysaccharide content of *C. arabica* at 43.0%–45.0% dmb and *C. robusta* at 46.9%–48.3% dmb is comparatively high. Mannose and galactose are the most abundant polysaccahrides present in green coffee beans. The acid hydrolysis of green coffee beans, during which the mono- and oligosaccharides are removed, yields the constituent sugars of the polysaccharide including galactose, glucose, mannose, arabinose, xylose, rhamnose, and at least one uronic acid. Most structural polysaccharides, like cellulose, hemicellulose, and pectins are either poorly or totally insoluble in water. The presence of cellulose in coffee beans was unequivocally demonstrated by Wolfrom et al. (1964) and Robinson (1980) at a level of approximately 5% dbm. The pectin levels were extracted in a range of 1%–4% dbm from the coffee beans using hot water, dilute acid (for primary cell wall pectins), and ammonium oxalate (for middle lamella pectins) (Plunkett 1956; Thaler and Arneth 1967). Extraction into alkali has yielded several hemicelluloses of variable composition but mannose is always present at a significant level. Thaler and Arneth (1967) indicated that during roasting the cellulose remained stable, the mannan was slightly affected, the galactan was partially destroyed, and the araban was greatly reduced in proportion to the severity of roast. The polysaccharide-containing fractions form 9.0% to 12.0% of roasted *C. arabica* and 10.0%–15.0% of similarly roasted *C. robusta* beans, and galactose, mannose, and arabinose could be released by hydrolysis.

Green coffee beans contain 3%–9% low-molecular-mass carbohydrates especially sucrose. There was more sucrose detected in *C. arabica* than in *C. robusta.* Small quantities of free glucose (0.5%–1.0%) are also present. Clifford (1975) indicated that raffinose (1-alpha-6-galactosylsucrose) and stachyose (1-alpha -6-galactosylraffinose) are also present, with these being higher in *C. robusta* than in *C. arabica*. Roasting caused a progressive and ultimately severe loss of these carbohydrates. Sometimes only small quantities of sucrose, glucose, and fructose remained in trace amounts, and the majority part is lost during roasting. Traces of arabinose, galactose, and in one case maltose, suggested that polysaccharides are degraded at high temperature degrees of roasting (Calzolari and Lokar 1967; Nakabayashi 1977). It is generally accepted that sugar degradation, with or without reaction with other components, yields many of the flavor producing substances of roasted coffee (Feldman et al. 1969; Amorim et al. 1974). However, Amorim et al. (1974) concluded that the differences in beverage quality could not be explained solely by differences in the sugar content in the green beans. Humic acids refers to the water-soluble high molecular mass fraction of roasted coffee beans from which sugars, and/or amino acids, and/or phenols can be released by hydrolysis. Clifford (1972) indicated that after water-soluble humic acids were purified by dialysis, yields of 12%–15% for these compounds in a mass range of 5,000–50,000 were observed.

13.3.2 Lipid Content of Green Coffee Beans

Most of the information about coffee bean lipids is based on the *C. arabica* species (Arabica), due to its commercial importance and popularity. For the same reason, considerable information is also available for *C. canephora*, the second most world widely cultivated coffee species. On this basis the lipid levels *Coffea sp.* may be divided into three groups: *C. arabica* contain 12%–18%, *C. canephora* 9%–13% and *C. liberica* 11%–12% (Carisano and Gariboldi 1964). In general, *C. arabica* beans have higher lipid content than *C. canephora*. However, depending on the origin and variety, large variations can be observed (Pinto and Carvalho 1961; Kroplien 1963; Tango and Carvalho 1963; Clifford 1985; Orsl and Dicházi 1989).

There are two reports which present the results of analysis carried out on coffee beans other than *C. arabica* and *C. canephora* (Wilbaux 1956; Chassevent et al. 1973). Chassevent et al. (1973) studied six species belonging to the *Mascarocoffea* of the *Coffea* genus, in which the main characteristic is to have little or no caffeine in the seeds and a narrow geographic distribution (Clifford et al. 1991). On average they have higher lipid content than *C. arabica* and *C. canephora*. Wilbaux (1956) investigated seeds from *C. eugenioides, dewevrei, congensis,* and *abeokutae.*

The major components of coffee oil are neutral triglycerides, in which the most abundant fatty acids are palmitic, stearic, oleic, and linoleic. The oil contains an unusually high level of unsaponifiable content which consists of sterols, sterol esters, diterpenes, wax, pigments, vitamins, and hydrocarbons (Folstar et al. 1975; Tiscornia

1979). They are present both in free-state and as mono-esters of long-chain aliphatic acids (Alcaide et al. 1971). Kulaba (1981) reported a possible connection between the content of kahweol and beverage quality (Kulaba 1981). He concluded that low kahweol and high oil content was associated with high beverage quality, that high kahweol and medium oil content was associated with medium quality, and that low kahweo and low oil content was associated with low quality.

Lipids are important components of coffee beverage and aroma, although the majority are lost when the grounds undergo the preparation process (Folstar 1985). Lipids are expelled to the bean surface during roasting, forming a layer which may trap volatile aromas and impairing the immediate loss of these compounds (Clifford 1985; Arnaud 1988). Coffee oil is also obtained from roasted coffee, from the spent grounds of roasted and ground coffee after brewing, or from the instant coffee industry. The most important commercial use for this oil is the aromatization of soluble coffee (Clarke 1985).

13.3.3 The Wax Content of Green Coffee

There is little research available on the wax content of green coffee, that are derivatives of serotonin, and have been blamed for digestive disorders (Van der Stegen 1979). The waxes are N-beta-alkanoyl-5-hydroxytryptamines (C-5-HT) containing primarily arachidic, behenic, and lignoceric acids (Folstar et al. 1975; Van der Stegen and Noomen, 1977).

13.3.4 Mineral Content of Coffee Beans

The mineral composition of different green coffees varies due to the different processing conditions that are used commercially in the extraction of roasted coffees. Generally, it is considered that the higher the yield of soluble material extracted from roasted coffee the lower the mineral or potassium content. It is believed that most of the minerals are chemically associated with the main constituents of coffee beans; part of the potassium is present in the salt of chlorogenic acids, and a further part is present in the salt of a loose caffeine-chlorogenic acid complex (Smith and Tola 1998). A magnesium-chlorogenic acid complex is reported to be responsible for the color of good quality green coffee beans (Northmore 1965, 1967). The magnesium content was the quality-limiting factor.

13.3.5 Amino Acids and Protein Content of Coffee Beans

Arabica coffee contains 2% of free amino acids (Walter 1970). Campos and Rodrigues (1971) used chromatographic and electrophoretic methods, and their findings indicated that most of the amino acids commonly found in plant tissues were also present in green coffee. However, traces of three unidentified amino acids were also detected. The study observed that there was varietal differences in the amino acid content. These differences were mainly in the arginine, beta-alanine, and pipecolic acid of *C. arabica* or *C. robusta*. Table 13.5 and 13.6, taken from Poisson (1977), summarizes the data from Wallter (1970) and Barbirolli (1965).

Amino acids are destroyed by heat, however, they were detected in roasted coffee and coffee brew in small quantities (Pereira and Pereira 1971). Also an uncharacterized peptide was reported to be of importance in roasted coffee aroma production (Russwurm 1970).

The crude protein content of coffee, estimated as Nx6.25, was reported to be 11—15.8 g per 100 g (Babirolli 1965; Streuli 1975) . However, the water-soluble protein, amounting to 3% of the bean, has a nitrogen content of 15% (Underwood and Deatherage 1952). They also reported that the water-soluble proteins of Santos and Colombia coffees had an iso-electric point of pH 4.6–4.7, indicating that there was a low content of basic amino acids. Amorim and Josephson (1975) studied the water-soluble nitrogen component of green coffee of Brazilian origin (Rio and Soft) using different methods of gel filtration and dialysis with membranes of different molecular mass cut-offs, and found that there was no significant differences in the protein content of Rio or Soft (good quality) coffees. They observed that there were numerous isoelectric proteins in the pH range of 5.7–6.3, and a few in the range of 4.4–4.7pH using non-urea gel contrary to previous reports. They were able to show that green coffee contains protein-chlorogenic acid complexes similar to those detected in sunflower seeds (Sabir et al. 1974). Poisson (1977), reviewing the work on the composition of proteins in coffee, observed that when proteins are degraded during roasting, a number of substances are produced concurrently with the formation of coffee aroma and color. The degradation of proteins causes loss of protein and the more severe the roast the lower the protein content. It was reported that when Santos coffee was roasted to six different degrees of roast, that is, 10, 12, 14, 16, 18, and 20 based on percentage loss in weight,there was a 6% loss in protein weight at the lowest level and a 14% loss in protein weight at the highest level (Fobe et al. 1967). When extracts of protein from green and roasted coffee beans were hydrolyzed they yielded 18 amino acids (Underwood and Deatherage 1952; Thaler and Gaigl 1963). Supporting this evidence, Centi-Grossi et al. (1969) showed that there was no difference between *C. arabica* and *C. robusta* (Centi-Grossi et al. 1969). Their amino acid analysis showed that individual protein-bound amino acids have a different roasting sensitivity. Glutamic acid, leucine, valine, phenylalanine, and proline increased on roasting (Roffi et al. 1971), whereas cystine, cysteine, methionine, lysine, serine, and threonine were destroyed (Thaler 1963). Clifford (1975) also commented that those amino acids that are destroyed during roasting do not have simple aliphatic side chains, whereas those that increase, with the exception of glutamic acid, have an aliphatic side chain.

13.3.6 Phenolic Acids and Chlorogenic Acids

Quinyl esters of hydroxycinnamic acids are generally known as chlorogenic acids (CGA) in green coffee beans and were first discovered by Robiquet and Boutron in 1837 (Sondheimer 1964). Chlorogenic acids are almost universal in all plants, and 5-CQA is usually the major component. Few tissues are as rich as coffee seeds, where the CQA level may exceed 10% dry matter basis (dmb). In some fruits, 4-p-coumaroylquinic acid seems predominant, whereas artichoke contains several isomers, 1,3-dicaffeoylquinic acid, (1,3-DiCQA), and 1,5-dicaffeoylquinic acid

(1,5-DiCQA) (Nichiforesco 1970), that are not found in coffee. Pineapple contains 1,4 -DCoQA (Sutherland and Gortner 1959).

CGA is present in many *Coffea* species (Clifford 1985a,b; Clifford et al. 1989; Rakotomalala et al. 1993; Anthony et al. 1993). In the two main cultivated species, *C. canephora* and *C. arabica,* CGA account for 7%–10% and 5%–8% of dry matter basis (dmb), respectively (Clifford, 1985b; Rakotomalala 1992). The three main groups of CGA are caffeoylquinic acids (CQAs), feruloylquinic acids (FQAs), and dicaffeoylquinic acids (diCQAs) (Clifford et al. 1977). The caffeoylquinic acids are the most abundently occurring (Arabicas 5.5%–7%, Robustas 8%), followed by DCQA (Arabicas 0.6%, Robustas 1.8%), and feruloylquinic acids (Arabicas 0.3%, Robustas 0.6%–1.2%). Each group contains three isomers based on the number and identity of the acylating residues (Clifford, 1985a,b). Roasting causes the progressive loss of the mono- and dicaffeoylquinic acids, but it appears that the FQA are more heat stable and become the largest occurring CGA in dark roasted coffee beans (Clifford 1972; Rees and Theaker 1977; Van der Stegen and Van Duijn 1980).

Phenolic compounds are antioxidants and can help reduce the risk of cardiovascular disease (Rice-Evans et al. 1996; Olthof et al. 2001). The most prevalent phenolic compounds in food are the hydroxycinnamic acids (Herrmann 1976; Kuhnau 1976), and the major component of this class is caffeic acid, which occurs in food mainly as esters called chlorogenic acid (CGA). The experimental procedure to estimate CGA content includes three steps: (1) extraction, (2) purification, and (3) separation and quantification of the different isomers by HPLC. The extraction, separation, and quantification of the different isomers are defined in terms of their optimal chemical reagents or solvents (Colonna 1979; Clifford et al. 1985; Trugo 1984; Van Der Stegen et al. 1980). A fourth purification procedure is also mentioned in these studies, and a fifth variation is the standard technique used in Germany.

13.4 EFFECT OF ROASTING ON THE ANTIOXIDANT ACTIVITY OF COFFEE BREWS

Since green coffee has a mild, green, bean-like aroma, the desirable aroma associated with coffee beverages develops during roasting. The quality of the coffee beverage depends on the selection of the raw beans and the roasting process—particularly the roasting time. During roasting, the coffee beans are heated to 200°C–250°C, and the roasting time can range from 0.75 to 25 min, the optimum time being 1.5–6 min, depending on the degree of roasting required (light, medium, or dark) (Belitz and Grosch 1987; Parliament 2000). Many complex physical and chemical changes take place during roasting, including the obvious change in color from green to brown.

Roasting of the coffee beans at different celsius temperatures affects the composition of coffee, which can be profiled using capillary electrophoresis (CE) (Parliament 2000; Ames et al. 2000). Although compounds with antioxidant properties (mainly CGA) are lost during the roasting of coffee beans (Parliment 2000), the overall antioxidant properties of the coffee brew can be maintained, or even enhanced, by the development of compounds possessing antioxidant activity including Maillard reaction products (Nicoli et al. 1997a; Nicoli et al. 1997b; Daglia et al. 2000). Maillard reaction products formed in both foods and model systems on heating are reported to possess various types of antioxidant activity and even pro-oxidant properties (Nicoli et al., 1999). The major compositional changes that occur due to roasting are decreases in protein, amino acids, arabinogalactan, reducing sugars, trigonelline, chlorogenic acid, sucrose, and water, and the formation of melanoidins (Parliment, 2000). Many of these changes are due to the Maillard reaction.

The antioxidant activity of fractions of the ethyl acetate in an extract of a dark-roasted coffee brew has been reported, but the effect of roasting on the antioxidant properties of the fractions has yet to be investigated. No links between levels of particular classes of compounds in coffee and antioxidant activity have been made. Therefore, the aim of this chapter is examine the different compositional extracts from coffee beans and their cumulative role on the Nrf2/ARE pathway, and the contribution of their components to the overall antioxidant activity of coffee.

13.5 COFFEE AND Nrf2/ARE PATHWAY

Many diseases such as cardiovascular, neurodegenerative, aging, diabetes, obesity, and some types of cancer are caused by poor nutrition and lifestyle behaviors. One of the most vital mechanisms to guard against such diseases is the protection of cells against reactive oxygen species (ROS)–induced damage. To protect from ROS–induced damage, cells possess different intracellular defense mechanisms. One way to shield cells and tissues from ROS, carcinogens, and carcinogenic metabolites is the activation of Phase II detoxifying and antioxidative enzymes. The most common Phase II detoxifying enzymes are glutathione S-transferase (GST), NAD (P) H: quinone oxidoreductase 1 (NQO1), γ-glutamylcysteine ligase (γGCL), and heme oxygenasel (HO1); and the antioxidative enzymes such as superoxide dismutase (SOD), catalase (CAT), and glutathione peroxidase (GPx) (Talalay et al. 1995; Kensler 1997; Wilkinson and Clapper 1997; Ishii et al. 2000; Talalay 2000; Zhang and Gordon 2004). These Phase II enzymes play a critical role in converting reactive electrophiles or xenobiotics into less toxic products. A deficiency in Phase II enzyme activity is associated with an increased risk in developing these diseases.

The expressions of many Phase II genes is regulated by the activation of the nuclear factor-Erythroid-2 p45 subunit (NE-E2)-related factor 2 (Nrf2)/ARE pathway. The expression of these Phase II genes are regulated by the activation of antioxidant response element (ARE) or electrophile response element (EpRE), and are found in the 5'- flanking region of the respective gene promoter of many of these Phase II genes (Favreau and Pickett 1991; Rushmore et al. 1991; Alam et al. 2000). ARE, a *cis*-active element which is activated via binding of the transcription factor Nrf2, is a member of the cap-and-collar family of the basic region in leucine zipper proteins. Increased nuclear levels of Nrf2 provoke gene transcription of Phase II detoxifying enzymes. In quiescent cells, Nrf2 is sequestered or retained in the cytoplasm associated with actin-anchored protein Keapl, an E3 ubiquitin ligase substrate adaptor.

Oxidative stress or electrophilic stimuli in cytoplasm causes dissociation of Nrf2 from Keapl, allowing Nrf2 to translocate to the nucleus, heterodimerize with Maf, and bind to ARE, eventually resulting in transcriptional regulation of target genes. Here, ROS or electrophilic stimuli cause oxidation of cysteine thiol groups located in the intervening region of Keap1, leading to the formation of disulfide bonds (between C273 and C288). This results in a conformational change that renders Keap1 unable to bind to Nrf2, thereby inducing translocation of Nrf2 to the nucleus. After translocation to the nucleus, Nrf2 may dimerize with small Maf proteins (MafG, MafK), large Maf proteins (c-Maf), or other basic leucine-zipper (bZIP) proteins (such as c-Fos, Fra1, p45-NF-E2, ECH, Bach1, and Bach2). The resultant Nrf2-Maf2 heterodimer binds to the ARE and recruits the general transcriptional machinery for up-regulation of ARE-driven genes, including GSTA2, NQO1, GCL, HO-1, UGT, and so on.

Coffee extracts like chlorogenic acid, kahweol, and N-methylpyridinium have the ability to modulate Nrf2-dependent transcription, controlling production of proteins involved in detoxification, antioxidant defence, protein degradation, and inflammation. Kahweol induces Nrf2-dependent transcription, probably through the PI3K and p38 signaling, and through increased nuclear translocation of Nrf2. Chlorogenic acid increases nuclear translocation of Nrf2 probably through PI3K, while N-methylpyridinium increases nuclear translocation of Nrf2, and also leads to an increase in the transcription of Nrf2.

Upon activation by ROS or electrophilic stimuli or upstream protein kinases, induce the translocation of Nrf2 into the nucleus, its binding to ARE/EpRE, and the onset of the transcription of Phase II enzymes such as glutathione S-transferases (GST), UDP-glucuronyltransferases (UGT), γ-glutamate cysteine ligases (γGCL), NAD(P)H-quinone oxidoreductase 1 (NQO1), or heme oxygenase 1 (HO1).

The diterpenes, cafestol and kahweol, have been found to interact with the Nrf2/ARE-pathway, increasing the nuclear Nrf2 protein level and modulating ARE-mediated gene expression (Venugopal and Jaiswal 1996; Yu et al. 1999; Balogun et al. 2003; Zhang and Hannink 2003; Chen et al. 2004; Huber et al. 2004; Jemal et al. 2005; Higgins et al. 2008; Itoh 1999).

Coffee and some of its some components have strong antioxidant capabilities that activate the Nrf2/ARE pathway and expression of important Phase II enzymes. This strong antioxidant capability of coffee is often attributed to its rich phytoconstituents including caffeine, chlorogenic acid, caffeic acid, and hydroxyhydroquinone (HHQ). The *in vitro* study of Boettler et al. (2011a) using human colon carcinoma cells (HT29) identified pyridinium derivatives like N-methylpyridinium ion (NMP) as even more potent activators of the Nrf2 nuclear translocation than the known Nrf2 activator chlorogenic acid (CGA) (Boettler et al. 2011a). Furthermore, N-methylpyridinium (NMP), a degradation product formed from trigonelline during roasting of coffee beans, was found to increase Phase II enzyme activities in rats (Somoza et al. 2003). Recently, Nadine et al. (2012) have identified NMP, as well as chlorogenic acid (CGA) a major polyphenol in raw coffee beans, as potent activators of the Nrf2/ARE pathway, activating nuclear Nrf2-translocation as well as gene expression of different Phase II enzymes in the colon carcinoma cell line HT29 (Boettler et al. 2011). Furthermore, caffeine and its metabolites help in proper cognitive functionality. Coffee lipid fraction containing cafestol and kahweol act as safeguards against some malignant cells by modulating the detoxifying enzymes.

In a subsequent human intervention study we observed an increase of transcripts of Phase II genes in peripheral blood lymphocytes (PBL) after 4-weeks of daily consumption of either a coffee rich in CGA or one rich in NMP (Boettler et al. 2011). Both CGA-rich coffee and NMP-rich coffee have the capability to activate the Nrf2/ARE pathway. The question arises whether it is the increased amount of green coffee bean constituents or the typical heavy roasting of green coffee beans that enhances the Nrf2/ARE-activating properties of a coffee beverage *in vitro* and *in vivo*. To this end, an Arabica-based coffee blend was produced with a considerable content in chlorogenic acids (580.1 mg/L) combined with an increased NMP concentration (71.4 mg/L) (Bakuradze et al. 2011). The coffee extract (CE) of this hybrid CGA/NMP-rich (CN) coffee contains amounts of NMP comparable to those recently reported in the NMP-rich coffee, but with a significantly higher concentration of CGA (Table 13.1). Because the degradation of CGA and formation of NMP showed an inverted progression in relation to the roasting time/temperature during the process of roasting, a mixture of two different coffees was necessary to maintain the desired characteristics in the resulting CN coffee brew (Bakuradze et al. 2011). This hybrid coffee was used to test the hypothesis whether a combination of raw coffee bean constituents with heavy roast characteristics enhances the Nrf2/ARE-activating potency of coffee. The study was performed in a two-step approach: (1) with respect to the underlying mechanism, Nrf2/ARE-activating properties of a respective coffee extract CN-CE were examined in HT29 colon carcinoma cells, a cell culture model that is well characterized in terms of cell signaling and known to be sensitive to the activation of Nrf2/ARE-dependent gene expression; (2) the relevance of these findings were observed *in vivo* in a human pilot intervention study, investigating the effect of 4-weeks of daily consumption of the hybrid coffee on the transcription of Nrf2-dependent genes in human peripheral blood lymphocytes (PBLs) of the participants.

Interpretation of experimental results are determined by performing the comparative experimental studies on animal models (rats, rabbits, monkies, etc.). The effects of any composition of the coffee are determined on the basis of the amount of doses used, the duration of coffee administration, and the metabolic characteristics of each animal species. The metabolism of coffee is complex. Its physiological effect can be explained in part by three mechanisms: antagonism of adenosine receptors, inhibition of phosphodiesterases, and mobilization of intracellular calcium. The only neurological effects that have been clearly demonstrated are increase in alertness and the delay in the onset of sleep. The caffeine contained in coffee elicits a constriction of cerebral blood vessels. For this reason, it is present in many pharmaceutical products used to treat migraine headaches. Caffeine also potentiates the analgesic effect of some medications. In healthy individuals, consumption of coffee in moderate amounts does not modify cardiovascular functions, or systolic, and diastolic blood pressure. The gastric or intestinal intolerances that are sometimes attributed to coffee are linked to individual sensitivities and could not be reproduced in experimental studies. Coffee exerts a cholecystokinetic (promoting emptying of the gallbladder) action and increases external secretion of the pancreas. Coffee consumption does not cause diseases of the respiratory apparatus. Endocrine functions are not modified by consumption of coffee. Consumption of coffee does not have any important effect on muscle function. There is no evidence that coffee consumption is a risk factor for bone fractures.

Coffee consumption increases energy metabolism in the hours following its ingestion but does not modify the total energy expenditure. Coffee consumption has no harmful effects on reproduction or fertility. Coffee in the usual amounts of human consumption does not have any teratogenic action (any agent that can disturb the development of an embryo or fetus. Teratogens may cause a birth defect in the child or a teratogen may halt the pregnancy outright). In the habitual amounts of human consumption, coffee does not have any genotoxic (a toxic agent that damages DNA molecules in genes, causing mutations, tumors, etc.), mutagenic, or carcinogenic potential.

Recently, we demonstrated that coffees are rich in either the raw bean constituents, with CGA as a lead compound, or the typical roasting products such as NMP enhanced Nrf2/-ARE-dependent gene transcription both *in vitro* and *in vivo*. On the basis of these findings, an Arabica coffee blend, rich in both CGA and NMP, was produced to determine the Nrf2-activating properties of a coffee beverage combining both characteristics. *In vitro* this hybrid coffee extract CN-CE clearly showed enhanced potency to increase nuclear Nrf2 translocation, indicating effective activation of Nrf2 signaling. The amounts of NMP in CN-CE (71.7 mg/L) and in the NMP-rich coffee extract NMP-CE (73.3 mg/L) were comparable and also in the range where the isolated constituent possesses strong Nrf2 activating properties. Thus NMP, a known activator of Nrf2 translocation, might contribute to the effects of both coffee extracts.

Furthermore, we addressed the question of whether the translocation of Nrf2 into the nucleus is reflected downstream by the induction of Nrf2/ARE-dependent gene expression. The *in vitro* data indicate that the presence of green coffee bean constituents suppresses the onset of HO1 transcription, whereas a high amount of dark roasted coffee compounds seems to be crucial for HO1 expression. The induction of NQO1 gene transcription by CN-CE appeared in the same concentration range where maximal Nrf2 nuclear translocation was observed, indicative for downstream transfer of Nrf2 signals. A report showed a significant decrease of NQO1 mRNA expression in Nrf 2(–/–) mice in comparison to wild type mice indicating the regulation of NQO1 gene transcription by Nrf2. Furthermore, Nrf 2(–/–) mice showed a weak response in terms of NQO1 induction after tertiary butylhydroquinone (tBHQ) treatment in the liver and intestine than in the respective wild type. In previous studies we demonstrated increased NQO1 transcript levels in HT29 cells after 24 h of incubation with 10 μM NMP.17 CN-CE concentrations inducing a significant NQO1 gene transcript induction (100 μg/mL CNCE) comprising of 5 μM NMP, thus within the effective range of this compound. However, the NMP-rich coffee extract itself failed to induce the NQO1 gene transcription after 24 h, indicating that green coffee constituents contribute substantially to the effects of CN-CE on NQO1 transcription. Yet, coffee high in only green coffee bean constituents such as CGA-CE displayed weak action in inducing the NQO1 gene transcription, supporting the hypothesis that a hybrid of both green and dark roast coffee constituents enhances the Nrf2/ARE-activating potential. Modulation of NQO1 has already been reported in other coffee constituents. Feng et al. (2005) determined an increased NQO1 activity in JB6 mouse epithelial cells after 18 h of treatment with 40 and 80 μM chlorogenic acid. Furthermore, the coffee-specific

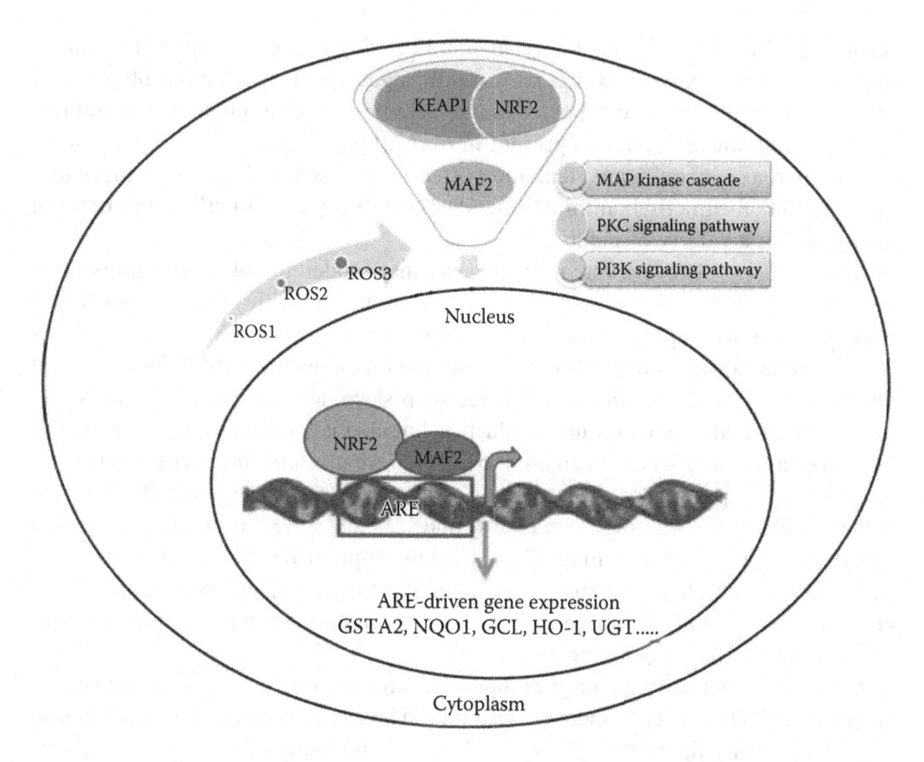

FIGURE 13.2 (See color insert.) ARE-driven gene expression by NRF2. ARE activation signals disassociate the NRF2-KEAP1 complex allowing NRF2 to translocate into the nucleus, where it binds to the ARE and transcriptionally activates downstream target genes. (PI3K = phosphatidylinositol 3-kinase, MAPK = mitogen-activated protein kinase, PKC = protein kinase C isoenzymes, ARE = antioxidant response element, NRF2 = NF-E2-related factor 2, KEAP1 = Kelch-like-ECH-associated protein 1, NQO1 = NAD(P)H:quinone oxidoreductase, GSTA2 = glutathione S-transferases 2, ROS = reactive oxygen species.)

diterpenes cafestol and kahweol have been reported to increase NQO1 mRNA, suggesting that coffee constituents other than NMP contribute to the observed effects. The ARE-driven gene expression by NRF_2 are presented in Figure 13.2.

13.6 THE IMPACT OF GREEN COFFEE ON HEALTH (IS COFFEE HARMFUL?)

There is a big question regarding the effect of coffee on human health. Perhaps the peak of the anti-coffee hysteria occurred during the nineteenth century, with coffee being blamed for every imaginable illness and disorder. It has been the subject of intensive research in the last few decades. However, the results of many studies have varied in terms of coffee's relative benefit (Kummer 2003). The current research is mixed. In general, coffee is known for its most famous component caffeine (1, 3, 7-trimethylxanthine), a bitter alkaloid stimulates the central nervous system (CNS), cardiovascular system (CVS), and perhaps mobilizes energy resources. Caffeine is a secondary metabolite which helps in the coffee plant's defense system, and it also acts as an antifungal agent, a selective phytotoxin, and a limited insectival chemosterilant. Caffeine is the psychoactive ingredient in coffee, tea, and cola, and is present in over 60 plant species of which the most well-known are cocoa-beans, tea, and coffee. The closely related substances theophylline (1, 3-dimethylxanthine) and theobromine (3, 7-dimethylxanthine) are also found in a variety of plants.

The majority of recent research suggests that moderate coffee consumption is benign or mildly beneficial in healthy adults. Caffeine is highly soluble in water, and is one of the first components to dissolve into the brewing coffee. Many of the effects of caffeine are obvious depending upon the quantity consumed including increased alertness, anxiety, irritability, interference with sleep, and jitteriness. It works as a mild diuretic. Caffeine can cause headaches, but also it can act as a vasoconstrictor, and in certain instances can been used to help relieve migraine headaches. Yet again, regular consumers of caffeine-containing products can suffer withdrawal symptoms if they suddenly stop taking them (Barry and Kenneth 1998). In this regard, coffee can be said to be habit-forming. Caffeine consumption has been linked to short-term increases in blood pressure, heart rate, and to occasional irregular heartbeat. However, studies linking coffee and caffeine to osteoporosis have been a matter of debate in the scientific community.

Caffeine is not coffee's only component; another component is diterpenes—cafestol and kahweol. They increase serum lipid levels, causing a rise in total cholesterol, low-density-lipoprotein (LDL) cholesterol, and triglycerides. Therefore, they may increase the risk of heart disease and affect liver function (RobUrgert et al. 1997; Cornelis and El-Sohemy 2007). The diterpenes cafestol and kahweol have been found to interact with the Nrf2/ARE-pathway, increasing the nuclear Nrf2 protein level, and modulating ARE-mediated gene expression. It has been found that coffee drinkers may have a lower risk for developing type 2 Diabetes, gallstones, colon cancer, and have a lower risk of liver damage. A study conducted on Dutch coffee drinkers (consuming seven or more cups a day) found that there are chances of halving the risk of developing type 2 Diabetes, but could not conclusively state that it was definitely coffee that lowered the risk or whether other factors are involved (Salazar-Martinez et al. 2004).

In this chapter, two studies linking coffee and cancer is reviewed. The first found a decreased risk of liver cancer (specifically, hepatocellular carcinoma, or HCC) resulting from daily consumption of coffee. According to the study, conducted by Manami Inoue at the National Cancer Center in Tokyo, the HCC rate among people who never drank coffee was 547.2 cases per 100,000 people over 10 years, and 214.6 cases per 100,000 people for daily coffee drinkers. Further, the risk decreased with the amount of coffee consumed. The second study, conducted by Karin B. Michels (2005), at Brigham and Women's Hospital in Boston, examined data from the Nurses' Health Study on women and the Health Professionals' Follow-up Study on men. The data indicated there was no association between consumption of caffeinated coffee and the incidence of colon or rectal cancer. Interestingly, the study found that those who regularly drank two or more cups per day of decaffeinated coffee had almost half the incidence of rectal cancer, 12 per 100,000 person-years (person-years refers to the number of people studied multiplied by the total observation time), compared to those who never drank decaffeinated coffee (19 per 100,000).

Green coffee beans (GCB) and GCB extracts are inexpensive natural ingredients with great potential to induce weight loss, as they contain high concentrations of caffeine and chlorogenic acids. Caffeine has been shown to promote lipolysis in both animals and humans. A small, short-term clinical trial conducted by Thom (2007) compared weight loss and body fat reduction in 30 subjects randomly assigned to receive instant coffee or chlorogenic acid-enriched instant coffee. Significant weight loss and body fat reduction from baseline was reported in the enriched coffee group, but not the regular instant coffee group. Chlorogenic acid along with caffeic and quinic acids were shown to inhibit α-amylase enzymes *in vitro*. Such inhibition could decrease the breakdown of starch into glucose and lower the caloric intake. More recently, Vinson et al. (2012) evaluated the efficacy of a commercial GCB extract in weight loss management. Significant reductions in body weight (-8.04 ± 2.31 kg), body mass index (-2.92 ± 0.85 kg/m^2), and percent body fat ($-4.44 \pm 2.00\%$) were observed in 16 overweight adults during 22-weeks of treatment.

Coffee is helpful in healing neurodegenerative disorders Bradykinesia, tremory rigidity, and Parkinson's disease. The putative mechanism for prevention of the degeneration of substantia nigra cells is mediation of Adenosine A2 receptor antagonist by caffeine. Similarly, coffee acts as NADPH (NADPH is nicotinamide adenine dinucleotide phosphate hydrogen or nicotinamide adenine dinucleotide phosphate [NADP] carrying electrons bonded with hydrogen [H] ion or simply the reduced form of NADP), a cofactor of glutatione reductase, which helps in the reduction of free radicals in substantia nigra and biosynthesis of dopamine. Coffee is beneficial for colon rectal cancer patients. The putative action of coffee and its other constituent is the inhibition of excretion of bile acids, which in turn increases the cholesterol level. Similarly, antioxidant activities of chlorogenic acids (cafeic, cinnamic, ferulic) and purine derivatives (caffeine) helps in the stimulation of the detoxification processes via glutatione S-transferases. Liver diseases can also be cured by moderate intake of coffee, which helps in the reduction of liver cirrhosis (5X) via serum glutamiltransferase.

13.7 FUTURE PROSPECTS

Since, coffee has a preventive effect on human health and is said to have antioxidant, antidiabetic, anti-inflammatory, and weight-reducing properties (Bakuradze et al. 2011; Larsson et al. 2006; van Dam et al. 2006; Bonita et al. 2007). Overweight and obesity issues represent serious health problems and are among the leading causes of death. Rates of obesity have more than doubled worldwide since 1980. Because of the relatively high cost and small number of prescription weight loss drugs, their limited effectiveness, and their potential adverse health effects, the use of dietary supplements is increasingly perceived by consumers as a safer and more natural way to treat weight management and obesity. Due to its positive influence on inflammation, coffee is of special interest when searching for physiologically functional food constituents. The main component of the phenolic compounds of coffee is chlorogenic acid (Farah et al. 2006; Shearer et al. 2003; Frost-Meyer and Logomarsino 2012). In healthy human beings ingredients of coffee are easily metabolized (Higdon and Frei 2006). Based on survey data, experimental results, and dose application, there is a serious need to combine all these elements on a molecular scale to investigate the potential of metabolites of coffee ingredients in modulating the cytokine signaling, the MAP kinases based cell signaling, the neurological synaptic signaling, and other complex metabolic networks.

13.8 CONCLUSION

The nuclear factor-E2-related (Nrf2) protein is the key regulator of the transcription of Phase II enzymes and antioxidant enzymes. Since, Phase II enzymes have the ability to neutralize dangerous species (electrophilic or oxidant species or highly reactive intermediates), they generate less reactive and more soluble substances that can be eliminated from the organisms. Simultaneously, Nrf2 protein acts on DNA promoters as a regulatory factor for the transcription of the antioxidant enzymes such as superoxide dismutase (SOD), catalase (CAT), and glutathione peroxidase (GPx). This in turn enhances the expression of SOD, CAT, and GPx resulting in a reduction of the levels of dangerous species such as O^{2-} (superoxide anion radical), H_2O_2 (hydrogen peroxide), and O_2^{2-} (peroxide anion). This enzymatic activity decreases the downstream formation of other reactive oxygen species (ROS), and neutralizes or reduces their deleterious actions. Therefore, there is a serious need to identify such bioactive substances that can modulate the transcription and increase the activity of these protective enzymes.

Under normal (reducing) condition, Nrf2 remains anchored to its inhibitor cytoplasmic complex Keapl–Nrf2 (Kelch-like ECH associated protein-1) for its poly-ubiquitination and subsequent 26S proteasome-mediated degradation. However, under oxidative stress or exposure to inducers, Nrf2 is disrupted from this complex, allowing its translocation to the nucleus of the cells, where it binds to the antioxidant response element (ARE) or to the electrophile response element (EpRE) present in the promoter region of the mentioned enzymes, increasing their transcription.

On the basis of these facts and information, we can conclude that intake of a coffee beverage is sufficient to modulate the protein Nrf2, increasing the activity of antioxidant enzymes, and improving the defense system against oxidative stress. Therefore, increased intake of green coffee could also affect the concentration and the expression of Nrf2 protein. Although, comparative studies involving a single dose and repetitive doses of coffee, shows that an accumulative effect can be considered as beneficial consequence for coffee drinkers.

This chapter mostly focuses on the effect of the administration of coffee on the activity of antioxidant enzymes and the transcription of phase II enzymes correlated to the Nrf2/ARE pathway. Therefore, it is important to quantify the levels of these bioactive substances in green coffee beverage which could eventually have a wide application in treating human health conditions. There are questions about the effect of coffee on human health system, and it has been a subject of intensive research in the last few decades.

REFERENCES

Akiyama, T., 2001. Coffee market liberalization since 1990. In *Commodity Market Reforms: Lessons of Two Decades*; Akiyama, T., J. Baffes, D. F. Larson, and P. Varangis (Eds.); World Bank: Washington, DC.

Alam, J., C. Wicks, D. Stewart, P. Gong, et al., 2000. Mechanisms of heme oxygenase-1 gene activation by cadmium in MCF-7 mammary epithelial cells. Role of p38 kinase and Nrf2 transcription factor. *J. Biol. Chem.* 275: 27694–27702.

Ames, J. M., L. Royle, G. W. Bradbury, 2000. Capillary electrophoresis of roasted coffee. In *Caffeinated Beverages: Health Benefits, Physiological Effects and Chemistry*; Parliment, T. H., C. T. Ho, P. Schieberle (Eds.); ACS Symposium Series 754; American Chemical Society: Washington, DC, 364–373.

Balogun, E., M. Hoque, P. Gong, E. Killeen, C.J. Green, R. Foresti, J. Alam, R. Motterlini, 2003. Curcumin activates the haemoxygenase-1 gene via regulation of Nrf2 and the antioxidantresponsive element. *Biochem. J.* 371: 887–895.

Belitz, H. D. and W. Grosch, 1987. Coffee, tea, cocoa. In *Food Chemistry*; Springer: New York, 681–688.

Bertrand, B., B. Guyot, F. Anthony, P Lashermes, 2003. Impact of the *Coffea canephora* gene introgression on beverage quality of *C.arabica*. *Theor. Appl. Genet.* 107: 387–394.

Calzolari, C., E. Cerma, 1963. Sulle sostanze grasse del caffè. *Riv. Ital. Sostanze Grasse* 40: 176–80.

Charrier, A. C. and J. Berthaund, 1985. Botanical classification of coffee. In *Coffee: Botany, Biochemistry and Production of Beans and Beverage*; Clifford, M. N., K.C. Willson (Eds); Croom Helm: London, 13–47.

Chassevent, F., G. Dalger, S. Gerwig, J. C. Vincent, 1974. Contribution 9 l'&de des Mascarocofia: Etude des fractions lipidiques et insaponifiables. Relation eventuelle entre les teneurs en cafeine et en acides chlorogeniques. *Cafe. Cacao. The.* 18: 49–56.

Chassevent, F., S. O. Gerwig, M. Bouharmont, 1973. Influence eventuelle de diverses fumures sur les teneurs en acides chlorogeniques et en cafeine de grains decafeiers cultives. In *Proc. 6th Int. Sci. Coll. Coffee (Bogotá)* ASIC, Paris, 57–60.

Chen, C., D. Pung, V. Leong, V. Hebbar, G. Shen, S. Nair, W. Li, A.N. Kong, 2004. Induction of detoxifying enzymes by garlic organosulfur compounds through transcription factor Nrf2: effect of chemical structure and stress signals. *Free Radical Biol. Med.* 37: 1578–1590.

Cornelis, M. C., A. El-Sohemy, 2007. Coffee, caffeine, and coronary heart disease. *Curr. Opin. Clin. Nutr. Metab. Care* 10(6): 745–751.

Daglia, M., A. Papetti, C. Gregotti, F. Berte, G. Gazzani, 2000. In vitro antioxidant and ex vivo protective activities of green and roasted coffee. *J. Agric. Food Chem.* 48: 1449–1454.

Davis, A. P., R. Govaerts, D. M. Bridson, P. Stoffelen, 2006. An annotated taxonomic conspectus of the genus *Coffea rubiaceae)*. *Bot. J. Linnean Soc.* 152: 465–512.

Enyan, F., B. K. B. Banful, P. Kumah, 2013. Physical and organoleptic qualities of coffee bean under different drying methods and depths of drying in a tropical environment. *Int. Res. J. Plant Sci.* 4(9):280–287.

Favreau, L. V., C. B. Pickett, 1991. Transcriptional regulation of the rat NAD(P)H:quinone reductase gene. Identification of regulatory elements controlling basal level expression and inducible expression by planar aromatic compounds and phenolic antioxidants. *J. Biol. Chem.* 266: 4556–4561.

Feng, R., Y. Lu, L. L. Bowman, Y. Qian, V. Castranova, M. Ding, 2005. Inhibition of activator protein-1, NF-B, and MAPKs and induction of phase 2 detoxifying enzyme activity by chlorogenic acid. *J. Biol. Chem.* 280(30): 27888–27895.

Friis-Hansen, E. (Ed.). 2000. CDR Policy Paper Series, Agricultural Policy in Africa After Adjustment. Centre for Development Research: Copenhagen.

Hartmann L, R. C. A. Lago, J. S. Tango, C. G. Teixeira, 1968. The effect of unsaponifiable matter on the properties of coffee seed oil. *J. Amer. Oil. Chem. Soc.* 45:577–579.

Hicks P. A. 2002. Post-harvest processing and quality assurance for specialty/organic coffee products. In *Asian Regional Round-Table on Sustainable, Organic and Speciality Coffee Production, Processing and Marketing*; Chiang Mai, Bangkok, Thailand.

Higgins, L., C. Cavin, K. Itoh, M. Yamamoto, J. D. Hayes, 2008. Induction of cancer chemopreventive enzymes by coffee is mediated by transcription factor Nrf2. Evidence that the coffee-specific diterpenes cafestol and kahweol confer protection against acrolein. *Toxicol. Appl. Pharmacol.* 226(3): 328–337.

Huber, W., H. Candee, B. Coles, R. King, et al., 2004. Potential chemoprotective effects of the coffee components kahweol and cafestol palmitates via modification of hepatic N-acetyltransferase and glutathione S-transferase activities. *Environ. Mol. Mutagen.* 44: 265–276.

Illy, A. and R. Viani, 1995. The plant. In *Espresso Coffee: The Chemistry of Quality*; Academic Press: San Diego, CA, 19–20.

Ishii, T., Itoh, K., Takahashi, S., Sato, H. et al., 2000. Transcription factor Nrf2 coordinately regulates a group of oxidative stress-inducible genes in macrophages. *J. Biol. Chem.* 275: 16023–16029.

Itoh, K., N. Wakabayashi, Y. Katoh, T. Ishii, K. Igarashi et al., 1999. Keapl represses nuclear activation of antioxidant responsive elements by Nrf2 through binding to the amino-terminal Neh2 domain. *Genes Dev.* 13: 76–86.

Jemal, A., T. Murray, E. Ward, A. Samuels, R.C. Tiwari, A. Ghafoor, E. J. Feuer, M. J. Thun, 2005. Cancer statistics. *CA Cancer J. Clin.* 55: 10–30.

Kensler, T. W., 1997. Chemoprevention by inducers of carcinogen detoxication enzymes. Environ. *Health Perspect.* 105(4), 965–970.

Keservani, R. K., R. K. Kesharwani, A. K. Sharma, 2015a. *Pulmonary and Respiratory Health: Antioxidants and Nutraceuticals*; CRC Press, Taylor & Francis Group: London, 279.

Keservani, R. K., R. K. Kesharwani, N. Vyas, S. Jain, R. Raghuvanshi, A. K. Sharma, 2010. Nutraceutical and functional food as future food: A Review. *Der Pharmacia. Lett.* 2: 106–116.

Keservani, R. K. and A. K. Sharma, 2014. Flavonoids: Emerging trends and potential health benefits. *J. Chin. Pharm. Sci.* 23(12): 815–822.

Keservani, R. K., S. Singh, V. Singh, R. K. Kesharwani, A. K. Sharma, 2015b. *Nutraceuticals and Functional Foods in the Prevention of Mental Disorder*; CRC Press, Taylor and Francis Group: London, 255.

Kroplien, U., 1963. *Green and Roasted Coffee Tests*, Gordian: Hamburg, p. 206.

Kummer, C., 2003. *The Joy of Coffee: The Essential guide to Buying, Brewing, and Enjoying*, Houghton Mifflin: Boston.

Mancha-Agresti, P. D. C., A. S. Franca, L. S. Oliveira, R. Augusti, 2008. Discrimination between defective and non-defective Brazilian coffee beans by their volatile profile. *Food Chem.* 106: 787–796.

McClumpha, A. D., 1988. The trading of green coffee. In *Coffee (volume 6): Commercial and Technico-Legal Aspects*; Clarke, R. J. and R. Macrae (Eds.); Elsevier Applied Science: London.

Nicoli, M. C., M. Anese, L. Manzocco, C. R. Lerici, 1997. Antioxidant properties of coffee brews in relation to roasting degree. *Lebensm. Wiss. -Technol.* 30: 292–297.

Nicoli, M. C., M. Anese, M. Parpinel, 1999. Influence of processing on the antioxidant properties of fruit and vegetables. *Trends Food Sci. Technol.* 10: 94–100.

Nicoli, M. C., M. Anese, M.T. Parpinel, S. L. Franceschi, C. R. Lerici, 1997. Loss and formation of antioxidants during food processing and storage. *Cancer Lett.*114: 71–74.

Parliment, T. H. 2000. An overview of coffee roasting. In *Caffeinated BeVerages: Health Benefits, Physiological Effects and Chemistry*; Parliment, T. H., C. T. Ho, P. Schieberle, Eds.; ACS Symposium Series 754; American Chemical Society: Washington, DC, 188–201.

Pendergrast, M., 2009. Coffee: Second to oil? *Tea Coffee Trade J.* 181(4): 38–41.

Ponte, S., 2002a. Brewing a bitter cup? Deregulation, quality and the re-organization of the coffee marketing chain in East Africa. *J. Agrarian Change* 2(2): 248–272.

Raikes, P., Jensen, M. F., Ponte, S. 2000. Global commodity chain analysis and the French filière approach: Comparison and critique. *Econ. Soc.* 29(3): 390–417.

Roburgert, N. E., G. van der Weg, T. G. Kosmeijer-Schuil, M. B. Katan, 1997. Separate effects of the coffee diterpenes cafestol and kahweol on serum lipids and liver aminotransferases. *American J Clinical Nutrition*. 65(2): 519–524.

Rushmore, T. H., M. R. Morton, C. B. Pickett, 1991. The antioxidant responsive element. Activation by oxidative stress and identification of the DNA consensus sequence required for functional activity. *J. Biol. Chem.* 266:11632–11639.

Salazar-Martinez, E., W. C. Willett, A. Ascherio, et al., 2004. Coffee consumption and risk for type 2 diabetes mellitus. *Ann Intern Med.* 140: 1–8.

Smith, B. D., K. Tola, 1998. Caffeine: Effects on psychological functioning and performance. I *Caffeine*; Spiller, G. A., Ed.; CRC Press: Boca Raton, FL, 251–300.

Talalay, P., 2000. Chemoprotection against cancer by induction of phase 2 enzymes. *BioFactors.* 12: 5–11.

Talalay, P., J. W. Fahey, W. D. Holtzclaw, T. Prestera, Y. Zhang, 1995. Chemoprotection against cancer by phase 2 enzyme induction. *Toxicol. Lett.* 82(83): 173–179.

Talbot, J. M., 2004. *Grounds for Agreement: The Political Economy of the Coffee Commodity Chain*. Rowman & Littlefield: Lanham, 50.

Thom, E., 2007. The effect of chlorogenic acid enriched coffee on glucose absorption in healthy volunteers and its effect on body mass when used long-term in overweight and obese people. *J. Int. Med. Res.* 35: 900–908.

Venugopal, R. and A. K. Jaiswal, 1996. Nrf1 and Nrf2 positively and c-Fos and Fral negatively regular the human antioxidant response elementmediated expression of NAD(P) H:quinone oxidoreductase 1 gene. *Proc. Natl. Acad. Sci. U.S.A.* 93: 14960–14965.

Wilkinson, J., M. L. Clapper, 1997. Detoxification enzymes and chemoprevention. *Proc. Soc. Exp. Biol. Med.* 216: 192–200.

Yu, R., W. Lei, et al., 1999. Role of a mitogen-activated protein kinase pathway in the induction of phase II detoxifying enzymes by chemicals. *J. Biol. Chem.* 274: 27545–27552.

Zhang, D. D., M. Hannink, 2003. Distinct cysteine residues in Keapl are required for Keapl-dependent ubiquitination of Nrf2 and for stabilization of Nrf2 by chemopreventive agents and oxidative stress. *Mol. Cell. Biol.* 23: 8137–8151.

Zhang, Y. and G. Gordon, 2004. A strategy for cancer prevention: stimulation of the Nrf2-ARE signalling pathway. *Mol. Cancer Ther.* 3, 885–892.

14 Metabolomics Study of Green Coffee Beans

Anh Hong Phan, Takuya Miyakawa, and Masaru Tanokura

CONTENTS

14.1 INTRODUCTION

Initially discovered in the late sixteenth century, coffee has become the world's most traded good and most consumed beverage.[1] As scientists became more aware of coffee's popularity in daily human life, they started to study the taste, flavor, and health benefits of coffee and why it tends to hold its value well over time. The identification of the organic compounds in green coffee beans has been the focus of researchers for many years. The amount and composition of these precursor compounds have been reported to contribute significantly to the taste and flavor of coffee.[2] Green coffee beans are first roasted in a process with varying time courses and temperatures in which new components and characteristics are generated.[3] The end result makes the beans ready for commercial sale and consumption.

Nuclear magnetic resonance (NMR) spectroscopy has been considered a powerful tool in food analysis due to its simplicity and speed in sample preparation without destroying the food, while being highly informative. Therefore, the technique has been successfully utilized in analyzing the compositional state of numerous foods such as potatoes,[4] mango juice,[5] milk,[6,7] and black garlic.[8] NMR spectral analysis not only provides metabolite profiles of certain food samples but also allows for both quantitative analysis and the detection of trace compositional changes. When combined with other multivariate analysis methods such as principal component analysis (PCA) or orthogonal partial least squares discriminated analysis (OPLS-DA), NMR is more effective in distinguishing foods of different species and origins and provides more data on the food sample being analyzed. This chapter mainly summarizes NMR-based metabolomics studies of green coffee beans. Special attention is first paid to the organic compounds in green coffee bean extract (GCBE) and then how these compounds evolve throughout the roasting process is explored. Finally, the NMR-based sensory evaluation of coffee is analyzed.

14.2 ANALYSIS OF THE ORGANIC COMPOUNDS IN GREEN COFFEE BEAN EXTRACT

With the aim of further understanding the chemical compositions of GCBE, many analytical techniques and methodologies using high-performance liquid chromatography (HPLC),[9] ultravoilet (UV)-visible spectrophotometry,[10] and liquid chromatography–mass spectrometry (LC–MS)[11] have been utilized. NMR spectroscopy, despite some drawbacks, analyzes food in an effective way due to its simplicity in nondestructive sample preparation, which causes fewer qualitative and quantitative changes to the original mixture compared with other methods. Therefore, NMR spectroscopy has been used to construct a comprehensive metabolite profile of GCBE. Figure 14.1 shows typical one-dimensional (1-D) ^{1}H and ^{13}C spectra of GCBE. The resulting signal assignment that was obtained by means of different types of two-dimensional (2-D) spectra demonstrated the presence of 16 water-soluble compounds in GCBE samples[12] of the two most common coffee species—*Coffea arabica* and *Coffea robusta*. The compounds identified are 3-CQA, 4-CQA, 5-CQA (isomers of caffeoylquinic acid; CQA), acetic acid, caffeine, choline, citric acid, L-glutamic acid, L-alanine, L-asparagine, L-glutamine, quinic acid, malic acid, *myo*-inositol, sucrose, and trigonelline. Overall, the assigned ^{1}H and ^{13}C NMR spectral patterns of the two typical GCBEs revealed no remarkable distinctions in the metabolite profiles between the species except for a slight fluctuation in the chemical shifts of caffeine and CQAs.[13] This variation was expounded by the relative concentrations of caffeine and chlorogenic acids (CGAs) including CQAs. These two components interact with each other to form a caffeine–chlorogenate complex in an aqueous solution.[14] Unlike ^{1}H NMR spectra, ^{13}C NMR spectra showed no such change in the chemical shifts. The reason for this result may be that the noncovalent correlations between the caffeine and the CGAs are only strong enough to affect the chemical environments in ^{1}H nuclei but not in the ^{13}C nuclei.

The most apparent differences between the two coffee species, in addition to the ^{1}H NMR spectra, were clearly observed from the compositional portions captured from the PCA and OPLS-DA models derived from the ^{13}C NMR spectra of all the GCBEs.[13] The dramatic variance in the amount of components identified is one significant criterion used to differentiate GCBEs according to their species and origins.

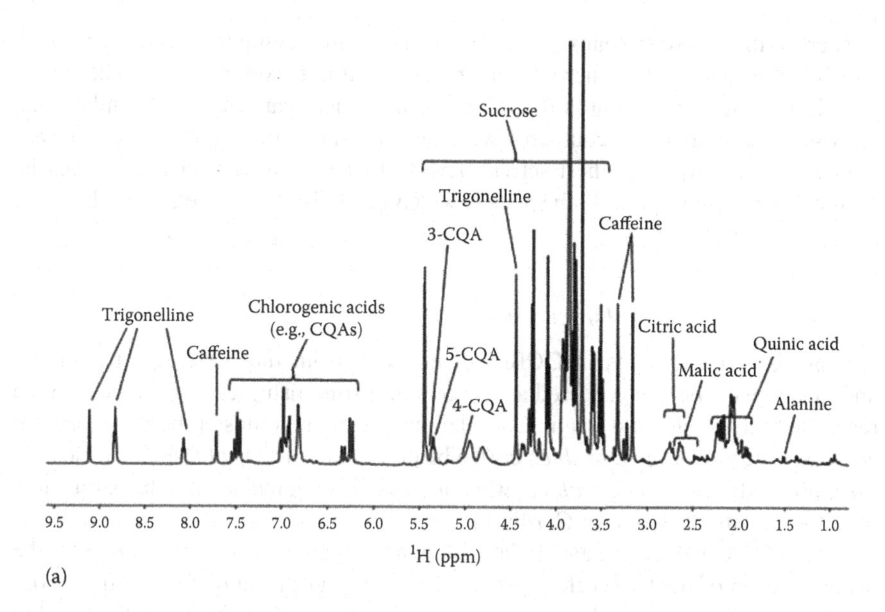

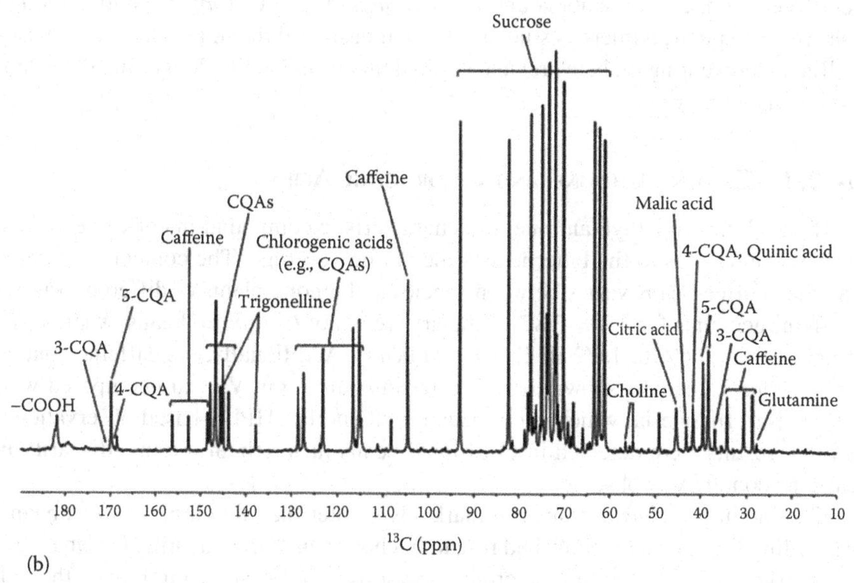

FIGURE 14.1 1D (a) ^{1}H and (b) ^{13}C NMR spectra of GCBE.

14.2.1 Sucrose

Sucrose, the carbohydrate accounting for the greatest portion in GCBEs, has been identified as an important precursor of coffee flavor and aroma compounds generated during roasting.[15] In regard to the taste, more sucrose accumulation in the coffee beans results in a better taste. This is why *C. arabica*, which has higher levels of sucrose in the green beans, is rather widely favored compared with *C. robusta*, which has a much lower sucrose content. A legitimate explanation for the difference in the sucrose amount is that *C. arabica* has less capacity for resynthesizing sucrose in the final stages compared with the early stages of *C. robusta* grain development. Moreover, the highest activity levels of sucrose synthase occur during the final development stage of both species, which gives rise to a large accumulation of carbohydrate.[16,17]

14.2.2 Citrate, Malate, and Trigonelline

Among the organic acids in GCBEs determined from the NMR spectra, citrate and malate have been considered as markers to distinguish green coffee beans with regard to both species and origin. Considerably greater amounts of these two organic acids were recorded in *C. arabica* coffee beans. Greater levels of these acids lead to the more acidic taste of *C. arabica*, whereas acidity is not included in the parameters used to evaluate the flavor of *C. robusta*.

Trigonelline, like citrate and malate, is counted as another possible marker for the differentiation of the two coffee species due to the significant difference in its content. Trigonelline is more abundant in *C. arabica* than in *C. robusta*. With regard to nutritional aspects, numerous studies have demonstrated the important role of trigonelline in preventing diabetes-related organ damage and aiding longer life expectancies in diabetic rats.[18]

14.2.3 Caffeine, Choline, and Chlorogenic Acids

Caffeine (1,3,7-trimethylxanthine) is a characteristic compound in coffee beans that greatly contributes to the bitterness of the coffee beverage. The content of caffeine in green coffee beans varies between species and among plants of different origins. Caffeine accounts for 2.2%–2.8% of the dry weight of *C. robusta* beans, whereas the range is from 0.6% to 1.2% in *C. arabica* beans. Additionally, the caffeine content in *C. robusta* beans is shown to be greater in beans from Vietnam compared with beans from Indonesia, which is consistent with another HPLC-based observation.[19] Similar results were detected in *C. arabica* beans in which an original disparity in caffeine content was observed.

Choline in *C. robusta* beans is remarkably greater than that in *C. arabica* beans. According to previously published research, choline has been identified as an essential nutrient required for methyl group metabolism and is shown to reduce the risk of breast cancer.[20]

CGAs are esters formed from the reaction between quinic acid and various types of transcinnamic acids, such as caffeic, *p*-coumaric, and ferulic acids. Although 18 types of CGAs in GCBEs have been reported, the most abundant forms are isomers of CQAs, which are the esters formed by quinic acid and caffeic acid including 5-*O*-CQA (5-CQA), 4-*O*-CQA (4-CQA), and 3-*O*-CQA (3-CQA). Greater amounts of CQAs were detected in *C. robusta* GCBEs, making these beans more resistant than *C. arabica* to phytopathogens, and to biological and mechanical stresses.[19]

14.2.4 Acetic Acid and Amino Acids

Acetic acid and amino acids are reliable markers to differentiate coffee beans. Although no species were distinguished from the other based on relative concentrations of acetic acid and amino acids, coffee beans of different geographical origins were possibly detected. Levels of acetic acid are greatest in Tanzanian coffee beans followed by beans from Brazil, Vietnam, Guatemala, Indonesia, and Colombia. As for amino acids, the content of free amino acids in GCBEs that were quantified on the basis of NMR spectra were on the order of 0.1–0.7 mM,[12] or 0.3%–0.6% on a dry weight basis.[21] Nonetheless, there is no evidence to support the link between the presence of free amino acids and the formation of coffee aroma during roasting.

14.3 EVOLUTION OF COFFEE COMPOSITION DUE TO ROASTING PROCESS AND ROASTING DEGREE

Roasting is an important process in coffee production because it leads to remarkable physical and chemical changes in the beans.[22,23] Therefore, roasted coffee beans contain many novel substances that green coffee beans lack.[3,24] Coffee at different roasting degrees has distinguishable sensory qualities and is hence enjoyable. The longer the coffee beans are held in the roaster and/or the higher the roasting temperature, the darker the coffee beans become. The roasting degrees can be measured by judging the bean's color with the naked eye, using a colorimeter, or by the weight lost as water during roasting.

Green coffee beans were roasted at three distinct times: 5, 7, and 9 min at 220°C, to obtain light, medium, and dark degrees of roast, respectively, prior to being subjected to signal assignment. Thirty compounds present in GCBEs and roasted coffee bean extracts (RCBEs) were determined,[22,23] including 3-CQA, 4-CQA, 5-CQA, acetic acid, caffeine, choline, citric acid, γ-aminobutyrate (GABA), L-alanine, L-asparagine, L-glutamic acid, quinic acid, malic acid, myo-inositol, sucrose, and trigonelline; and the compounds formed during the roasting process are 5-hydroxymethylfurfural, γ-quinide, *syllo*-quinic acid, α-(1-3)-L-arabinofuranose, α-(1-5)-L-arabinofuranose, β-(1-3)-D-galactopyranose, β-(1-6)-D-galactopyranose, β-(1-4)-D-mannopyranose, γ-butyrolactone, 2-furylmethanol, formic acid, lactic acid, *N*-methylpyridinium, and nicotinic acid. Figure 14.2 shows comparative ^1H NMR spectra of GCBEs and RCBEs at the three roasting stages.[23] A difference in the components in the roasted coffee bean was also observed in the spectra. The evolution of coffee bean components during the roasting process was also assessed by quantifying the relative concentrations of each individual identified compound. General changes were primarily shown by the degradation of polysaccharides, oligosaccharides, CGAs, and trigonelline, the rapid disappearance of free amino acids, and the formation of aromatic compounds.

14.3.1 Evolution of Saccharides

Among saccharides, sucrose is the most abundant simple carbohydrate occurring in the GCBE mixture on a by-mole basis.[12] Sucrose is rapidly degraded when coffee

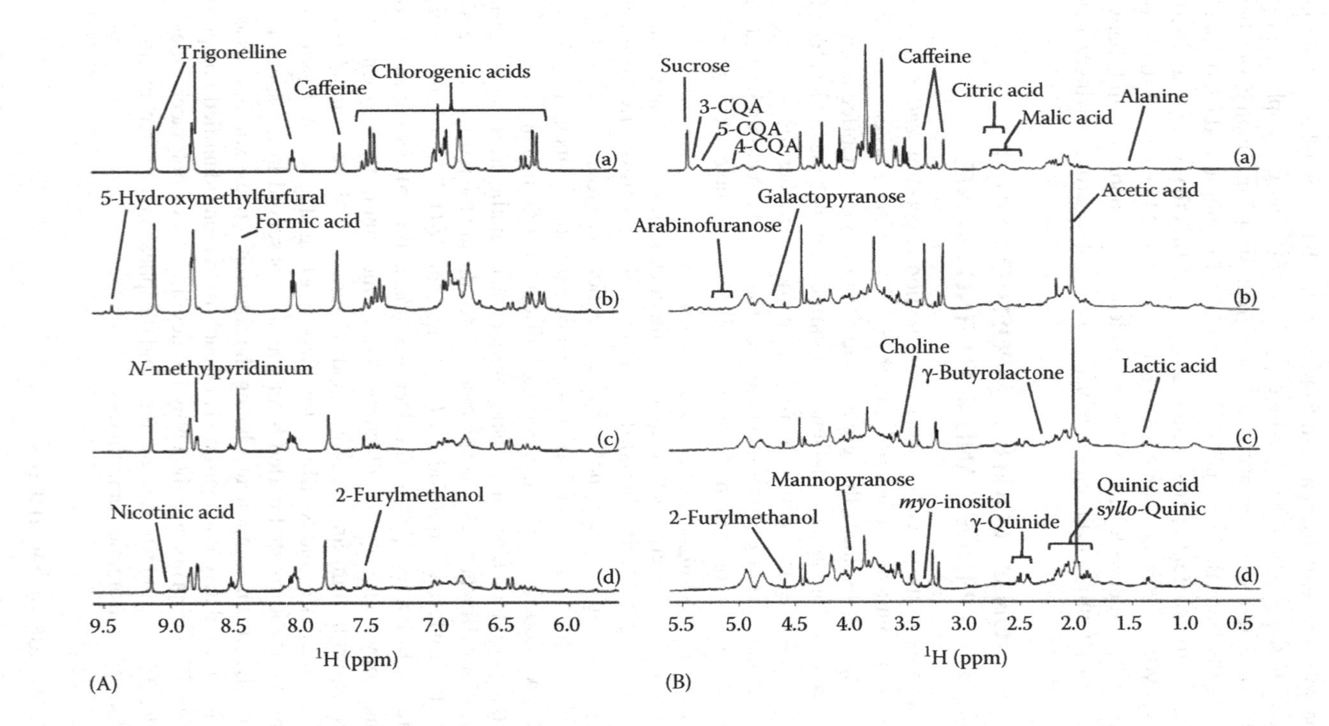

FIGURE 14.2 (A) Low-field and (B) high-field ^1H NMR spectra of (a) green coffee bean extract and coffee bean extracts with (b) light, (c) medium, and (d) dark degrees of roast.

beans are roasted at 220°C. After 5 min of roasting (light roast), sucrose was no longer detectable. Sucrose is important as it acts as an aroma precursor due to its significant contribution to the formation of numerous classes of compounds that affect the flavor of coffee beverages.[25,26] These compounds or classes of compounds include furans, aldehydes, aliphatic acids, organic acids (acetic acid, formic acid, and lactic acid), aroma compounds (2-furylmethanol and γ-butyrolactone), and 5-hydroxymethylfurfural. 5-Hydroxymethylfurfural, a common compound present in heat-processed foods, unlike the rest of the newly generated compounds, showed the highest levels of concentration after a slight roasting before being degraded rapidly upon further roasting.

Polysaccharides (including cellulose, mannan, and arabinogalactan), which were not determined by NMR in either green or roasted coffee beans, have been detected using high-resolution gas chromatography mass spectrometry (GC-MS) and make up half of the dry weight of green coffee beans.[27] These polysaccharides are retained in the cell wall of green coffee beans as part of the insoluble polysaccharide complex, which causes them to be undetectable in the NMR spectra. During the roasting process, the high temperature aids in losing the cell wall, which increases the solubility of both arabinogalactans and mannans. The degradation of α-(1-3)-L-arabinofuranose, α-(1-5)-L-arabinofuranose, β-(1-3)-D-galactopyranose, and β-(1-6)-D-galactopyranose units from arabinogalactans after light roasting could be attributed to the greater thermal lability of arabinogalactans compared with that of β-(1-4)-D-mannopyranose from mannan, which was less susceptible to degradation even after a dark roast.[28] Changes in polysaccharides were plainly backed by PCA score plots, which had high statistical values for Rx^2: 63.8% for PC1 and 17.3% for PC2. The PCA shows that β-(1-4)-D-mannopyranose, which contributes to the negative side of PC1, formed during roasting, whereas α-(1-3)-L-arabinofuranose, α-(1-5)-L-arabinofuranose, β-(1-3)-D-galactopyranose, and β-(1-6)-D-galactopyranose contribute to the positive side of PC2, which means there was a formation followed by a degradation (Figure 14.3).[23] Polysaccharides in coffee beans, especially β-(1-4)-D-mannopyranose, may be used as chemical markers during the roasting process. The water-soluble polysaccharides that appear after roasting, which play an important role in the retention of volatile substances, contribute to the viscosity of the coffee brew and, thus, to the sensation known as "body" in the mouth.[29]

14.3.2 Evolution of Chlorogenic Acids and Trigonelline

Among the 30 CGAs reported to be present in coffee beans, the three most abundant isomers that were detected in both GCBEs and RCBEs by NMR are 3-CQA, 4-CQA, and 5-CQA. However, the content of CGAs, including these three isomers, decrease considerably with longer roasting times and could be considered an index of roasting degrees. As opposed to the case of CGAs, the levels of quinic acid, γ-quinide, and syllo-quinic increase notably. Known as a dominant acid in roasted coffee beans, quinic acid increases remarkably during roasting. This could be interpreted as being caused by the degeneration of CGAs. γ-Quinide and syllo-quinic, consequently, were formed as an internal ester and isomeric product of quinic acid, respectively. Interestingly, while CGAs have an astringent taste, its decomposition products, such as quinic acid and quinide, contribute to the bitterness of roasted beans.[29,31] In

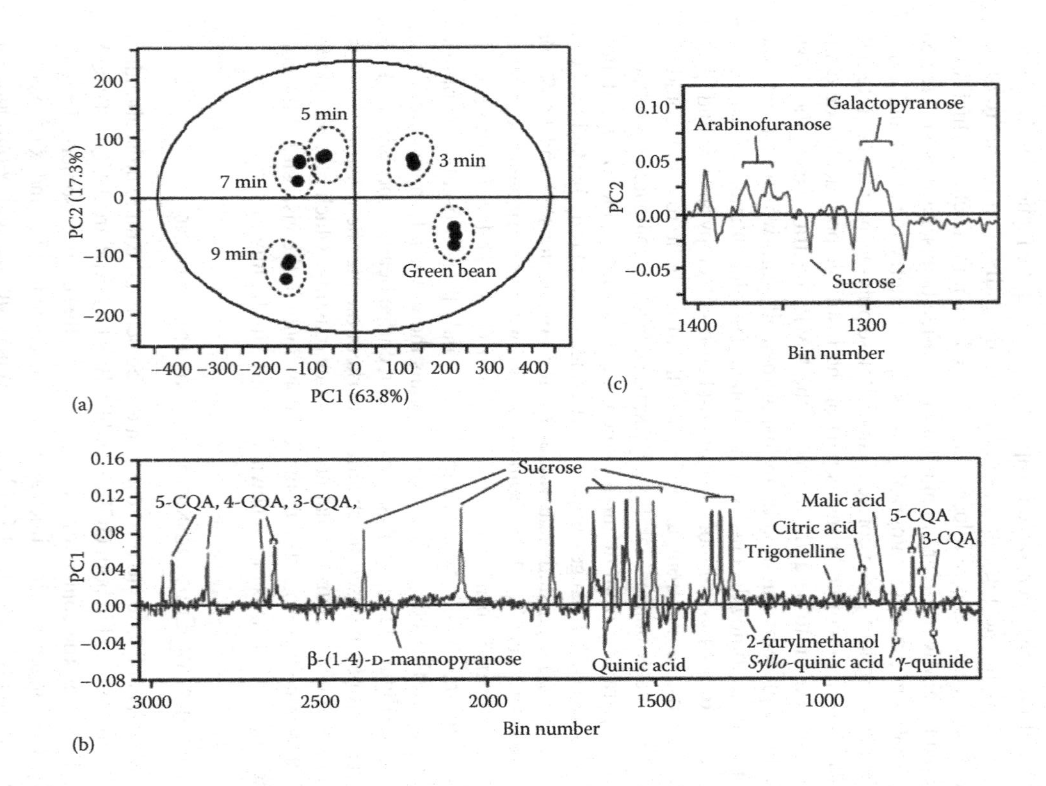

FIGURE 14.3 (a) PCA score, (b) loading plots for PC1, and (c) loading plots for PC2 derived from the ^{13}C NMR spectra of coffee bean extracts with different degrees of roast. Green bean, 3, 5, 7, and 9 min represent the green coffee bean extract and coffee bean extracts roasted for 3, 5, 7, and 9 min, respectively. The fitness and predictability of the models are indicated by Rx^2 values of 63.8% and 17.3% for PC1 and PC2, respectively, and have a Q^2 of 0.99.

addition to the increasing amounts of quinic acid, γ-quinide, and *syllo*-quinic, the formation of cinnamic acids is due to the thermal degradation of CGAs.

Studies of trigonelline show the important contribution it has to flavor and aroma, as well as its beneficial nutritional factors.[32,33] Despite its high level in GCBEs, trigonelline is continuously degraded by thermolysis at high temperatures during roasting, which leads to the gradual accumulation of two thermal decomposition products: *N*-methylpyridinium as a major product, and nicotinic acid. The decrease in the *N*-methylpyridinium level after 7 min of roasting is attributable to further degeneration and/or interaction with other thermolytic products. Trigonelline and its thermal degradation products have direct and indirect effects on other physicochemical properties of a cup of coffee, such as the flavor and aroma.

14.3.3 Evolution of Free Amino Acids

As identified by NMR, there are four main free amino acids (L-glutamic acid, L-alanine, L-asparagine, and GABA) present in GCBEs at low concentrations of 0.1–0.7 mM.[20] The time frame of changes in amino acid composition was monitored using NMR spectroscopy. The results showed that free amino acids decreased notably during the first minutes of roasting and completely disappeared 4 min after roasting.

14.3.4 Formation of Aroma Compounds

During the roasting process, coffee beans undergo many physical changes such as temperature-related changes in color and chemical changes, as well as developing characteristic aromas. There are several principal classes of aroma compounds in roasted coffee that are listed in Table 14.1.[3] Although the degradation of sucrose is a notable contributor to the generation of a number of aroma compounds, there is still a wide range of factors that impact these chemical changes, such as the breakdown of sulfur-containing amino acids, hydroxyl-amino acids, proline and hydroxyproline, trigonelline, quinic acid moiety, carotenoids, and minor lipids.[3,34] The mechanism underlying this formation has received little investigation. Future research efforts will likely focus on the elucidation of mechanistic and kinetic parameters for the formation and deterioration of key aroma compounds.

14.4 NMR-BASED SENSORY PREDICTION OF COFFEE

The development of artificial tongues to mimic the chemical sense of taste has received a great deal of attention.[35] Based on the idea that NMR spectroscopy could be a very useful "magnetic tongue" for the characterization and prediction of the taste of foods, which originated from the successful correlation of NMR metabolomic fingerprints and the sensory features of sour cherry juice[36] and tomatoes[37], the use of an NMR spectroscopic approach to analyze the taste of coffee bean extracts has been investigated. The use of NMR-based metabolomics coupled with the multivariate method of orthogonal projection to latent structures (OPLS) was demonstrated to be effective and successful in predicting the taste of four types of commercial roasted coffee beans, including both the *C. arabica* and *C. robusta* species at light and dark roasted levels.[2]

TABLE 14.1
Classes of Volatile Compounds Identified in Roasted Coffee Beans

Sulfur Compounds
Thiols
Hydrogen sulfide
Thiophenes (esters, aldehydes, and ketones)
Thiazoles (alkyl, alkoxy, and acetal derivatives)
Pyrazines
Pyrazine itself
Thiol and furfuryl derivatives
Alkyl derivatives (primarily methyl and dimethyl)
Pyridines
Methyl, ethyl, acetyl, and vinyl derivatives
Pyrroles
Alkyl, acyl, and furfuryl derivatives
Oxazoles
Furans
Aldehydes, ketones, esters, alcohols, acids, thiols, sulfides, and in combination with pyrazines and pyrroles
Aldehydes and Ketones
Aliphatic and aromatic species
Phenols

Source: Buffo et al., *Flavour and Fragrance Journal*, 2004, 19: 99–104.

14.4.1 Correlations between Chemical Components Detected by NMR and Sensory Descriptors

The chemical compositions of *C. arabica* and *C. robusta* beans at dark and light roasts were accurately identified by the assignment of ^{1}H NMR spectra. A sensory evaluation performed in a human trial, suggested that different tastes showed remarkable distinctions dependent on either the coffee species or the roasting level. Among seven tastes, umami, however, was the only taste that was not taken into account in the human sensory test due to its seemingly insignificant impact on the taste of coffee roasted to various degrees. The score plot of the standard OPLS model revealed considerable distinctions in the sensory characteristic of all four types of RCBEs. In general, light roasted *C. arabica* extracts are characterized by sourness as well as saltiness; dark roasted *C. arabica* extracts feature a more marked astringency and bitterness. In contrast, dark roasted *C. robusta* extracts are dominated by bitter, body, and sweet tastes. However, none of the descriptors were found in the sensory characteristic of the light roasted *C. robusta* beans, which indicates their relatively plain or mild features compared with other samples.

Table 14.2 summarizes the correlations between the compounds detected in the ^{1}H NMR spectra and the analyzed sensory descriptors.[2] The body taste of the coffee drink positively corresponds to the contents of polar lipids, mannose, quinide, and quinic acids, while it negatively corresponds to arabinose, galactose, and trigonelline.

TABLE 14.2

Correlation between Compounds in Coffee Beans and Sensory Descriptors Highlighted by the OPLS Models[a]

	Sweetness		Bitterness		Sourness		Astringency		Saltiness		Body	
Compound	*p*	*p* (corr)	*p*	*p* (corr)	*p*	*p* (corr)	*p*	*p* (corr)	*p*	*p* (corr)	*p*	*p* (corr)
3-CQA	−.13	−.87	−.11	−.88	.13	.89	−.09	−.75	−.07	−.53		
4-CQA	−.14	−.88	−.12	−.70	.14	.91	−.11	−.78	−.06	−.59		
5-CQA	−.18	−.87	−.13	−.90	.11	.56	−.10	−.58	−.14	−.58		
Acetate					.07	.50			.19	.56		
Caffeine									−.18	−.85		
Citrate	−.07	−.56	−.05	−.64	.07	.59	−.06	−.71	.05	.63		
Formate	−.09	−.57			.09	.58			.10	.51		
Lactate									.09	.54		
Lipids	.08	.57	.09	.74	−.08	−.60	.09	.74			.09	.73
Malate	−.11	−.70	−.08	−.74	.11	.75	−.08	−.73	.13	.87		
N-Methylpyridinium			.05	.60								
Quinic acid	.12	.65	.12	.79	−.12	−.69	.12	.75			.12	.78
syllo-Quinic acid	.13	.66	.16	.94	−.13	−.67	.17	.98			.16	.93
γ-Quinide	.10	.56	.13	.83	−.10	−.56	.13	.89			.13	.83
Trigonelline	−.13	−.76	−.12	−.78	.14	.82	−.10	−.66			−.12	−.77
α-(1-3)-L-arabinofuranose	−.06	−.65			.06	.70			.06	.53		
α-(1-5)-L-arabinofuranose	−.07	−.63	−.08	−.90	.05	.61	−.09	−.92	.06	.61	−.08	−.87
β-(1-3)-D-galactopyranose	−.14	−.85	−.13	−.87	.08	.70	−.10	−.79	.10	.72	−.10	−.54
β-(1-6)-D-galactopyranose	−.16	−.50	−.10	−.52	.16	.54	−.11	−.75	.10	.50	−.13	−.86
β-(1-4)-D-mannopyranose	.09	.58	.14	.82			.17	.94			.09	.56

Note: The *p*(corr) value shows the correlation of a spectral bin, which represents each compound, toward sensory descriptors. Blank shows the value of $p < .05$ and $p(\text{corr}) < .5$ in the S-plots for the OPLS models.

[a] The *p* value represents the magnitude of a spectral bin.

A sour taste, negatively relates to the amounts of lipids, quinide, and quinic acids, and positively relates to CGAs, citrate, malate, formate, acetate, trigonelline, arabinose, and galactose. Coffee drink sweetness positively correlates with lipids, quinic acids, mannose, and quinide, and it negatively correlates with CGAs, citrate, formate, malate, trigonelline, arabinose, and galactose. An astringent taste is positively associated with lipids, quinic acid, mannose, and quinide, while it is negatively associated with CGAs, malate, trigonelline, arabinose, and galactose. Saltiness positively correlates with most of the acids and with all of the polysaccharides except mannose, and it negatively correlates with CGAs and caffeine. The bitterness of coffee negatively correlates with CGAs.

14.4.2 NMR-Based Sensory Predictions

Similarities in the chemical composition and sensory features of dark roasted *C. arabica* extracts and four types of commercial coffee bean extracts (Mokha Taste, Mild Taste, Kilimanjaro Taste, and Dark Roast Taste) were demonstrated in a predictive OPLS model (Figure 14.4).[2] As shown in the scatter plots from the model, the sourest was Mokha Taste, whereas Dark Roast Taste was the mildest. In terms of bitterness, Dark Roast Taste had the highest level, followed by Kilimanjaro Taste, Mild Taste, and Mohka Taste, which is identical to the sensory features of commercial coffee beans. The accuracy of the predictive OPLS model utilizing NMR spectra, with or without a human sensory test, has demonstrated the potential application of NMR-based metabolomics in combination with multivariate statistical analysis in the sensory prediction of roasted coffee bean products.

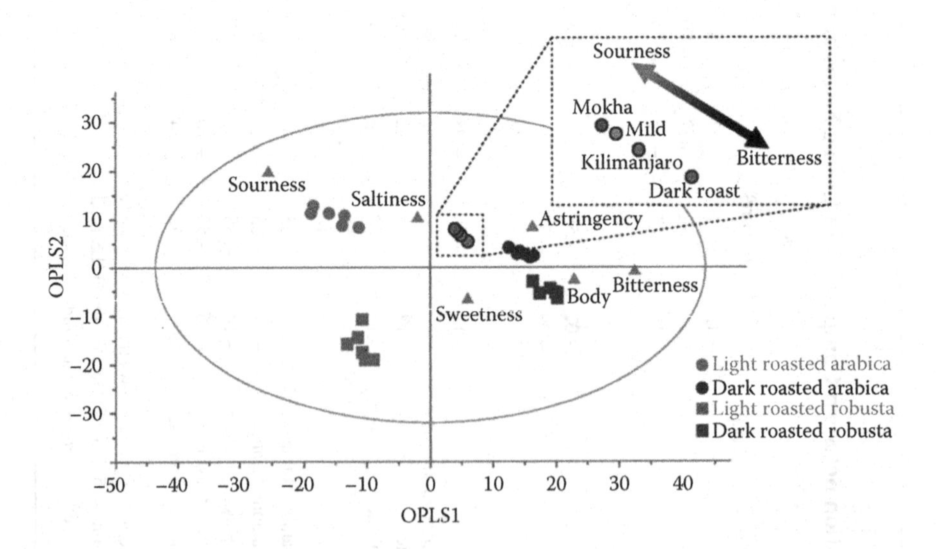

FIGURE 14.4 Score and scatter plots of the predictive OPLS model, including the four commercial roasted coffee bean samples.

14.5 CONCLUSION

In summary, a global metabolite profile of GCBEs has been established utilizing NMR combined with multivariate analysis methods (PCA and/or OPLS-DA). The evolution of the NMR-visible components in coffee bean extracts during the roasting process was also observed. This evolution not only accurately identifies the distinction among coffee beans at different degrees of roasting but also offers an excellent holistic method, together with significant chemical markers, to control and characterize the coffee bean roasting process.

By taking advantage of NMR as a "magnetic tongue," a methodology to evaluate the taste of coffee bean extracts was established based on the detailed NMR spectral assignments using a predictive OPLS model. Accordingly, NMR has the potential to detect in-depth sensory descriptions of coffee bean extracts due to its efficiency and high level of accuracy.

REFERENCES

1. Ellis, M. 2011. *The Coffee-House: A Cultural History.* London: Hachette UK.
2. Wei, F., Furihata, K., Miyakawa, T., and Tanokura, M. 2014. A pilot study of NMR-based sensory prediction of roasted coffee bean extracts. *Food Chemistry* 152: 363–369.
3. Buffo, R. A., and Cardelli-Freire, C. 2004. Coffee flavour: An overview. *Flavour and Fragrance Journal* 19: 99–104.
4. Pacifico, D., Casciani, L., Ritota, M., Mandolino, G., Onofri, C., Moschella, A., Parisi, B., Cafiero, C., and Valentini, M. 2013. NMR-based metabolomics for organic farming traceability of early potatoes. *Journal of Agricultural and Food Chemistry* 61: 11201–11211.
5. Koda, M., Furihata, K., Wei, F., Miyakawa, T., and Tanokura, M. 2012. Metabolic discrimination of mango juice from various cultivars by band-selective NMR spectroscopy. *Journal of Agricultural and Food Chemistry* 60: 1158–1166.
6. Hu, F., Furihata, K., Ito-Ishida, M., Kaminogawa, S., and Tanokura, M. 2004. Nondestructive observation of bovine milk by NMR spectroscopy: Analysis of existing states of compounds and detection of new compounds. *Journal of Agricultural and Food Chemistry* 52: 4969–4974.
7. Hu, F., Furihata, K., Kato, Y., and Tanokura, M. 2007. Nondestructive quantification of organic compounds in whole milk without pretreatment by two-dimensional NMR spectroscopy. *Journal of Agricultural and Food Chemistry* 55: 4307–4311.
8. Liang, T., Wei, F., Lu, Y., Kodani, Y., Nakada, M., Miyakawa, T., and Tanokura, M. 2015. Comprehensive NMR analysis of compositional changes of black garlic during thermal processing. *Journal of Agricultural and Food Chemistry* 63: 683–691.
9. Ky, C. L., Louarn, J., Dussert, S., Guyot, B., Hamon, S., and Noirot, M. 2001. Caffeine, trigonelline, chlorogenic acids and sucrose diversity in wild *Coffea arabica* L. and *C. canephora* P. accessions. *Food Chemistry* 75: 223–230.
10. del Castillo, M. D., Ames, J. M., and Gordon, M. H. 2002. Effect of roasting on the antioxidant activity of coffee brews. *Journal of Agricultural and Food Chemistry* 50: 3698–3703.
11. Clifford, M. N., Johnston, K. L., Knight, S., and Kuhnert, N. 2003. Hierarchical scheme for LC-MS n identification of chlorogenic acids. *Journal of Agricultural and Food Chemistry* 51: 2900–2911.

12. Wei, F., Furihata, K., Hu, F., Miyakawa, T., and Tanokura, M. 2010. Complex mixture analysis of organic compounds in green coffee bean extract by two-dimensional NMR spectroscopy. *Magnetic Resonance in Chemistry* 48: 857–865.
13. Wei, F., Furihata, K., Koda, M., Hu, F., Kato, R., Miyakawa, T., and Tanokura, M. 2012. ^{13}C NMR-based metabolomics for the classification of green coffee beans according to variety and origin. *Journal of Agricultural and Food Chemistry* 60: 10118–10125.
14. D'Amelio, N., Fontanive, L., Uggeri, F., Suggi-Liverani, F., and Navarini, L. 2009. NMR reinvestigation of the caffeine-chlorogenate complex in aqueous solution and in coffee brews. *Food Biophysics* 4: 321–330.
15. De Maria, C. A. B., Trugo, L. C., Moreira, R. F. A., and Werneck, C. C. 1994. Composition of green coffee fractions and their contribution to the volatile profile formed during roasting. *Food Chemistry* 50: 141–145.
16. Geromel, C., Ferreira, L. P., Guerreiro, S. M. C., Cavalari, A. A., Pot, D., Pereira, L. F. P., Leroy, T., Vieira, L. G., Mazzafera, P., and Marraccini, P. 2006. Biochemical and genomic analysis of sucrose metabolism during coffee (*Coffea arabica*) fruit development. *Journal of Experimental Botany* 57: 3243–3258.
17. Privat, I., Foucrier, S., Prins, A., Epalle, T., Eychenne, M., Kandalaft, L, Caillet, V., Lin, C., Tanksley, S., Foyer, C., and McCarthy, J. 2008. Differential regulation of grain sucrose accumulation and metabolism in *Coffea arabica* (Arabica) and *Coffea canephora* (Robusta) revealed through gene expression and enzyme activity analysis. *New Phytologist* 178: 781–797.
18. Hamden, K., Mnafgui, K., Amri, Z., Aloulou, A., and Elfeki, A. 2013. Inhibition of key digestive enzymes related to diabetes and hyperlipidemia and protection of liver-kidney functions by trigonelline in diabetic rats. *Scientia Pharmaceutica* 81: 233.
19. Alonso-Salces, R. M., Serra, F., Reniero, F., and Héberger, K. 2009. Botanical and geographical characterization of green coffee (*Coffea arabica* and *Coffea canephora*): Chemometric evaluation of phenolic and methylxanthine contents. *Journal of Agricultural and Food Chemistry* 57: 4224–4235.
20. Xu, X., Gammon, M. D., Zeisel, S. H., Lee, Y. L., Wetmur, J. G., Teitelbaum, S. L., Bradshaw, P. T., Neugut, A. I., Santella, R. M., and Chen, J. 2008. Choline metabolism and risk of breast cancer in a population-based study. *The FASEB Journal* 22: 2045–2052.
21. Arnold, U., Ludwig, E., Kühn, R., and Möschwitzer, U. 1994. Analysis of free amino acids in green coffee beans. *Zeitschrift für Lebensmittel-Untersuchung und Forschung* 199: 22–25.
22. Wei, F., Furihata, K., Hu, F., Miyakawa, T., and Tanokura, M. 2011. Two-dimensional ^{1}H-^{13}C nuclear magnetic resonance (NMR)-based comprehensive analysis of roasted coffee bean extract. *Journal of Agricultural and Food Chemistry* 59: 9065–9073.
23. Wei, F., Furihata, K., Koda, M., Hu, F., Miyakawa, T., and Tanokura, M. 2012. Roasting process of coffee beans as studied by nuclear magnetic resonance: Time course of changes in composition. *Journal of Agricultural and Food Chemistry* 60: 1005–1012.
24. Murkovic, M., and Bornik, M. A. 2007. Formation of 5-hydroxymethyl-2-furfural (HMF) and 5-hydroxymethyl-2-furoic acid during roasting of coffee. *Molecular Nutrition & Food Research* 51: 390–394.
25. Sanz, C., Maeztu, L., Zapelena, M. J., Bello, J., and Cid, C. 2002. Profiles of volatile compounds and sensory analysis of three blends of coffee: Influence of different proportions of *Arabica* and *Robusta* and influence of roasting coffee with sugar. *Journal of the Science of Food and Agriculture* 82: 840–847.
26. Ginz, M., Balzer, H. H., Bradbury, A. G., and Maier, H. G. 2000. Formation of aliphatic acids by carbohydrate degradation during roasting of coffee. *European Food Research and Technology* 211: 404–410.

27. Bradbury, A. G., and Halliday, D. J. 1990. Chemical structures of green coffee bean polysaccharides. *Journal of Agricultural and Food Chemistry* 38: 389–392.
28. Redgwell, R. J., Trovato, V., Curti, D., and Fischer, M. 2002. Effect of roasting on degradation and structural features of polysaccharides in *Arabica* coffee beans. *Carbohydrate Research* 337: 421–431.
29. Illy, A., and Viani, R. (Eds.). 1995. *Espresso Coffee: The Chemistry of Quality.* London, UK: Academic Press.
30. Rubico, S. M., and McDaniel, M. R. 1992. Sensory evaluation of acids by free-choice profiling. *Chemical Senses* 17: 273–289.
31. Frank, O., Zehentbauer, G., and Hofmann, T. 2006. Bioresponse-guided decomposition of roast coffee beverage and identification of key bitter taste compounds. *European Food Research and Technology* 222: 492–508.
32. Taguchi, H., Sakaguchi, M., and Shimabayashi, Y. 1985. Trigonelline content in coffee beans and the thermal conversion of trigonelline into nicotinic acid during the roasting of coffee beans. *Agricultural and Biological Chemistry* 49: 3467–3471.
33. Viani, R., and Horman, I. 1974. Thermal behavior of trigonelline. *Journal of Food Science* 39: 1216–1217.
34. Stadler, R. H., Varga, N., Hau, J., Vera, F. A., and Welti, D. H. 2002. Alkylpyridiniums. 1. Formation in model systems via thermal degradation of trigonelline. *Journal of Agricultural and Food Chemistry* 50: 1192–1199.
35. Savage, N. 2012. The taste of things to come. *Nature* 486: S18–S19.
36. Clausen, M. R., Pedersen, B. H., Bertram, H. C., and Kidmose, U. 2011. Quality of sour cherry juice of different clones and cultivars (*Prunus cerasus* L.) determined by a combined sensory and NMR spectroscopic approach. *Journal of Agricultural and Food Chemistry* 59: 12124–12130.
37. Malmendal, A., Amoresano, C., Trotta, R., Lauri, I., De Tito, S., Novellino, E., and Randazzo, A. 2011. NMR spectrometers as "magnetic tongues": Prediction of sensory descriptors in canned tomatoes. *Journal of Agricultural and Food Chemistry* 59: 10831–10838.

Index

D

E

F

Q

R

S

T

U

V

W

Printed in the United States
by Baker & Taylor Publisher Services